Alison Kew. 9/91 Heffers.

50-00

new

WENNER-GREN CENTER
INTERNATIONAL SYMPOSIUM SERIES

VOLUME 55

NEUROBIOLOGY OF EARLY INFANT BEHAVIOUR

NEUROBIOLOGY OF EARLY INFANT BEHAVIOUR

Proceedings of an International Wallenberg Symposium
at the Wenner-Gren Center, Stockholm, August 28–September 1, 1988

Edited by

Curt von Euler
*Nobel Institute for Neurophysiology, Karolinska Institute,
S-104 01 Stockholm*

Hans Forssberg
*Department of Pediatrics, Karolinska Hospital,
S-104 01 Stockholm*

and

Hugo Lagercrantz
*Nobel Institute for Neurophysiology, Karolinska Institute, and
Department of Pediatrics, Karolinska Hospital,
S-104 01 Stockholm*

Managing Editor

Vanja Landin
*Nobel Institute for Neurophysiology, Karolinska Institute,
S-104 01 Stockholm*

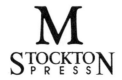

M
STOCKTON
PRESS

First published 1989

Published by
THE MACMILLAN PRESS LTD
Houndmills, Basingstoke, Hampshire RG21 2XS
and London
Companies and representatives
throughout the world

Printed in Great Britain by
Camelot Press, Southampton

British Library Cataloguing in Publication Data
Neurobiology of early infant behaviour.
1. Children. Behaviour. Neurobiological aspects
I. Euler, Curt Von   II. Forssberg, Hans, *1949–*   III.
Lagercrantz, Hugo
612'.8
ISSN 0083–7989
ISBN 0–333–48893–8

Published in the United States and Canada by
Stockton Press, 15 East 26th Street, New York, NY 10010
Library of Congress Cataloging-in-Publication Data available
ISBN 0–935859–70–5

Contents

IV. Sensory Systems

*m·F
differences in
maturation*

V. Psychobiology

List of Active Participants

Heidelise Als
Enders Main, Rm. M-29
The Children's Hospital
320 Longwood Avenue
Boston, MA 02115, USA

Anne C. Bekoff
Department of EPO Biology
University of Colorado
Boulder, Colorado 80309, USA

Colin Blakemore
University Laboratory of
Physiology
Parks Road
Oxford OX1 3PT, UK

Elliott M. Blass
Department of Psychology
Johns Hopkins University
Baltimore, MD 21218, USA

Oliver J. Braddick
Dept of Experimental Psychology
University of Cambridge
Cambridge, UK

Paul Casaer
Dev. Neurol. Res. Unit &
Div. of Paediatric Neurology
Dept Paediatrics and Neonatal
Medicine
K.U. Leuven University Hospital
Gasthuisberg
3000 Leuven, Belgium

Peter de Chateau
Dept of Paediatric Psychiatry
S:t Görans Hospital
S-112 81   Stockholm, Sweden

Harry T. Chugani
Division of Nuclear Medicine &
Biophysics
Dept of Radiological Sciences
UCLA School of Medicine
Los Angeles, CA 90024, USA

Giovanni Cioni
Istituto Scientifico
I-56018 Calambrone/Pisa, Italy

Staffan Cullheim
Department of Anatomy
Karolinska Institute
S-104 01   Stockholm, Sweden

Frank H. Duffy
Children's Hospital
300 Longwood Ave.
Boston, Mass 02115, USA

Curt von Euler
Nobel Institute for Neurophysiology
Karolinska Institute
S-104 01   Stockholm, Sweden

Edda Farnetani
Centro di Fonetica del CNR
Università di Padova
Via Oberdan, 10
I-35100 Padova, Italy

William P. Fifer
New York State Psychiatric
Institute
722 West 168th Street
New York, N.Y. 10032, USA

Hans Forssberg
Department of Pediatrics
Karolinska Hospital
S-104 01 Stockholm, Sweden

Patricia Goldman-Rakic
Sect. of Neuroanatomy
Yale Univ. School of Medicine
333 Cedar St.
New Haven, CT 06510, USA

Sten Grillner
Nobel Inst. for Neurophysiology
Karolinska Institute
S-104 01 Stockholm, Sweden

Richard M. Held
Massachusetts Institute of
Technology
79 Amherst Street - E10-145
Cambridge, MA 02139, USA

Claes von Hofsten
Department of Psychology
University of Umeå
S-901 87 Umeå, Sweden

David H. Ingvar
Dept of Clinical Neurophysiology
University Hospital
S-221 85 Lund, Sweden

Jan K.S. Jansen
Institute of Physiology
University of Oslo
Karl Johans gt 47
Oslo, Norway

Ingemar Kjellmer
Department of Pediatrics
Östra Sjukhuset
S-416 85 Göteborg, Sweden

Norman A. Krasnegor
Center for Research for Mothers
and Children
National Inst. of Child Health
and Human Development
National Institute of Health
Bethesda, Maryland 20892, USA

Hugo Lagercrantz
Nobel Institute for Neurophysiology
Karolinska Institute and
Department of Pediatrics
Karolinska Hospital
S-104 01 Stockholm

David N. Lee
Department of Psychology
University of Edinburgh
Edinburgh, EH8 9J2, Scotland

Gunnar Lennerstrand
Department of Opthalmology
Huddinge Hospital
S-141 86 Huddinge, Sweden

Björn Lindblom
Deparment of Linguistics
University of Stockholm
S-106 91 Stockholm, Sweden

Hans C. Lou
John F. Kennedy Institute
Department of Neuropediatric,
Gl. Landevej 7
DK-2600 Glostrup, Denmark

Keiko Mizukami
Developmental Psychology Research
Laboratory
National Children's Medical Research
Center
3-35-31, Taishido, Setagaya-ku,
Tokyo 154, Japan

Lars Olson
Dept of Neurobiology
Karolinska Institute
S-104 01 Stockholm, Sweden

Hanus Papousek
Max-Planck Inst. for Psychiatry
Kraepelin Str. 10 - EPB
D-8000 Munich 40, FRG

Michael E. Phelps
Division of Nuclear Medicine &
Biophysics
Dept of Radiological Sciences
UCLA School of Medicine
Los Angeles, CA 90024, USA

Heinz F.R. Prechtl
Dept of Developmental Neurology
University Hospital
Oostersingel 59
NL-9713 EZ Groningen,
The Netherlands

Pasko Rakic
Section of Neuroanatomy
Yale Univ. School of Medicine
New Haven, CT 06510, USA

Scania de Schonen
Lab. Neurosciences Cognitives
LNF1, C.N.R.S.
31 Chemin J. Aiguier
F-13009 Marseille, France

Henk Spekreijse
The Netherlands Ophthalmic
Research Institute
P.O. Box 12141
NL-1100 AC Amsterdam-Zuidoost,
The Netherlands

Elisabeth S. Spelke
Department of Psychology
Cornell University
Ithaca, New York 14853, USA

Michael Studdert-Kennedy
Haskins Laboratories
270 Crown St.
New Haven, CT 06511, USA

Nils W. Svenningsen
Department of Paediatrics
Neonatal Intensive Care Unit
University Hospital
S-221 85 Lund, Sweden

Esther Thelen
Department of Psychology
Indiana University
Bloomington, IN 47405, USA

Colwyn Trevarthen
Department of Psychology
University of Edinburgh
7 George Square
Edinburgh EH8 9JZ, Scotland

Joseph J. Volpe
St. Louis Children's Hospital
400 S. Kingshighway
St. Louis, Missouri 63110, USA

Rolf Zetterström
Department of Pediatrics
S:t Görans Hospital
S-112 82 Stockholm

Acknowledgements

The transdisciplinary conference, on which this book is based had brought together an elite of scientists, working in different fields of neurosciences, developmental neuropsychology and psychobiology, radiology, brain metabolism, pediatrics and neonatology, to discuss the many important problems on the relationships between normal and perturbed brain development on the one hand, and the development of cognitive functions and behaviour in full term and prematurely born babies on the other.

The Symposium was made possible through generous support from Marcus Wallenberg's Foundation for International Scientific Cooperation. Financial support was obtained also from the Swedish Medical Research Council, the Swedish Council for Research in the Humanities and Social Sciences, "Stiftelsen Sven Jerrings Fond", and AB Astra for which we want to express our sincere gratitude.

The Organizing Committee:

Curt von Euler, Hans Forssberg,
Claes von Hofsten, Hugo Lagercrantz,
Rolf Zetterström

Introductory Remarks

Curt von Euler

Perhaps the single most important and challenging issue in neuroscience concerns the manner in which the brain relates to mind and behaviour. Thus, a fundamental problem is the identification and elucidation of brain events underlying cognitive operations and generation of action and behaviour. The last decades have seen a rapidly increasing interaction between basic neurobiology and the cognitive and behavioural sciences that has spawned the fields of modern neuropsychology and psychobiology, the aims of which are to constrain hypotheses and models of perceptive and cognitive processes and behavioural control by neurobiological facts and principles. This interdisciplinary interaction has proven especially fruitful in the study of the changing linkages during ontogeny between brain structure, and brain metabolism on the one hand, and cognition and motor functions on the other. This developmental approach provides increased possibilities to study dynamically structure/function relationships during fetal, neonatal and infant development, with respect to growth of perceptive functions, information processing, motor skills, learning capabilities, memory, and social and affective behaviour.

Recent advances in this area, some of which are reported here, are providing new knowledge about the astounding perceptive, cognitive and learning capacities already attained at preterm ages. Important new insights have also been gained into the time dependence of many developmental processes underlying the various "critical" or "sensitive" periods, for instance in the ontogeny of the visual system (e.g. Hubel & Wiesel, 1970; LeVay et al., 1980 and several chapters in this volume), and we have learned from the work of Patricia Goldman-Rakic and her associates (e.g. Goldman, 1978) that the architectural reorganization that a brain, consequential to a lesion, may undergo in midgestation cannot occur in a fetus which is only a few weeks older. Furthermore, investigations of infant's abilities to discriminate speech sounds suggest that human newborns are equipped with a great panoply of information analyzers which will become functional only if stimulated before a certain time during development; those channels which are not being used before that time will be functionally extinguished (Cutting & Eimas, 1975; Mehler, 1982). Ample evidence has been reported on the occurrence, at certain ages, of "dips and drops" in performance, for instance, in various perceptual functions, motor performances, and language learning (see e.g. several papers in Bever, 1981, and in this volume). However, we still have only a scanty knowledge about the neuro-biological bases of these apparent regressions, their biological significance and the timing mechanisms determining their appear-ances. The evidence at hand suggests, however, that during these regressions the neural mechanisms involved are being subject to a developmental alteration and reorganization, probably to provide for new, more mature and adaptable modes of operation.

The sequential order in which functions are acquired seems to exert important influences both on their development and on their structural underpinnings. An example of this can be taken from work by Ursula Bellugi and her collaborators (1988; see also Studdert-Kennedy in this volume) and by Helen Neville (1985, 1989) who have demonstrated stable differences in language processing of the American sign language between individuals who learn it as their first language and those who acquire it after they have learned another language. This leads us to the important issue of to what extent biological determinants exert critical influences on the structural organization of the hardware. For instance, could it be, as Jacous Mehler once asked (1982), that language when developed sufficiently to become a means for coding informa-tion, exerts an influence on the structure and "wiring" of the neural mechanisms for other cognitive functions, e.g. some memory functions, or does the rate of development of these functions procede along a preset time course, with its accelerations, dips and drops, independent of language? In general, the problems on the fostering effects during development of the multidirectional interrelations among perception, action and cognition and their neurobiological counterparts are receiving heightened attention.

Increased knowledge about the neurobiological basis of the development of perception, cognition, motor control and behaviour is not only of great theoretical interest, but is also of high clinical relevance. The very rapid progress in neonatology and the technology of intensive care of preterm babies has made it possible to save a high proportion of even very prematurely born babies. Superficially, most of the preterm babies, who are not victims of perinatal asphyxia or brain hemorrhages, seem to develop fairly normally, not differing significantly from babies born at full term. This may be an illusion, however, caused by our scanty knowledge about the influences exerted on brain development by the different physical, mechanical, chemical and hormonal factors of the intrauterine environment and about the effects of deprivation of these factors at an abnormally early stage combined with an untimely exposure to the extrauterine environment (see e.g. Als in this volume). It would seem obvious that alterations of any of the large number of processes involved in neural development and brain maturation could lead to a series of events that ultimately give rise to altered synaptic density, neural connectivity and transmitter biochemistry in many parts of the brain, and consequently to altered functions. The recent rapid advancements in the fields of developmental neuropsychology and psychobiology are constantly providing more and more sophisticated and sensitive diagnostic methods and tools, allowing detection of anomalies in cognitive and behavioural development which could not, or cannot be revealed before sufficiently refined methods are, or will be, available. It may be recalled that it was not many decades ago that hardly any effects of transection of the corpus callosum could be detected and the functional significance of its 800 000 nerve fibers was questioned. Likewise the astounding advancements in the fields of developmental neuroanatomy, neurochemistry, neurophysiology as well as in the biophysics and technology of measuring and visualization of regional brain metabolism, blood flow and electrical activity now makes it possible to detect, with increasing sensitivity and resolution, the anomalies in brain development underlying functional disturbancies.

It is our hope that this Symposium, and the ensuing symposium volume, with its fairly unique constellation of contributors from many different scientific fields, reporting on some of the most important new advances and perspectives, may serve as a thought-provoking and inspiring avenue to new insigths into the intricate problems how the innately and experientially controlled development of brain mechanisms determine, in an interactive manner, the growth of cognitive and behavioural abilities.

REFERENCES

Bellugi, U., Klima, E. & Poizner, H. (1988). Sign language and the brain. In Language, Communication, and the Brain. (ed. F. Plum). Raven Press, New York, pp 30-56.

Bever, T.G. (ed.) (1981). Regressions in Development, Basic Phenomena and Theoretical Alternatives. MIT Press, Cambridge, Mass.

Cutting, J. & Eimas, P. (1975). Phonetic feature analyzers and the processing of speech in infants. In The Role of Speech in Language (eds. J.F. Kavanagh & J.E. Cutting). MIT Press, Cambridge, Mass.

Goldman, P. (1978). Neuronal plasticity in primate telencephalon. Anomalous projections induced by prenatal removal of frontal cortex. Science, 202, 768-770.

Hubel, D.H. & Wiesel, T.N. (1970). The period of susceptibility to the physiological effects of unilateral eye closure in kittens. J.Physiol. (London), 206, 419-436.

LeVay, S., Wiesel, T.N. & Hubel, D.H. (1980). The development of ocular dominance columns in normal and visually deprived monkeys. J.comp.Neurol., 191, 1-51.

Mehler, J. (1982). Studies in the development of cognitive processes. In U-Shaped Behavioral Growth (ed. S. Strauss). Academic Press, New York, pp 271-294.

Neville, H.J. (1985). Effects of early sensory and language experience on the development of the human brain. In Neonate Cognition. (eds. J. Mehler & R. Fox). Lawrence Erlbaum Associates, Hillsdale, N.J., pp 349-363.

Neville, H.J. (1989). Whence the specialization of the language hemisphere? In Modularity and the Motor Theory of Speech Perception. (eds. I.G. Mattingly & M. Studdert-Kennedy). Lawrence Erlbaum Associates, Hillsdale, N.J., in press.

I. Brain Development

1

Principles of Development in the Nervous System

Colin Blakemore

INTRODUCTION

The nervous system is an instrument of connexion. Perception, thought, language, movement - all of them presumably depend on the precise organization of circuits of neurons. Surely the most formidable task to be accomplished during the development of a human body is the construction of the nervous system, with its 10^{11} or so neurons linked together by perhaps 10^{14} synapses.

Broadly speaking, the aspects of connectivity to be achieved during neural development fall into three classes:

1) Topography. The majority of axon systems not only terminate in specific target structures but also have some kind of ordered arrangement of projection within each target. In the visual system, for instance, axons innervating the superior colliculus (SC), lateral geniculate nucleus (LGN) and primary visual cortex terminate in specific layers and arrange themselves to produce 'maps' of the retina and thus of the visual field.

2) Registration. When two or more fibre systems innervate a single structure, they usually distribute themselves to form particular spatial arrangements with respect to each other, either terminating together on neurons of similar type, or, more often, segregating from each other into separate layers, bands, patches, etc.. In the primate visual system, a good example is provided by

----

Much of the research described in this chapter was done in collaboration with W.M. Cowan, L.J. Garey, Z. Henderson, R. Insausti, D.J. Price, N.V. Swindale, F. Vital-Durand and T.J. Zumbroich. Work performed at Oxford was supported by grants from the Medical Research Council, the Wellcome Trust and the Science and Engineering Research Council.

the separation of axons carrying signals from the two eyes into different layers, at the level of the LGN, and into a pattern of 'stripes' within layer IVc of the visual cortex (see LeVay et al., 1980).

3) Specificity. Neurons can have remarkably specific properties within a particular domain of responsibility - for instance, upper motor neurons controlling a limited group of motor units in a particular muscle or sensory neurons responding best to a particular stimulus from within the full range of sensitivity of a sense organ. For vision, the distinctive selectivity of most cells in the cat and monkey striate cortex for the orientation of lines or edges in the visual field (see Hubel and Wiesel, 1977) is a well-known example of such specificity.

The achievement of all these characteristics during development reduces to the problem of how growing axons find their way to their target cells and how they arrange themselves to form synapses to generate the properties of those cells.

The major conclusion that emerges from research on this topic during the past twenty years (much of it on the visual system) is that a variety of factors and mechanisms are involved in the attainment of the final pattern of connectivity. Some aspects of connectivity appear to be determined completely by genetic instructions, or at least by inherent mechanisms independent of the presence of impulses in the developing pathway. Others seem to rely on the pattern of impulses, either spontaneous or evoked by functional use, but the activity is needed only to promote the formation or validation of connexions, which are ultimately specified by inherent instructions. And yet others are even more directly guided by the way in which the developing system is used.

Some specific examples, all taken from the development of the mammalian visual system, will illustrate the diversity of mechanisms involved in development and the way in which they can interact.

DEATH OF GANGLION CELLS PARTLY DEPENDENT ON CENTRAL COMPETITION

The developmental death of neurons, a process first described by Studnicka in 1905, is now known to occur on a substantial scale: in many structures, half or more of all nerve cells die before maturity. In all mammalian species so far examined, the number of ganglion cells born during development and the number of their axons entering the optic nerve considerably exceed the number that finally survive in the adult: cell death is undoubtedly responsible for most if not all of this loss (see Williams and Herrup, 1988). Estimates of the proportion of mammalian ganglion cells dying vary between 80% for the cat (Williams et al., 1986) and about 60% for rhesus monkey (Rakic and Riley, 1983a), human (Provis et al., 1985) and rat (Crespo et al., 1985).

In some species, massive ganglion cell death starts to occur **before** optic axons have reached their central targets and therefore is likely to be initiated either by an intrinsic genetic timetable or by interactions in the retina itself. However, in mammals with frontal vision and hence a considerable binocular overlap of the visual fields of the two eyes, some fraction of cell death appears to depend on a competitive battle for territory of innervation in central target structures, or some other form of interaction dependent on the presence of both sets of axons.

The LGN and the SC of binocular mammals are innervated by both eyes; initially, terminal axons from the two eyes are widely intermingled in both structures, but they gradually segregate from each other, forming distinct monocular layers in the LGN and separating in laminar, topographic and distributions in the SC (see Rakic, 1977; Williams and Chalupa, 1982; Insausti et al., 1985).

Part, at least, of this process of segregation involves and regulates selective death of ganglion cells and their axons. If one eye is removed before optic axons reach their targets (i.e. prenatally in cat or monkey), the number of surviving ganglion cells in the remaining eye is much higher than normal (though less than the total number of cells born) and the optic axons of the remaining eye do not become restricted within the target structures in the normal way. This implies that some component of ganglion cell death is dependent on competitive interaction between axons from the two eyes in central target structures.

The projection from the eye to the ipsilateral SC provides a particularly striking example of competitive regulation of cell death. In adult rodents, the retina sends a small projection, arising almost entirely from a patch of ganglion cells lying in the extreme temporal crescent of the retina (which views the small binocular portion of the visual field), to terminate in a few segregated clumps in the rostral part of the ipsilateral SC (representing the middle of the visual field).

At birth, however, when optic axons are still invading the SC in rodents, fibres from the ipsilateral eye extend exuberantly over the entire rostro-caudal extent of this nucleus and a distinct population of 'aberrant' ganglion cells, scattered over the whole retina outside the temporal crescent, contributes to this projection. The cells of origin of this initial projection, including its aberrant component, can be labelled by injection into the ipsilateral SC of retrogradely-transported dyes.

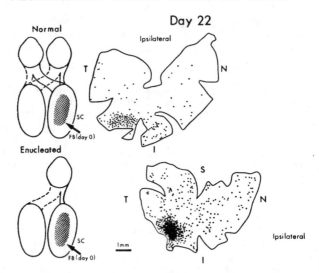

Figure 1   Insausti et al (1984) used the long-lasting dye FB to test whether the normal loss of the aberrant population of ipsilaterally-projecting nasal ganglion cells in the hamster is due to cell death. The right SC in a number of animals was filled by a single pressure injection of 15 nl of FB on the day of birth (day 0), as indicated on the schematic diagram of the retino-collicular pathway. Then on day 22 a whole mount of the retina of the ipsilateral eye was examined by fluorescence microscopy; the upper diagram shows the whole mount for a typical animal (T,N,I = temporal, nasal, inferior retina) with the position of every cell labelled with FB marked as a dot. The distribution of cells **retaining** the FB picked up at birth is indistinguishable from the normal, diminished population characteristic of the adult, with very few cells outside the temporal crescent. On the other hand, for animals in which the left eye was removed at birth (which retain an exuberant projection from the remaining eye to the ipsilateral SC), the population of FB-labelled ganglion cells is greater and contains a substantial number of aberrant nasal cells, 'rescued' by the removal of competing influences from the other eye. (Modified from Insausti et al., 1984).

The exuberant projection of ipsilateral axons over the SC largely disappears during the first two weeks of postnatal life in the hamster (Insausti et al., 1985) and it is clear that this involves the loss of input from most of the aberrant population of nasal ganglion cells.   Fig. 1 shows results from a study by Insausti et al. (1984) in which a long-lasting fluorescent retrograde tracer, fast blue (FB), was used to discover whether the removal of this initial projection is due to the death of these aberrant nasal ganglion cells or to the withdrawal of axons without the explicit elimination of their cell bodies. FB was injected into the right SC, filling most of the nucleus, on the day of birth, and the distribution of labelled ganglion cells was examined in a whole mount of the ipsilateral (right) eye at day 22 (at which stage in normal hamsters the projection from cells outside the temporal crescent of the retina has largely disappeared). In the normal animal (top half of Fig. 1) the distribution of cells still labelled with FB is indistinguishable from the pattern of cells labelled by an injection of retrograde tracer **at that age.** This strongly suggests that the substantial numbers of nasal ganglion cells that initially sent axons to the ipsilateral SC (and therefore picked up the FB when it was injected) have actually died. In the enucleated animal (lower half of Fig. 1) these aberrant nasal cells are still present, rescued as a result of the elimination of competitive interactions between the two eyes' axons.

SEGREGATION OF AFFERENT INNERVATIONS IN THE GENICULO-CORTICAL PATHWAY

Many structures in the nervous system are innervated by several afferent systems. In a number of cases these different, but all appropriate, inputs are locally segregated from each other into layers, clumps or bands. Some of these characteristic patterns emerge during development from an immature arrangement of overlapping termination, like that already described for ipsilateral and contralateral optic axons innervating the rodent SC.

When axons from the two optic nerves first enter the LGN in cat and monkey, the primordial nucleus is not layered but is a single mass of cells (see Rakic, 1977). Fibres from the two eyes are intermingled and probably even innervate the same individual neurons (see Shatz and Kirkwood, 1984). However, they then proceed to segregate from each other and the typical layered structure of the nucleus emerges. This process certainly involves changes in the distribution and branching patterns of individual axons, but it is also accompanied by a component of ganglion cell death. Competitive interactions dependent on the presence of the two sets of axons, and probably on spontaneous activity in them, seem to be involved, since removal of one eye prior to the complete innervation of the LGN and SC causes a failure of lamination and segregation, and the rescuing of a significant number of ganglion cells in the remaining eye (see Chalupa et al., 1984; Rakic, 1977; Rakic and Riley, 1983b).

Abolition of spontaneous impulse activity in the fibres innervating the cat LGN, starting prior to segregation, interferes with the normal restriction of axon termination and the formation of layers (Sretavan et al., 1988). Thus, **activity** in the two sets of fibres seems to influence the normal competitive reorganization of terminals. But since this process takes place prenatally in cat and monkey, the activity involved is not visually elicited and does not relate to the animal's own visual experience.

A superficially similar process takes place **after** birth in the monkey's visual cortex. When the axons of cells in right-eye and left-eye laminae of the LGN first arrive in the cortex, before birth, they are initially mixed together in layer IVc (Rakic, 1977). The two sets of axons gradually segregate from each other to form a distinctive pattern of alternating bands, each about 0.3 mm wide. Although this process starts before birth, it mainly occupies a 'sensitive period' during the first six weeks of postnatal life and it is indubitably influenced by visually-elicited activity in the two sets of axons: deprivation of one eye by closure of the lids biases the process of segregation so that the axons carrying signals from that eye come to occupy small patches of territory within layer IVc, while the terminal territory of the non-deprived eye is proportionately enlarged (LeVay et al., 1980).

Competitive axon redistribution and synaptogenesis can occur remarkably rapidly: reverse deprivation (opening a previously deprived eye and closing the other), as long as it takes place within the sensitive period, causes the shrunken patches to re-expand completely over the course of only a week or so (Swindale et al., 1981), with parallel changes in the physiological properties of neurons in the cortex (Blakemore et al., 1981).

In this case, then, the control of innervation is dependent on competitive interaction reflecting the relative strength of visually-driven activity of the two eyes, and it seems to be accomplished through local axon pruning, within layer IVc, without significant cell death in the LGN (Williams & Rakic, 1988).

EXUBERANCE OF CORTICO-CORTICAL CONNEXIONS

By the day of birth, in cats, all the major fibre systems into and out of the primary visual cortex (area 17) are quite well established, are reasonably mature in their laminar distributions and are at least roughly appropriate in their topographic arrangements (Henderson & Blakemore, 1986). Apart from such anatomically minor errors as the intermixing of left-eye and right-eye LGN axons in layer IV (as in the newborn monkey), there is little evidence of gross inappropriateness of connexion in these ascending and descending projections, all of which must have been constructed and guided without the benefit of visual experience.

On the other hand, there is a great deal of evidence that cortico-cortical interconnexions are highly exuberant when they first appear. For instance, Innocenti (1981) showed that, at the time of birth in cats, cells scattered throughout the whole of area 17 send axons across in the corpus callosum to reach the opposite hemisphere, whereas in the adult there is no interhemispheric projection from or to area 17 itself. Innocenti also showed that after an injection of FB into the occipital lobe of one hemisphere early in life, many cells in area 17 of the opposite hemisphere remain labelled some weeks later, after the exuberant projection has been removed. This implies that withdrawal of axons from targets that are inappropriate for the adult, without the **death** of the cells themselves, plays a large part in sculpting this particular cortico-cortical pathway.

There is also gross exuberance of the cortico-cortical projections within the same hemisphere in the young cat. For instance, the primary visual cortex initially receives a strong projection from the **auditory** cortex on the same side - a projection that is not present in the adult (see Innocenti et al., 1988). Many features of the initial cortico-cortical projections out of area 17 are also highly unusual. Price and Zumbroich (1989) have shown that, in young kittens, each region within area 17 sends a mass of axons into a plexus in the white matter under the cortical plate. These fibres from the striate cortex extend over the whole occipital region, including areas of cortex that will never be innervated by those axons. This wide-ranging subplate projection gradually disappears, leaving only the 'appropriate' fibre bundles invading topographically related regions of extrastriate visual cortex.

Even the topographically appropriate projection from area 17 to the grey matter of the neighbouring area 18 initially arises from an aberrant arrangement of neurons within area 17 (Price and Blakemore, 1985a). In the adult cat, the cells of origin of this 17-to-18 pathway lie mainly in distinct clusters in the upper layers of the cortex; but injection of retrograde tracers into area 18 of very young kittens shows them to lie in two continuous bands of roughly equal cell density, one in the upper layers and the other, highly anomalously, in the lower layers.

Price and Blakemore (1985b) used the FB technique to analyse the mechanisms involved in the elimination of the aberrant components of this projection. They found that after injection of FB into area 18 within a few days of birth the cells that remained labelled with the dye in area 17 at 3-4 weeks of age were still distributed as two continuous bands but the density of labelled cells in the lower layers was enormously reduced compared with those in the upper layers. The conclusion is that axon withdrawal from area 18 without cell death is primarily responsible for creating the gaps between the typical clusters of upper-layer cells but that cell death plays a major part in eliminating the aberrant lower-layer projection (Fig. 2).

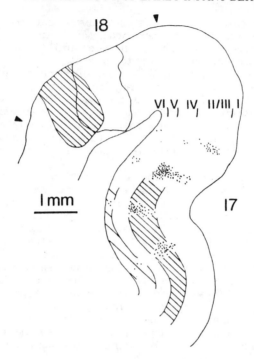

Figure 2   This camera lucida drawing shows a coronal section through the lateral gyrus of the left hemisphere of a 30-day old kitten, in which a small injection of FB had been made into area 18 (whose borders are indicated by arrow heads) on day 2. The central core of this injection site is represented by the hatched shape within area 18. The overlapping unfilled shape, centred more medially, shows the side of an injection of another fluorescent dye, daimidino yellow (DY), made on day 29. Within area 17, the dots show individual cells labelled with DY (indicating the state of the 17-to-18 projection at day 29). They lie mainly in distinct clusters in layers II/III, with very few cells in the lower layers. The cells labelled with FB (retaining the dye that they had picked up 4 weeks earlier) lie densely in a continuous band in layer II/III (indicated by the heavily hatched area) with a much sparser but continuous band in the lower layers. Double-labelled cells were found in regions of overlap of DY and FB containing neurons. This result suggests that axon withdrawal without cell death creates the gaps between the upper-layer clusters, while the elimination of initial very dense lower-layer population is partly due to cell death. (From Price, 1985; results described by Price & Blakemore, 1985b).

Although these major rearrangements of the 17-to-18 projection take place between about 10 and 20 days of age, directly after eye-opening, they do not seem to depend crucially on visual stimulation. Certainly the characteristic adult pattern, with the cortico-cortical cells in area 17 distributed mainly in clusters in the upper layers, emerges even in cats that have been reared in darkness. It remains to be seen whether competitive interactions between the terminals of axons innervating area 18 are responsible for the regulation of the regressive events in this cortico-cortical pathway and, if so, whether the competition is dependent on spontaneous impulse activity.

THE EMERGENCE OF STIMULUS SPECIFICITY

One of the most remarkable examples of precisely-organized connectivity in the entire nervous system is the arrangement of afferent input to individual neurons of the primary visual cortex of higher mammals, which creates their selectivity for the orientation of visual stimuli as well as for the direction of motion, colour, etc. (see Hubel & Wiesel, 1977). We still do not know how these properties are constructed by the integration of excitatory and inhibitory inputs to and between the cells, but obviously it must require a very specific ensemble of synaptic innervation of each neuron. Interestingly, although many of these properties of the receptive fields emerge without visual experience in some visual cortical cells (implying that the basic regulation of connectivity forming them is innately determined), visual stimulation is essential for the completion and maintenance of selective properties and various deliberate manipulations of early visual experience result in corresponding changes in the selectivity of the overall population of cortical cells (see Movshon & Van Sluyters, 1981).

Thus it appears that the regulation of neuronal connectivity, exemplified by that of the visual pathway, is accomplished through a variety of mechanisms. Innate mechanisms (presumably genetic instructions, promoting selective growth and guidance) result in the construction of the major fibre pathways and the basic pattern of innervation of target structures, without which local competitive and activity-dependent interactions would be impossible. The initial overproduction of neurons and the exuberance of axonal projection, especially in cortico-cortical pathways remains a mystery. Does it simply represent irreducible errors or lack of specificity in genetic instruction? Or could it be that the exuberance of the immature nervous system serves some essential purpose at that stage in development, quite different from the function of the refined system of the adult?

REFERENCES

Blakemore, C., Vital-Durand, F. and Garey, L.J. (1981). Recovery from monocular deprivation in the monkey: 1. Reversal of physiological effects in the visual cortex. Proc. Roy. Soc. Lond. B., 213, 399-423.

Chalupa, L.M., Williams, R.W. and Henderson, Z. (1984). Binocular interaction in the fetal cat regulates the size of the ganglion cell population. Neuroscience, 12, 1139-1146.

Crespo, D., O'Leary, D.D.M. and Cowan, W.M. (1985). Changes in the number of optic nerve fibers during late prenatal and postnatal development in the albino rat. Dev. Brain Res. 19, 129-134.

Henderson, Z. and Blakemore, C. (1986). Organization of the visual pathways in the newborn kitten. Neurosci. Res., 3, 628-659.

Hubel, D.H. and Wiesel, T.N. (1977). Functional architecture of macaque monkey visual cortex. Proc. Roy. Soc. Lond. B., 198, 1-59.

Innocenti, G.M. (1981). Growth and reshaping of axons in the establishment of visual callosal connections. Science, 212, 824-827.

Innocenti, G.M., Berbel, P. and Clarke, S. (1988). Development of projections from auditory to visual areas in the cat. J. comp. Neurol., 272, 242-259.

Insausti, R., Blakemore, C. and Cowan, W.M. (1984). Ganglion cell death during development of ipsilateral retino-collicular projection in golden hamster. Nature, 308, 362-365.

Insausti, R., Blakemore, C. and Cowan, W.M. (1985). Postnatal development of the ipsilateral retinocollicular projection and the effects of unilateral enucleation in the golden hamster. J. comp. Neurol., 234, 393-409.

LeVay, S., Wiesel, T.N. and Hubel, D.H. (1980). The development of ocular dominance columns in normal and visually deprived monkeys. J. comp. Neurol., 191, 1-51.

Movshon, J.A. and Van Sluyters, R.C. (1981). Visual neuronal development. Ann. Rev. Psychol., 32, 477-522.

Price, D.J. (1985). The Organization and Development of Area 18 of the Cat's Visual Cortex. University of Oxford, D.Phil. thesis.

Price, D.J. and Blakemore, C. (1985a). The postnatal development of the association projection from visual cortical area 17 to area 18 in the cat. J. Neurosci., 5, 2443-2452.

Price, D.J. and Blakemore, C. (1985b). Regressive events in the postnatal development of association projections in the visual cortex. Nature, 316, 721-724.

Price, D.J. and Zumbroich, T.J. (1989). Postnatal development of cortico-cortical efferents from area 17 in the cat's visual cortex. J. Neurosci. (in the press).

Provis, J., van Driel, D., Billson, F.A. and Russel, P. (1985). Human fetal optic nerve: overproduction and elimination of retinal axons during development. J. comp. Neurol. 238, 92-101.

Rakic, P. (1977). Prenatal development of the visual system in rhesus monkey. Phil. Trans. Roy. Soc. Lond. B., 278, 245-260.

Rakic, P. and Riley, K.P. (1983a). Overproduction and elimination of retinal axons in the fetal rhesus monkey. Science, 219, 1441-1444.

Rakic, P. and Riley, K.P. (1983b). Regulation of axon number in primate optic nerve by prenatal binocular competition. Nature, 305, 135-137.

Shatz, C.J. and Kirkwood, P.A. (1984). Prenatal development of functional connections in the cat's retinogeniculate pathway. J. Neuroscience, 4, 1378-1397.

Sretavan, D.W., Shatz, C.J. and Stryker, M.P. (1988). Modification of retinal ganglion cell axon morphology by prenatal infusion of tetrodotoxin. Nature, 336, 468-471.

Studnicka, F.K. (1905). Die Parietalorgane. In Lehrbuch der vergleichende mikroskopischen Anatomie der Wirbeltiere Vol.5 (ed. A. Oppel). Fischer, Jena.

Swindale, N.V., Vital-Durand, F. and Blakemore, C. (1981). Recovery from monocular deprivation in the monkey: 3. Reversal of anatomical effects in the visual cortex. Proc. Roy. Soc. Lond. B., 213, 435-450.

Williams, R.W. and Chalupa, L.M. (1982). Prenatal development of retinocollicular projections in the cat: an anterograde tracer transport study. J. Neurosci., 2, 604-622.

Williams, R.W. and Herrup, K. (1988). The control of neuron number. Ann. Rev. Neurosci., 11, 423-453.

Williams, R.W. and Rakic, P. (1988).   Elimination of neurons from the rhesus monkey's lateral geniculate nucleus during development. J. comp. Neurol., 272, 424-436.

Williams, R.W., Bastiani, M.J., Lia, B. and Chalupa, L.M.   (1986). Growth cones, dying axons, and developmental fluctuations in the fiber population of the cat's optic nerve.   J. comp. Neurol. 246, 32-69.

2

Neurochemical Modulation of Fetal Behaviour and Excitation at Birth

Hugo Lagercrantz

INTRODUCTION

Although several papers in this volume describe active fetal behaviour such as reactions to sensory stimulation and fetal movements, there are also indications that expressions of fetal behaviour are to some extent suppressed. Maybe this inhibition of neural pathways is of importance for normal maturation (see Als, this volume). According to video-tape recordings of the fetal sheep, the fetus is never or very seldom awake (Rigatto 1987). Breathing movements are actively inhibited from a suprapontine level (see Dawes 1984). During stress e.g. the fetus responds with paralysis, apnea and bradycardia in contrast to the adult fight-and-flight response with marked tachycardia.

The inhibition of some fetal behaviours might be very appropriate for the adaptation to the low oxygen tension in utero, particularly during asphyxia. This inhibition seems to be immediately reversed at birth, when the newborn baby is aroused, starts to breathe continuously and becomes independent of maternal heating and nutrition by the umbilical cord. However, the infant mammal might still continue to react with some kind of inhibited behaviour e.g. with paralysis, apnea and bradycardia instead of agitation, tachypnea and tachycardia (Kaada 1987).

The partially inhibited state of the fetus, immediately reversed after birth, is assumed to be due to neurohormonal mechanisms, particularly the inhibition of the fetus during asphyxia. This paper is a somewhat provocative attempt to correlate the development of some behaviours during early development. However, our knowledge about the relationship between chemical neurotransmission and behaviour is very limited particularly in the fetus and the newborn. As an example, the breathing behaviour will be mainly discussed, since this type of behaviour has been relatively easy to quantitate in relation to the administration of neurohormones and their antagonists.

SOME NOTES ON THE DEVELOPMENT OF NEUROCHEMICAL MECHANISMS

The development of neuronal pathways, projections of dendrites and organization of synapses is far from complete in the central nervous system at birth. Although most of the known neurotransmitters and -modulators occur early during ontogenesis and even reach peak concentrations before birth, they are probably more important for the development of the connectivity in the brain than for synaptic transmission per se (Parnavelas & Cavanagh 1988).

Inhibitory neurotransmitters seem to dominate before birth. Morphological studies have shown that the flat synaptic vesicles which are supposed to contain inhibitory neurotransmitters dominate over the spherical ones with excitatory neurotransmitters in the newborn kitten (see Cullheim & Ulfhake, this volume). Inhibitory neurotransmitters like GABA, taurin, endorphins and somatostatin occur in relatively higher concentrations than excitatory neurotransmitters like glutamate, aspartate and acetylcholine (Fig. 1).

Circulating neurohormones might play a relatively more important role in the fetus and the infant than later in life. In the periphery the sympathetic nervous system is not functioning in the newborn rat which is completely dependent on circulating catecholamines from the adrenal medulla during asphyxia. Also in the human newborn infant circulating catecholamines play a relatively greater functional role than the sympathetic nervous system (see Lagercrantz & Slotkin 1986). Fetal plasma catecholamines are normally very low before birth (Jones 1980), but increase considerably during labour and at birth (vidae infra).

Circulating substances with neurohormonal action like the prostaglandins are formed in the placenta and transferred to the fetus particularly during the end of gestation (Thorburn & Rice 1987).

The low oxygen tension in the fetus particularly during asphyxia can stimulate the formation and release of neuroactive substances like adenosine (Winn et al 1981).

NEUROCHEMICAL INHIBITION OF FETAL BREATHING BEHAVIOUR?

Although breathing behaviour is considered to be' a mainly autonomic activity it is also driven by a forebrain drive during awakefulness and by subconscious dreaming activity during rapid eye movement (REM) sleep (Euler 1987). Breathing movements are relatively easy to quantitate in the fetus and the newborn and there is some information regarding its nature of modulation by neurohormones.

Fig. 1 Tentative scheme of the relative innervation with some excitatory (stippled) and inhibitory (blank) neurotransmitters in the brain during development. When no human data has been available, extrapolation from studies in the rat has been performed. Glutaminergic markers peak after birth in the rat brain (Greenamyre et al 1987), but possibly before birth in the human (Barks et al 1988). Aspartate concentrations increase successively after birth in the human brain (Man et al 1987). Fetal data not available. GABA concentrations increase rapidly before birth and peaks at about one year (Johnston & Coyle 1981). Cholinergic markers (ACh) increase rapidly in the human cortex after birth (see Johnston & Coyle 1981). Noradrenergic neurons innervate the rat cerebral cortex extensively at an early stage in the rat (Felten et al 1982). Endorphine (met-enkephalin) concentrations in the medulla from Gingras & Long (1988). Extensive somatostatin (SRIF) innervation has also been found to occur transiently (Parnavelas & Cavanagh 1988) in the rat brain. Substance P data from Bergström et al (1984).

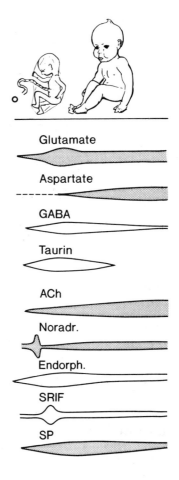

Glutamate

Aspartate

GABA

Taurin

ACh

Noradr.

Endorph.

SRIF

SP

Fetal breathing movements appear early during the gestation. Extensive studies in the chronically instrumented fetal sheep have demonstrated that the breathing movements are episodic and occur only during low-voltage electrocortical activity corresponding to REM-sleep. During high voltage electrocortical activity or non-REM-sleep, breathing seems to be actively inhibited (see Dawes 1984). Pinching, auditory or visual stimulation do not elicit breathing during this state. These periods of inhibition increase towards the end of gestation corresponding to the maturation and differentiation of state dependent brain activities. The term fetus nearly ceases to breathe a few days before birth (see Bryan et al 1986).

A number of inhibitory neurotransmitters/modulators have been proposed to mediate this inhibition: e.g. endorphines, GABA, adenosine and somatostatin (see Gluckman & Bennet 1986). The evidences for such an inhibitory role is the finding of relatively higher concentrations in the brain stem of these neurohormones in the fetus than in the adult and the demonstration of continuous breathing after pharmacological blockade of endogenous activity. For example relatively higher concentrations of met-enkephalin has been found in brain stem nuclei controlling respiration in fetal than in adult rabbits (Gingras & Long 1988) and fetal breathing has been reported to be stimulated by the endorphin antagonist naloxone (see Moss et al 1986).

    It is probably not so simple that just a single neuro-transmitter inhibits fetal breathing movements; but there may possibly be a dominance of synapses with inhibitory neurotrans-mitters/modulators converging at the central respiratory neurons and increasing the threshold for neuronal firing (see Cullheim & Ulfhake, this volume and Lagercrantz 1987).

    An alternate possibility is that the placenta produces some inhibitory neurohormone, which depresses fetal breathing move-ments. If the fetus is artificially ventilated with air in utero and the umbilical cord occluded, spontaneous breathing movements occur continuously, which stop when the occlusion is lifted (Adamson et al 1987). The possible humoral agent mediating this respiratory inhibitory effect could be prostaglandins. By blocking the prostaglandin synthesis with indomethacine fetal breathing is stimulated and occurs continuously (Wallen et al 1986). It is interesting to note that fetal breathing stops a few days before birth, corresponding to the surge of prostaglandins before labour (Thorburn & Rice 1987).

    The fetal response to stress e.g. asphyxia is inhibitory in its nature while it is not so in later postnatal life. While the adult generally reacts with a fight-and-flight response with increased muscular blood flow, increased breathing and tachy-cardia, the fetus becomes paralysed with decreased muscular blood flow, stops breathing and becomes bradycardic. This so called fetal diving response is probably a very adequate response to save oxygen consumption (Fig. 2).

    The neurochemical mechanism behind this inhibitory response is not clear. There is certainly a substantial release of excita-tory amino acids as seen in the fetal sheep (Hagberg et al 1987) and of catecholamines (Jones 1980) which could be expected to cause more excitatory responses. However, more noradrenaline than adrenaline has been found to be released in the human fetus than in adults during asphyxia (Lagercrantz & Slotkin 1986). Noradrena-line decreases muscle blood flow. There might be a difference in receptor responses. Inhibitory alpha-d_2 receptors occur more frequently in early age (Marcus et al 1987).

    Another important possibility is the release of inhibitory

neurotransmitters and -modulators which might overcome the excitatory effects and inhibit the release of excitatory neurotransmitters. Adenosine is such a neuromodulator which is released in very high concentrations during hypoxia or ischemia. Adenosine is formed in increasing concentrations in the brain at a PO_2-level of about 30 torr (Winn et al 1981), the normal PO_2 of the fetus! If PO_2 drops down to 10-15 torr a substantial increase of tissue adenosine levels could be expected to be released (and has in fact been found by collecting extracellular fluid with a microdialysis probe inserted into the fetal sheep brain). Adenosine has a number of inhibitory actions like causing sedation and hypotonia inhibiting brown fat activation and lipolysis (see Berne 1986). It also inhibits respiration probably mainly at a central level (see Lagercrantz et al 1987). It is interesting to note that while adenosine or its stable analogue has been reported to inhibit respiration in the fetal sheep (Szeto & Umans 1985) and young rabbit pups it stimulates adult breathing (see Runold et al 1986).

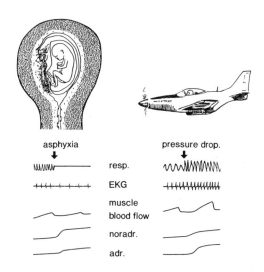

asphyxia   pressure drop.

resp.

EKG

muscle
blood flow

noradr.

adr.

Fig. 2   The fetus usually reacts with an inhibitory behaviour during hypoxic stress, in contrast to the adult fight-and-flight response.

EXCITATION AT BIRTH

At birth there is a substantial neurohormone surge particularly of catecholamines (CA). The plasma CA level in the fetal sheep has been found to be very low and so also in the human fetus the CA level is normally lower than in the resting adult. During labour the plasma CA levels increase several-fold in normal vaginal deliveries as indicated by analyses of fetal scalp blood samples (Bistoletti et al 1983). If the fetus is asphyxiated (scalp pH <7.25) the CA concentration can increase up to 100-fold. Infants delivered by elective cesarean section have considerably lower CA-levels. This indicates that the vaginal delivery as such triggers the CA surge, possibly by the squeezing and squashing of the fetal head (Lagercrantz & Slotkin 1986). Intermittent hypoxia due to uterine compressions or sustained fetal asphyxia can further potentiate the CA release.

There is also a surge of other neurohormones at birth like endorphines (see Moss et al 1982), neuropeptide Y (Lundberg et al 1986), TRH (Gluckman et al 1988) some gastro-intestinal hormones (Marchini et al 1988) and adenosine (Irestedt et al 1989). To what extent can this neurohormonal surge affect neonatal adaptation and the behaviour of the newborn?

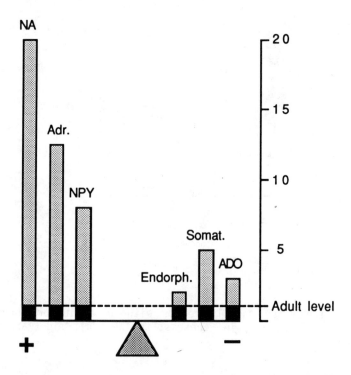

Fig. 3   Neurohormone surge at birth. Noradrenaline (NA) and adrenaline (Adr.) levels (see Irestedt et al 1984), neuropeptide Y (NPY) (Lundberg et al 1986), endorphine (Endorph.) (Moss et al 1982), somatostatin (Somat.) (Marchini et al 1988), adenosine (ADO) (Irestedt et al 1989).

By comparing vaginally born infants with infants delivered by elective cesarean section, we had a clinical experimental situation with a high (vaginal) and low CA group (cesarean section) of infants. The former were found to have better lung function, higher levels of glucose and free fatty acids and better pooling of blood towards the most vital organs (see Lagercrantz & Slotkin 1986). Furthermore asphyxiated infants (defined as pH <7.20) with high CA levels were found to have higher Apgar scores than infants with lower score but the same pH (Irestedt et al 1984). Recent studies have demonstrated that infants delivered by elective cesarean section were found to be less alert and to have a lower neurological score than vaginally delivered infants (Leijon et al 1988). This could not be related to analgesia. Most of the cesarean sections were performed under epidural analgesia which often also is given to women delivering vaginally. It is more likely that the difference in CA surge could be responsible for these behavioural differences.

It is well established that e.g. adrenaline given to adults in such high concentrations as seen after birth has substantial arousal and alerting effects and normally leads to a feeling of well-being provided the environmental circumstances are good (Frankenhaeuser 1971). Thus the CA release in the plasma from the sympatho-adrenal system can cause these effects. However, it is also possible that the noradrenaline rich structure locus coeruleus is activated simultaneously and is involved in causing this arousal (Svensson 1987).

CONCLUSIONS

Fetal breathing behaviour is partially inhibited before birth, tentatively due to some dominance of synapses with inhibitory neurotransmitters at the central respiratory neurons and circulating inhibitory neurohormones like adenosine and prostaglandines possibly of placental origin.

The fetal stress response reactions result in an inhibitory behaviour - the paralysis reflex. This difference in fetal stress reaction versus the adult might be due to release of more noradrenaline than adrenaline in the fetus than in the adult and a surge of adenosine and other inhibitory modulators which depress fetal behaviour.

The relatively depressed state of the fetus is immediately reversed at birth. The surge of catecholamines might be of importance for this reaction. However, the newborn infant still retains fetal inhibitory mechanisms which could be activated for example during hypoxia.

ACKNOWLEDGEMENTS

Supported by the Swedish Medical Research Council (Project No. 19X-5234) and Expressen's Prenatal Research Foundation.

REFERENCES

Adamson, S.L., Richardson, B.S. and Homan, J. (1987). Initiation of pulmonary gas exchange by fetal sleep in utero. J. Appl. Physiol., 62(3), 989-998.

Barks, J.D., Silverstein, F.S., Sims, K., Greenamyre, J.T. and Johnston, M.V. (1988). Glutamate recognition sites in human fetal brain. Neurosci. Letters, 84, 131-136.

Bergström, L., Lagercrantz, H. and Terenius, L. (1984). Post-mortem analyses of neuropeptides in brains from sudden infant death victims. Brain Res., 323, 279-285.

Berne, R.M. (1986). Adenosine: An important physiological regulator. NIPS, 1, 163-167.

Bistoletti, P., Nylund, L., Lagercrantz, H., Hjemdahl, P. and Ström, H. (1983). Fetal scalp catecholamines during labor. Am. J. Obst. Gyn., 147, 785-788.

Bryan, A.C., Bowes,, G. and Maloney, J.E. (1986). In Handbook of Physiology. The Respiratory System, 621-647.

Dawes, G.S. (1984). The central control of fetal breathing and skeletal muscle movements. J.Physiol., 346, 1-18.

Euler, C. von (1987). Breathing behavior. In Neurobiology of the Control of Breathing (eds. C. von Euler and H. Lagercrantz). Raven Press, New York.

Felten, D., Hallman, H., and Jonsson, G. (1982). Evidence for a neurotrophic role of noradrenaline neurons for the postnatal development of rat cerebral cortex. J.Neurocytol., 11, 119-135.

Frankenhaeuser, M. (1971). Behavior and circulating catecholamines. Brain Res., 31, 241-262.

Gingras, J.L. and Long, W.A. (1988). Chronic maternal hypoxia. Dev. Neurosci., 10, 180-189.

Gluckman, P.D. and Bennet, L. (1986). Neuropharmacology of fetal and neonatal breathing. In Reproductive and Prenatal Medicine (III). Respiratory Control and Lung Development in the Fetus and Newborn (eds. B.M.Johnston and P.D.Gluckman). Perinatology Press, Ithaca, N.Y.

Gluckman, P.D., Cook, C., Williams, C., Bennet, L. and Johnston, B. (1988). Electrophysiological, neuromodulator and neurotransmitter development of the late gestation fetal brain. In Fetal and Neonatal Development. (ed. C.T. Jones). Perinatology Press, Ithaca, N.Y.

Greenamyre, T., Penney, J.B., Young, A., Hudson, C., Silverstein, F.S. and Johnston, M.V. (1987). Evidence for transient perinatal glutamatergic innervation of globus pallidus. J.Neurosci., 7(4), 1022-1030.

Hagberg, H., Andersson, P., Kjellmer, I., Thiringer, K. and Thordstein, M. (1987). Extracellular overflow of glutamate, aspartate, GABA and taurine during hypoxia-ischemia. Neurosci. Lett., 78, 311-317.

Irestedt, L., Dahlin, I., Hertzberg, T., Sollevi, A. and Lagercrantz, H. (1989). Adenosine concentration in umbilical cord blood of newborn infants after vaginal delivery and cesarean section. Pediatr. Res. (in press).

Irestedt, L., Lagercrantz, H. and Belfrage, P. (1984). Causes and consequences of maternal and fetal sympathoadrenal activation during parturition. Acta Obst. Gynecol. Scand., 118, 111-115.

Johnston, M.V. and Coyle, J. (1981). Development of central neurotransmitter systems. Ciba Foundation Symposium 86, 251-270.

Jones, C.T. (1980). Circulating catecholamines in the fetus, their origin, action and significance. In Biogenic Amines in Development. (ed. H.Parvez and S.Parvez).

Kaada, B. (1987). The sudden infant death syndrome induced by 'the fear paralysis reflex'? Med. Hypotheses, 22, 347-356.

Lagercrantz, H. (1987). Neuromodulators and respiratory control during development. TINS, 10(9), 368-372.

Lagercrantz, H., Runold, M., Yamamoto, Y. and Fredholm, B. (1987). Adenosine: A putative mediator of the hypoxic ventilatory response of the neonate. In Neurobiology of the Control of Breathing. (eds. C. von Euler and H.Lagercrantz). Raven Press, New York.

Lagercrantz, H. and Slotkin, T. (1986). The stress of birth. Sci. Amer., 254, 100-107.

Leijon, I., Berg, G., Finnström, O. and Otamiri, G., (1988). Europ. Congr. in Perinatology. Abstracts, Rome.

Lundberg, J.M., Hemsén, A., Fried, G., Theodorsson-Norheim, E. and Lagercrantz, H. (1986). Co-release of neuropeptide Y (NPY)-like immunoreactivity and catecholamines in newborn infants. Acta

Physiol. Scand., 126, 471-473.

Man, E.H., Fisher, G.H., Payan, I.L., Cadilla-Perezrios, R., Garcia, N.M., Chemburkar, R., Arends, G. and Frey, W.H. (1987). D-aspartate in human brain. J.Neurochem. 48, 510-515.

Marchini, G., Lagercrantz, H., Winberg, J. and Uvnäs-Moberg, K. (1988). Fetal and maternal plasma levels of gastrin, somatostatin and oxytocin after vaginal delivery and elective cesarean section. Early Human Dev., 18, 73-79.

Marcus, C., Karpe, B., Bolme, P., Sonnenfeld, T. and Arner, P. (1987). Changes in catecholamine induced lipolysis in isolated fat cells during the first year of life. J. Clin. Invest., 79, 1812-1862.

Moss, I.R., Conner, H., Yee, W.F.H., Iorio, P. and Scarpelli, M. (1982). Human beta-endorphin-like immunoreactivity in the peri-natal/neonatal period. J. Pediatr., 101(3), 443-446.

Moss, I.R., Denavit-Saubié, M., Eldridge, F.L., Gillis, R.A., Herkenham, M. and Lahiri, S. (1986). Neuromodulators and trans-mitters in respiratory control. Fed. Proc., 45(7), 2133-2147.

Parnavelas, J.G. and Cavanagh, M.E. (1988). Transient expression of neurotransmitters in the developing neocortex. TINS, 11(3), 92-93.

Rigatto, H. (1987). Fetal state and control of breathing. In Neurobiology of the Control of Breathing. (eds. C. von Euler and H.Lagercrantz). Raven Press, New York.

Runold, M., Lagercrantz, H. and Fredholm, B.B. (1986). Ventilatory effect of an adenosine analogue in unanesthetized rabbits during development. J. Appl. Physiol. 61, 255-259.

Svensson, T.H. (1987). Brain norepinephrine neurons in the locus coeruleus and the control of arousal and respiration: implications for sudden infant death syndrome. In Neurobiology of the Control of Breathing. (eds. C. von Euler and H.Lagercrantz), Raven Press, New York.

Szeto, H.H. and Umans, J.G. (1985). The effects of a stable adenosine analogue on fetal behavioural, respiratory and cardio-vascular functions. In The Physiological Development of the Fetus and Newborn. (ed. C.T. Jones). Academic Press, London.

Thorburn, G.D. and Rice, G.E. (1987). Fetal maturation and the timing of parturition: a comparative analysis. Proc. Australian Physiol. Pharmacol. Soc. 18(2).

Wallen, L.D., Murai, D.T., Clyman, R.I., Lee, C.H., Mauray, F.E. and Kitterman, J.A. (1986). Regulation of breathing movements in fetal sheep by prostaglandin E2. J. Appl. Physiol., 60, 526-531.

Winn, R., Rubio, R. and Berne, R.M. (1981). Brain adenosine concentration during hypoxia in rats. Am. Sci. Physiol., 241, H235-H242.

3
On Innate and Extrinsic Determinants of Brain Development: Lessons from the Eye Chamber

Lars Olson, Maria Eriksdotter-Nilsson and Ingrid Strömberg

INTRODUCTION

By taking the early developing central nervous system apart and then following development of the isolated parts grafted e.g. to the anterior chamber of the eye, it becomes possible to evaluate the relative importance of intrinsic, genetic determinants of development in relation to the importance of connections between any given defined area of the brain and the rest of the central nervous system. Clearly, as pointed out by Blakemore (this volume), innate instructions are important for the early development of the basic cytoarchitecture. This is illustrated in anterior chamber grafting experiments (see Olson et al. 1984) where very immature isolated anlage of e.g. the hippocampal formation or cerebellum are able to develop organotypical lamination and other structural features characteristic of their normal mature counterparts. It is equally clear, however, that there must be epigenetic influences on the further development and synaptic organization of the brain. The one area of the central nervous system that appears to be most dependent upon appropriate connections with the rest of the central nervous system and the outer world is the cerebral cortex. In the eye chamber, isolated grafts of cerebral cortex will develop several abnormal features including a lack of appropriate inhibitory neuronal circuits and gliosis. Cortical grafts placed in contact with previously grafted brain tissue in the eye chamber will in many cases develop much more normally, suggesting trophic interactions between the two grafts. While the nature of such interactions has not been established, we know that physical contact between the "stimulating" and the "stimulated" graft is necessary (Björklund et al. 1983).

The trophic experiments described above emphasize the importance of membrane-bound, non-diffusible compounds such as surface recognition molecules and cell adhesion molecules for proper development. However, also hormones, hormone-like compounds and growth factors such as nerve growth factor, NGF, which may all act after being released from their sites of synthesis are crucial for normal brain development. Recent studies by Rakic et al. (1986) have emphasized an interesting isochronic course of synaptogenesis in several different areas of the primate cerebral cortex and the authors suggest that perhaps a single genetic or humoral signal might be operating (Rakic et al. 1986).   Our own studies in the anterior chamber of the eye indicate one such factor, NGF, to be important for cortical development. Thus, both cerebral cortex and cerebellar cortex will stop growing significantly earlier in the eye chamber following NGF treatment, leading to smaller, but otherwise undisturbed, transplants (Eriksdotter-Nilsson et al. 1988). Perhaps in this case NGF induces precocious maturation. We know that cortical areas contain and produce NGF normally. Thus, we have recently demonstrated that the β-nerve growth factor gene is indeed expressed in hippocampal neurons (Ayer-LeLievre et al. 1988). It is unlikely that this effect of excessive NGF on cortical areas is an unspecific toxic effect, since treatment with the same doses of NGF of basal forebrain transplants containing cholinergic neurons will instead result in increased growth of the transplants and survival of a larger number of cholinergic neurons.

Important differences between the primate and the rodent brain necessitate studies of development in primates. For studies of developmental aspects, an alternative approach has recently become available based on xenografting human tissues to rodent hosts. Using approaches approved of by the Ethical Committee of the Karolinska Institute, small tissue fragments recovered after elective routine abortions in the seventh to eleventh week of gestation can be grafted to the anterior chamber of the eye or into the central nervous system of rats or mice whose immune system is either suppressed by ciclosporin or to athymic, nude rats and mice. Many different areas of the early developing human nervous system such as the spinal cord, monoamine neurons from locus coeruleus, substantia nigra and the raphe nuclei, as well as cortical areas such as cerebellar cortex, the hippocampal formation and the cerebral cortex all survive and develop in rodent hosts. Basic cytoarchitectural and electrophysiological features develop in isolation in the eye chamber. However, development proceeds according to a human rather than a rat timetable; thus long survival times are necessary in order to even approach adult features. Nevertheless, the technique offers possibilities to study a wide window of human development. Xenografts of human fetal substantia nigra dopamine neuroblasts to striatum of dopamine-denervated rat hosts will lead to dopaminergic reinnervation of the host with restitution of functional deficits (Strömberg et al. 1986).

The importance of the "trauma" of vaginal delivery has been pointed out by Lagercrantz (this volume). Thus, there are marked differences in levels of catecholamines and various measures of arousal between children delivered normally and children delivered by caesarian section. One hypothesis proposed by Lagercrantz is that the prenatal fetus is in a state of inhibition from which it is released by birth. By grafting appropriate areas of brainstem tissue (such as respiratory centers and other formatio reticularis areas) to the eye chamber so that development proceeds from prenatal to postnatal and mature without a stress of birth, it might be possible to evaluate the relative involvement of the central nervous system vs. the peripheral nervous system and the endocrine system for these birth-induced changes.

To conclude, brain development proceeds from initial stages dominated by genetic determinants into stages when influences from the local surroundings as well as the outer world become increasingly important. Molecular communication by both membrane-bound and released components such as e.g. NGF, appear critical. Finally, the adult central nervous system seems to retain a considerable degree of plasticity enabling even structural rearrangements at the synaptic level. By learning more about factors that regulate development and plasticity in the adult organism, we might better understand how these processes are impaired in aging and how some of the deleterious effects of aging might be counteracted.

ACKNOWLEDGEMENTS

Supported by the Swedish Medical Research Council, Magnus Bergvalls Stiftelse, and the "Expressen" Prenatal Research Foundation.

REFERENCES

Ayer-LeLievre, C., Olson, L., Ebendal, T., Seiger, Å.and Persson, H. (1988). Expression of the β-nerve growth factor gene in hippocampal neurons. Science, 240, 1339-1341.

Björklund, H., Seiger, Å., Hoffer, B. and Olson, L. (1983). Trophic effects of brain areas on the developing cerebral cortex: I. Growth and histological organization of intraocular grafts. Dev. Brain Res., 6, 131-140

Eriksdotter-Nilsson, M., Skirboll, S., Ebendal, T., Olson, L. (1988) Differential effects of nerve growth factor on growth of cortex cerebri, hippocampus and cerebellum: Evidence from intraocular grafts. Manuscript for *Neuroscience*.

Olson , L., Björklund, H. and Hoffer, B. (1984). Camera bulbi anterior: New vistas on a classical locus for neural tissue transplantation. In Neural Transplants, Development and Function (eds. J. Sladek and D. Gash). pp. 125-165. Plenum Press, New York.

Palmer, M., Björklund, H., Olson, L. and Hoffer, B. (1983). Trophic effects of brain areas on the developing cerebral cortex: II. Electrophysiology of intraocular grafts. Dev. Brain Res., 6, 141-148.

Rakic, P., Bourgeois, J.-P., Eckenhoff, M.F., Zecevic, N. and Goldman-Rakic, P.S. (1986). Concurrent overproduction of synapses in diverse regions of the primate cerebral cortex. Science, 232, 232-235.

Strömberg, I., Bygdeman, M., Goldstein, M., Seiger, Å., Olson, L. (1986). Human fetal substantia nigra grafted to the dopamine-denervated striatum of immunosuppressed rats: evidence for functional reinnervation. Neurosci. Lett., 71, 271-276.

II. Muscle Tone and Postural Mechanisms

4

The Development of Neuromuscular Junctions as a Model of the Generation of Neuronal Circuitry

J. K. S. Jansen

The developmental processes which generate the neural machinery have been difficult to study in the vertebrate brain with its overwhelmingly intricate structure. The neuromuscular system is much simpler and more accessible. Several of the major events in neural development were first demonstrated for the innervation of the skeletal muscles, and this information has to a considerable extent guided later studies of brain development. In this short account I shall review some selected features of neuromuscular development which probably are relevant also for the generation of brain circuitry. Several recent reviews give more exhaustive coverage of the field (Betz, 1987; Van Essen, 1982; Bennett, 1983).

Cell death. About the time the motor axons have reached their primordial muscle mass the first major regressive event during development is initiated. Motor neurons (MNs) start to degenerate. Over the next week about 50% of the original complement of MNs die. Some support from the target determines the survival of the MNs. If a limb is amputated in the early embryo, virtually all the corresponding MNs degenerate. If the target is expanded, as with the transplantation of an extra limb, more MNs will survive. It is as if the MNs are competing for available target or perhaps for a trophic substance produced by the target in limiting amounts (Hamburger & Oppenheim, 1982). Paralysis of the muscle over the relevant period virtually prevents the cell death altogether (Laing & Prestige, 1978; Pitman and Oppenheim, 1979) suggesting that the trophic support may be activity-dependent.

Formation of synapses   The assembly of functional
synapses is obviously a complicated process. A large
number of components is required, both presynaptically,
for transmitter synthesis, storage and release, and
postsynaptically, for appropriate alignment of
receptors and enzymes. At the neuromuscular junction
(n.m.j.) the whole complex is assembled within an hour
after the early motor axons reach the myotubes of the
immature muscles (Kullberg et al., 1977).

    The acetylcholine receptor (AChR) is the
participant that is best known. The receptors are
expressed in the surface membrane already at the
myoblast stage. In the early myotubes the AChRs are
evenly distributed over the entire surface membrane.
Slightly later some of the receptors aggregate in much
denser small clusters (hot spots) randomly distributed
over the myotube surface (Vogel et al., 1972). When
MNs are added to cultures their emerging processes soon
establish contact with the myotubes, and grow along
their surface. Remarkably, the contact site is
independent of the preformed AChR aggregates, but very
rapidly, new aggregates are induced along the contact
path of the axon (Anderson et al., 1977; Frank &
Fischbach, 1977). Initially, the nerve induced AChR
aggregates consist of preformed receptors. These
receptors initially freely diffuse in the membrane but
appear to be trapped and aggregated along the nerve
contact path. As the neuronally induced aggregates
accumulate, the diffusely distributed AChRs are
reduced. This is not only due to the "trapping" effect
of the nerve, but also to a suppression of the
synthesis of the extrajunctional receptors
(Moody-Corbett & Cohen, 1982).

    These remarkable effects on the distribution of the
AChRs is not a general contact induction. Motoneuronal,
or at least cholinergic, processes are required.
Sensory ganglion cell processes, for instance, will
grow in intimate contact with the myotubes without
affecting the distribution of the AChRs (Cohen &
Weldon, 1980).

    Formation of ectopic junctions. The examination of
synapse formation after regeneration of motor nerves in
adult animals has provided valuable additional insights
into synaptogenesis. This applies particularly to the
second, "maturational" stage in formation of nmjs which
has been examined most effectively during ectopic
innervation from foreign nerves transplanted to
skeletal muscles. In many respects such ectopic
synapse formation reproduces the essential events of

the first innervation of embryonic muscles (Lømo,
1987).

An intact adult skeletal muscle will not accept
additional innervation. If, however, the muscle is
denervated or if the muscle is paralyzed a transplanted
motor nerve will start forming synapses ectopically on
virgin regions of the muscle fibers (Jansen et al.,
1973). The permissive state develops within a day or
two and can be prevented by maintaining activity by
stimulating the muscle directly. Interestingly, such
direct stimulation of the muscle will not prevent
reinnervation of the original end plate sites.

One advantage of studying ectopic junctions in
adult muscle is that their generation can be accurately
timed from the section of the original nerve. After
the early subsynaptic receptor aggregates are
established the further development of the n.m.j.
proceeds more slowly, taking several weeks. As the
nerve terminals increase their contact area by further
growth and arborization the post-synaptic receptor
aggregates expand accordingly. At the same time the
synaptic AChRs are stabilized. For the nmjs proper
synaptic function also requires a short duration of
channel opening and rapid removal of transmitter
effects. Within a few days the enzyme responsible for
this, acetylcholine-esterase (AChE), is deposited in
the subsynaptic membrane, and an additional reduction
in the open time of the AChRs further limits the
duration of the transmitter effect (Michler & Sakmann,
1980). Among the processes contributing the maturation
of the postsynaptic part of the n.m.j., some require
the continuous presence of the nerve terminal, whereas
muscle activity alone is necessary and sufficient for
others (Lømo, 1987).

As during normal development, the ectopically
innervated muscle fibers are initially superinnervated
by the transplanted nerve. With time many of the
redundant terminals are eliminated. The loss largely
affects terminals closely spaced along the muscle
fibers (Kuffler et al., 1980). Hence, there are
mechanisms which regulate the density of innervation of
the fibers.

The reinnervation of mature skeletal muscle has
provided important additional clues to our
understanding of synaptogenesis. The original endplate
sites are the preferred targets for the regenerating
axons. Surprisingly the muscle fibers themselves are
not the immediate and only element involved. Sanes and

coworkers (1978) were able to selectively destroy the
muscle fibers while leaving their basal lamina intact.
In such preparation the regenerating axons still found
the original end-plate sites and differentiated to
presynaptic terminals with active sites aligned with
the "postsynaptic" clefts as in normal junctions.
Pursuing this they have been able to identify and
partly purify a component of the junctional basal
lamina which enhances the aggregation of AChR and AChE
in cultured myotubes. The substance is produced by
motor neurons and may normally be involved in the
assembly of the critical elements of the n.m.j. (Reist
et al. 1987).

     Mechanisms of neuro-muscular interactions. With
its precision and accurate timing, the formation of
n.m.j.s is a closely regulated process which depends on
reciprocal exchange of signals between the MNs and
their targets. A trophic substance produced by the
muscle was suggested already by Hamburger to explain
his observations of the target dependence of early
motoneurons. More recently several groups have
obtained analogous results in vitro (see Henderson,
1987). Addition of muscle extract or conditioned
medium from cultured myotubes increase the survival of
cultured MNs. In other approaches the stimulation of
axonal outgrowth from MNs has been used to identify
putative trophic target-to-neuron effects.

     Most of the thinking about the retrograde
target to-neuron effect has been strongly influenced by
the identification of NGF and its spectrum of effects.
Nerve growth factor is produced by the target tissues
of sympathetic ganglion cells. It is required for the
survival of these cells both in vivo and in cell
culture. In the targets NGF is taken up by nerve
terminals and transported over the axons to the cell
bodies. It stimulates axonal outgrowth and through its
trophic effects and local availability it can determine
the distribution of processes generated by the neurons
(Campenot, 1982). A substance with such effects could
significantly contribute also to the development of
somatic MNs. For these the relevant substances have so
far eluded identification and it is still open whether
the various retrograde trophic effects are due to a
single substance or rather a combination of substances
with different effects on the MNs (Berg, 1984).

     Orthograde trophic effects from nerve to muscle are
equally striking. The early clustering of AChR in the
subsynaptic membrane has attracted particular attention
among the innervation induced effects. As already

described it goes along with the suppression of
perijunctional receptors and this takes place even in
paralyzed preparations (Davey & Cohen, 1986). However,
for other of the putative orthograde trophic effects it
may be difficult to distinguish between a strictly
trophic effect and the consequences of the activity in
the muscle fibers which follows innervation.

The postnatal loss of synapses. For some unexplained
reason synaptogenesis in the developing skeletal
muscles consistently overshoots its mark. Each of the
early muscle fibers gets innervated by branches from
several different motor axons. Even though many MNs
die from the time the muscles are first innervated the
polyneuronal innervation continues to increase. Soon
after birth the process is reversed, and over the next
few weeks synaptic terminals are eliminated until only
a single terminal remains on each muscle fiber. This
all happens while the number of MNs, and in some
muscles the number of muscle fibers, remain constant.
Hence, the essential change is a loss of terminal
branches from each MN, ie. a reduction in the size of
the motor unit (MU) (Brown et al., 1976).

The survival of only a single axon terminal to each
muscle fibre is a striking feature of the elimination
process. This apparently takes place without a
complete denervation of any fibers, even transiently.
Hence, it is not a question simply of a random loss of
terminals in the muscle. The single survivor suggests
that a competitive interaction between terminals
innervating the same muscle fiber is a prominent part
of the process (Brown et al., 1976).

The effect of removing competitors is the obvious
test for a competitive process. This has been done in
newborn rat and mouse muscles, and the result is clear.
The remaining MUs retain about twice as many terminals
as they do after normal development. This demonstrates
the competitive component of the elimination (Betz,
1987; Brown et al., 1976). A more controversial
question is whether a competitive process alone can
fully account for the neonatal loss of terminals
(Willshaw, 1981). After partial denervation of the
newborn mouse soleus the remaining MUs are appreciably
reduced from their initial size. This reduction is
more than can be accounted for by residual competition
between the few remaining MUs. Hence, in addition to
the competition between terminals innervating the same
muscle fiber, there is a noncompetitive component which

appears to be independent of the state of innervation of the muscle (Fladby & Jansen, 1987). There is an upper limit to the number of terminal branches that a MN can maintain. This "capacity" is reduced over the first few weeks of postnatal life and accounts for the noncompetitive component of synapse elimination. This might be due to the increasing demands on the individual terminals over the neonatal period. For example, as the muscle fibers grow in size, the amount of transmitter required to activate them increases correspondingly. Structurally this is seen as an expansion of the synaptic area, and the limited resources of each MN has to be restricted to fewer terminals.

Selective innervation of fast and slow fibers. Most skeletal muscles consist of functionally different types of fibers which can be classified as fast (F) or slow (S) on the basis of their characteristic mechanical, biochemical, and histological properties. Each MU contains exclusively fast (F) or slow (S) muscle fibers (Burke, 1981). When this was first established it was commonly thought that the differentiation of muscle fibers was induced at a moderately late stage by the innervating MN, for instance by its pattern of activity. This explained the homogeneity of the composition of the MUs. Now, however, it is clear that muscle fibers differentiate into F and S types quite early during development (Rubinstein and Kelly, 1981). Hence, the possibility came up that perhaps the neonatal elimination of synapses was an essential process for the generation of homogeneous mature MUs.

Thompson and coworkers (1984) approached this issue and found, in line with Gordon and Van Essen (1985), that MUs were largely homogeneous while muscle fibers were still polyinnervated. However, the neonatal rat lumbrical muscle has been reported to have MUs consisting of a random mixture of F and S muscle fibers (Jones et al. 1987), suggesting that the generation of functionally homogeneous MUs here is due to selective elimination of terminals from inappropriate muscle fibers. This motivated a recent study of the mouse soleus muscle which demonstrated a high degree of selectivity in the innervation of the muscle while the density of innervation is still maximal (Fladby and Jansen, 1988). Hence, the neonatal synapse elimination is not a decisive factor in the generation of homogeneous F and S MUs. A recent study of reinnervation of neonatal muscle also suggests a selective recognition process between appropriate

terminals and slow or fast fibers in the neonatal rat
soleus (Soileau et al., 1987).

Segmental preferences in muscle innervation. For
certain segmental muscles Wigston and Sanes (1985)
demonstrated a weak but definite segmental preference
for reinnervation by preganglionic sympathetic fibers.
Some other muscles, all with a wide segmental origin,
are innervated in a definite segmentotopic pattern.
Moreover, the pattern is concealed in the exuberant
neonatal innervation, and is only clearly manifest
after synapse elimination has taken place (Brown &
Booth, 1983). Hence, segmentally inappropriate
neonatal terminals are preferentially eliminated in
these muscles and the elimination process contributes
to a refinement of the innervation of the muscle.

MU size. There is a limit to the number of
synaptic terminals that a MN can sustain (Thompson &
Jansen, 1977). If a muscle is partially denervated,
the remaining MUs sprout and expand their field of
innervation in the muscle. Once reinnervation occurs
the regenerating MUs regain their territory at the
expence of the expanded remaining units (Thompson,
1978).If cross- or reinnervation is allowed to proceed
in competition with another muscle nerve, the two
nerves will share the available muscle fibres between
them, and each will reproduce its distribution of MU
sizes scaled to the size of the field available to the
particular nerve (Taxt, 1983). Hence, each neuron has
a "competitive vigor" according to the ratio between
its capacity to maintain terminals and the number of
terminals it is actually supporting at any time.

Effects of activity. The most intriguing of the
factors which influence competitive interactions in
muscle is the level of activity in the system. Motor
nerve block prevents the competitive loss of synaptic
terminals in neonatal muscles (Thompson et al., 1979)
and increased levels of activity accelerates the loss
of terminals (O'Brien et al., 1978). Prevention of
synapse elimination has also been obtained by pharmacological blocking of the AChR, suggesting the essential feature of the situation is the inactivity of the
muscle itself rather than the inactivity of the motor
nerve fibers (Ding et al.,1983). In addition to retaining redundant terminals at individual endplate sites
paralyzed muscle induced the formation of additional
synaptic sites on focally innervated fibers. Moreover,
the efficiency of synaptic transmission is significantly increased in such muscles (Ding et al., 1983).

Hence, inactivity of the muscle itself has striking effects on neuromuscular connectivity. It has been more difficult to determine whether there are additional effects governed by the level of activity in the presynaptic fibers. This requires differential control of the activity in separate groups of axons to the same muscle. This experiment was first performed during competitive reinnervation of the rat lumbrical muscle (Ribchester and Taxt, 1983). Blocking the impulse activity of the main nerve to the muscle demonstrated that the active minor nerve had a competitive advantage over the inactive axons.

A competitive advantage of presynaptic activity is also relevant for the normal neonatal loss of synapses as reported Ridge and Betz (1984). However, in a recent paper Callaway et al (1987) report the opposite results. They blocked the impulse activity in one of the spinal roots supplying the neonatal rabbit soleus muscle, and found, surprisingly, that the inactive MUs lost significantly fewer terminals and ended up appreciably larger than during normal development. More experiments are needed to settle the important question of the competitive advantage or disadvantage of presynaptic activity in the synapse elimination process.

Mechanisms of elimination. Several proposals have been advanced to explain the mechanisms underlying synapse elimination (see Van Essen, 1982). Essentially the models are based on a dynamic balance between effects of postulated substances which respectively promote or reverse terminal growth and maintenance. The simplest hypothesis is based on the MN growth factor postulated to be essential also for motoneuronal survival (see above). As already mentioned its production by muscle fibers appears to be repressed by muscle activity. Hence as the level of activity in the system increases a favoured terminal might exhaust the supply of the substance at the expence of its competitors which would be insufficiently supplied (Jansen et al., 1978; Brown et al., 1978). In this scheme the favoured terminal would be one belonging to the MN which has the highest "competitive vigor" in the group innervating the particular muscle fiber.

An alternative group of models is more complicated and introduces a terminal-destructive factor as the crucial element for the elimination of terminals. Recently, suggestive evidence has been presented for a key role of Ca^{++} activated proteases (Connold et al., 1986). However, at present our insight does not permit

a critical distinction between the various hypothesis.
New techniques, permitting repeated visualization of
pre- and postsynaptic parts of the same endplate over
the period of terminal competition may well provide
important relevant information (Balice-Gordon &
Lichtman, 1987).

Epilogue The message of this account of the establishment of neuromuscular connections is that important
developmental events are shaped by reciprocal cellular
interactions between pre- and postsynaptic elements.
The outcome of the two major regressive events are
influenced by competitive interactions among the
participants. Neuronal activity figures prominently in
the final outcome of the processes. These events are
instrumental for the epigenetic tuning of the final
motor output according to functional requirements.

    Analogous processes appear to be equally prominent
in the refinement of central connections. Also for
these overproduction followed by death of excess
neurons occur regularly. Again target dependence and
competition for targets acts as a decisive driving
force (see Cowan et al., 1984). However, while
numerical matching of MNs to fibers in the target
appears to be the main purpose of the normal
motoneuronal death, weeding out of abberantly
projecting neurons is a prominent feature of the
developmental death in central pathways. The
exuberance of early connections is also frequently
encountered in central pathways. Presumably the
striking analogies in the development of peripheral and
central pathways reflect fundamental similar ties in
the underlying cellular processes.

References

Anderson, M.J., Cohen, M.W., and Zorychta, E. (1977).
Effects of innervation on the distribution of acetyl-
choline receptors on cultured muscle cells. J.
Physiol. 268, 731-756.

Balice-Gordon, R.J. & Lichtman, J.W. (1987). The
relationship between pre- and postsynaptic competition
at developing neuromuscular junctions.
Soc.Neurosci.Abstr. 13, 375.

Bennett, M.R. (1983). Development of neuromuscular
synapses. Physiol. Rev., 63, 915-1048.

Berg, D.K. (1984). New neuronal growth factors. Ann. Rev. Neurosci. 7, 149-170.

Betz, W.J. (1987). Motoneuronal death and synapse elimination in vertebrates. In The Vertebrate Neuromuscular Junction. (ed. M. Salpeter) Alan Liss N.Y.

Brown, M.C. and Booth, C.M. (1983). Segregation of motor nerves on a segmental basis during synapse elimination in neonatal muscles. Brain Res., 273, 188-190.

Brown, M.C., Holland, R.L. and Hopkins W.H. (1981). Excess neuronal inputs during development. In Development in the Nervous System (eds. Dr. Garrod and J.D. Feldman) Cambridge Univ. Press, pp. 245-260.

Brown, M.C., Jansen, J. and Van Essen, D. (1976). Polyneuronal innervation of skeletal muscle in newborn rats and its elimination during maturation. J.Physiol. 261, 387-422.

Burke, R.E. (1981). Motor units: Anatomy, physiology and functional organization. Handb. of Physiol.sec. I, 345-422.

Callaway, E.M., Soha, J.M. and Van Essen, D.C. (1987). Competition favouring inactive over active motor neurones during synapse elimination. Nature, 328, 422-426.

Campenot, R.B. (1982). Development of sympathetic neurons in compartmentalized cultures. II. Local control of neurite survival by nerve growth factor. Dev. Biol., 93, 13-21.

Cohen, M.W. and Weldon, P.R. (1980). Localization of acetylcholine receptors and synaptic ultrastructure at nerve-muscle contacts in culture: Dependence on nerve type. J. Cell. Biol., 86, 388-401.

Connold, A.L., Evers, J.V. and Vrbova G. (1986). Effect of low calcium and protease inhibitors on synapse elimination during postnatal development in the rat soleus muscle. Dev. Brain Res., 28, 99-107.

Cowan, W.M., Fawcett, J.W., O'Leary, D.D.M. and Stanfield, B.B. (1984). Regressive events in neurogenesis. Science, 225, 1258-1265.

Davey, D.F., and Cohen, M.W. (1986). Localization of acetylcholine receptors and cholinesterase on nerve-contacted and noncontacted muscle cells grown in the presence of agents that block action potentials. J. Neurosci., 6, 673-680.

Ding, R., Jansen, J.K.S., Laing, N.G. and Tønnesen, H. (1983). The innervation of skeletal muscle in chickens curarized during early development. J. Neurocytol., 12, 887-919.

Fladby, T. and Jansen, J.K.S. (1987). Postnatal loss of synaptic terminals in the partially denervated mouse soleus muscle. Acta physiol.scand., 129, 239-246.

Fladby, T. and Jansen, J.K.S. (1988). Selective inner- vation of neonatal fast and slow muscle fibers before net loss of synaptic terminals in the mouse soleus muscle. Acta physiol.scand. 134, 561-562.

Frank, E. and Fischbach, G.D. (1977). ACh receptors accumulate at newly formed nerve-muscle synapse in vitro. In Cell and Tissue Interactions. (eds. J.W. Larsh and M.M. Burger) Raven Press, New York.

Gordon, H. and Van Essen, D. (1985). Specific inner- vation of muscle fiber types in a developmentally poly- innervated muscle. Dev. Biol., 11, 42-50.

Hamburger, V. and Oppenheim, R.W. (1982). Naturally occurring neuronal death in vertebrates. Neurosc. Comm., 1, 39-55.

Henderson, C.E. (1987). Activity and the regulation of neuronal growth factor metabolism. In The Neural and Molecular Basis of Learning (ed. J.P. Changeux and M. Konishi) Wiley & Sons.

Jansen, J.K.S., Lømo, T., Nicolaysen, K. and Westgaard, R.H. (1973). Hyperinnervation of skeletal muscle fibers: Dependence on muscle activity. Science, 181, 559-561.

Jansen, J.K.S., Thompson, W. and Kuffler, D.P. (1978). The formation and maintenance of synaptic connections as illustrated by studies of the neuromuscular junction. Progr. Brain Res., 48, 3-18.

Jones, S.P., Ridge, R.M.A.P. and Rowlerson, A. (1987). The non-selective innervation of muscle fibres and mixed composition of motor units in a muscle of neonatal rat. J. Physiol., 386, 377-394.

Kuffler, D.P., Thompson, W. and Jansen, J.K.S.   (1980).
The fate of foreign endplates in cross-innervated rat
soleus muscle. Proc. R. Soc. B., _208_, 189-222.

Kullberg, R.W., Lentz, T.L. and Cohen, M.W. (1977).
Development of the myotomal neuromuscular junction in
Xenopus laevis: An electrophysiological and fine-struc-
tural study. Dev. Biol., _60_, 101-129.

Laing, N.H. and Prestige, M.C. (1978). Prevention of
spontaneous motoneuron death in chick embryos. J.
Physiol., _282_, 33-34 P.

Lømo, T. (1987). Formation of ectopic neuromuscular
junctions: Role of activity and other factors. In _The
Neural and Molecular Basis of Learning_ (eds. J.-P.
Changeux and M. Konishi), Wiley & Sons Ltd.

Michler, A. and Sakmann, B. (1980). Receptor stability
and channel conversion in the subsynaptic membrane of
the developing mammalian neuromuscular junction. Dev.
Biol., _80_, 1-17.

Moody-Corbett, F. and Cohen, M.W. (1982). Influence of
nerve on the formation and survival of acetylcholine
receptor and choline esterase patches on embryonic
Xenopus muscle cells in culture. J. Neurosci., _2_,
636-646.

O'Brien, R.A.D., Østberg, A.J.C. and Vrbova, G. (1978).
Observations on the elimination of polyneuronal inner-
vation in developing mammalian skeletal muscle. J.
Physiol., _282_, 571-582.

Pittman, R. and Oppenheim, R.W. (1979). Cell death of
MNs in the chick embryo spinal cord. IV. Evidence
that a functional neuromuscular interaction is involved
in the regulation of naturally occurring cell death and
the stabilization of synapses. J. Comp. Neurol., _187_,
425-446.

Reist, N.E., Magill, C. and McMahan U.J. (1987).
Agrin-like molecules at synaptic sites in normal,
denervated and damaged skeletal muscle. J. Cell Biol.,
_105_, 2457-2469.

Ribchester, R.R. and Taxt, T. (1983). Motor unit size
and synaptic competition in rat lumbrical muscles
reinnervated by active and inactive motor axons. J.
Physiol., _344_, 89-111.

Ridge, R.M.A.P. and Betz, W.J. (1984). The effect of selective, chronic stimulation on MU size in developing rat muscle. J. Neurosci., 4, 2614-2620.

Rubinstein, N.A. and Kelly, A.M. (1981). Development of muscle fiber specialization in the rat hind limb. J. Cell Biol., 90, 128-144.

Sanes, J.R., Marshall, L.M. and McMahan, U.J. (1978). Reinnervation of muscle fiber basal lamina after removal of myofibers. Differentiation of regenerating axons at original synaptic sites. J. Cell Biol., 78, 176-198.

Soileau, L.C., Silberstein, L., Blau, H.M. and Thompson, W.J. (1987). Reinnervation of muscle fiber types in the newborn rat soleus. J. Neurosci., 7, 4176-4194.

Taxt, T. (1983). Motor unit numbers, motor unit sizes and innervation of single muscle fibers in hyperinnervated mouse soleus muscle. Acta physiol. scand., 117, 571-580.

Thompson, W.J. and Jansen, J.K.S. (1977). The extent of sprouting of remaining motor units in partly denervated immature and adult rat soleus muscle. Neurosci., 2, 523-535.

Thompson, W.J. (1978). Reinnervation of partially denervated rat soleus muscle. Acta physiol. scand., 103, 81-91.

Thompson, W.J., Kuffler, D.P. and Jansen, J.K.S. (1979). The effect of prolonged, reversible block of nerve impulses on the elimination of polyneuronal innervation of new-born rat skeletal muscle fibers. Neurosci., 4, 271-281.

Thompson, W.J., Sutton, L.A. and Riley, D.A. (1984). Fiber type composition of single motor units during synapse elimination in the neonatal rat soleus muscle. Nature, 309, 709-711.

Van Essen, D.C. (1982). Neuromuscular synapse elimination. In: Structural, functional and mechanistic aspects. In Neuronal Development (ed. N. Spitzer) Plenum Press N Y.

Vogel, Z., Sytkowski, A.J. and Nirenberg, M.W. (1972).
Acetylcholine receptors of muscle cells grown in vitro.
Proc.Nat.Acad. Sci., 69, 3180-3184.

Wigston, D.J. and Sanes, J.R. (1985). Selective
reinnervation of intercostal muscles transplanted from
different segmental levels to a common site. J.
Neurosci. , 5, 1208-1221.

Willshaw, D.J. (1981). The establishment and the subsequent elimination of polyneuronal innervation in the
developing muscle: Theoretical considerations. Proc.
R. Soc. B., 212, 233-252.

5
Postnatal Synaptic Reorganization of Cat Motoneurons

Staffan Cullheim and Brun Ulfhake

INTRODUCTION

The ability to stand, walk and run is gradually acquired by the kitten during the first six to eight postnatal weeks. Spinal α-moto-neurons (MNs) are of obvious importance for motor functions, since they constitute the "final common path" from the central nervous system (CNS) to the skeletal muscles. Like all CNS neurons, a MN receives information from a large number of neurons via synaptic connections. A prerequisite for a proper function of the MN is that the synaptic connections are established adequately. During the early postnatal period in the cat there is a loss of polyneuronal innervation of muscle fibers (Bagust et al., 1973), about half of the number of synapses on the cell body (Conradi and Ronnevi, 1975) and all synapses on the initial axon segment (Conradi and Ronnevi, 1977) of α-MNs disappear. Thus, previous studies on the synaptic connectivity of spinal α-MNs have indicated the occurrence of regressive events postnatally. By use of intracellular injections with horseradish peroxidase (HRP) in physiologically identified neurons (e.g. Cullheim and Kellerth, 1976) we have extended the synaptological analysis to also include the recurrent axon collaterals and dendritic trees of cat hind limb MNs from birth to the adult stage.

RECURRENT AXON COLLATERALS

The recurrent axon collaterals of α-MNs make up the first part of the neuronal chain mediating the recurrent inhibition of MNs (Eccles et al., 1954). During the first postnatal weeks there is a significant postnatal decrease in the number of end branches and suspected synaptic contacts within the collateral trees of the triceps surae α-motor axon (Cullheim and Ulfhake, 1982, 1985). This loss of branches occurs within a constant relative volume of the spinal cord. Detailed analysis of the changes in branching pattern and branch length has revealed that the loss of collateral branches is restricted to distal parts of the collateral trees (Remahl et al., 1985). Preliminary results from physiological studies on the re- current inhibition of MNs at different postnatal stages have indicated the same precision in the distribution of the recurrent effects between different motor pools (Cullheim and Ulfhake, unpublished observations). Thus, there are strong indications that the postnatal reduction in number of axon collateral terminals reflects a diminishing number of synaptic contacts with an unchanged population of target cells.

DENDRITIC TREES

In the newborn kitten, the α-MN dendrites show the same complexity as in the adult stage (Ulfhake et al., 1988). Thus, in triceps surae α-MNs, an average of 12 primary dendrites give rise to about 160 end branches in both kittens and adult cats. The spatial distribution differs, however, in that the dendrites are mainly oriented in the transverse plane at birth, while the adult triceps surae α-MN has a radial dendritic distribution. Thus, new territories are invaded by the dendrites postnatally along the rostro-caudal axis of the spinal cord. Topological analysis of the dendritic branching pattern has indicated that there is a remodeling of the dendrites postnatally, with a formation of new branches as well as a resorption of existing ones. These events seem to be balanced so that no significant net change in the number of dendritic branches occurs postnatally.

Peripheral dendritic branches in newborn kittens are equipped with numerous growth-associated morphological features, like growth cones and filopodia (Ulfhake and Cullheim, 1988a). Electron micro- scopic observations have revealed an almost obligate relationship between filopodial tips and vesicle-filled bouton-like neuronal profiles (Fig. 1). Also, the base of the filipodium is usually surrounded by synaptic boutons. Thus, the role for filopodia in vivo may be not only to form new dendritic branches but also to search for relevant synaptic inputs. After establishing a contact with such an input the filopodia may retract to place the synapse on the parent dendritic shaft (Fig. 2A).

The total receptive membrane area of a triceps surae α-MN increases from about 0.1 mm^2 at birth to 0.5 mm^2 in the adult (Ulfhake and Cullheim, 1988b). The dominance of the dendritic versus the somatic membrane area is pronounced already at birth (dendrite/soma ratio= 20) but is further strengthened from six weeks of age up to the adult stage when the dendrite/soma ratio is about 50. Calculations based on the postnatal changes in membrane area and synaptic density (Conradi and Skoglund, 1969) give a total number of synaptic boutons covering an α-MN of about 50,000 both in the newborn kitten and in the adult cat (Ulfhake and Cullheim, 1988b). This constant number of synapses should then be the result of a balance between the removal of some synaptic inputs and the

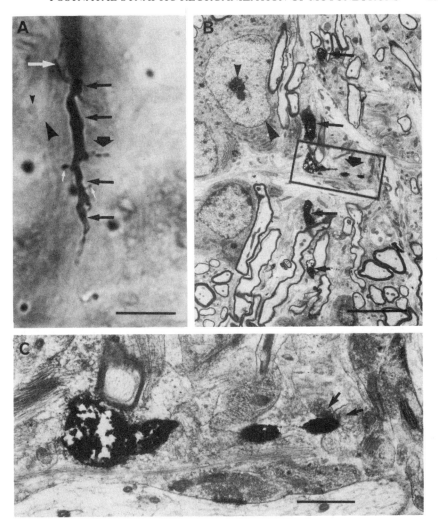

Fig. 1 A. Light micrograph of a 30 μm thick section showing a filopodial growth cone on a terminal α-motoneuron dendritic branch of
a 3 weeks old kitten (Bar= 10 μm). B. Electron micrograph of a
single ultrathin section from the thick section shown in A. Structures evident in both A and B have been labeled with the same symbols (Bar= 5 μm). The framed area in B is shown in an adjacent
ultrathin section (Bar= 1 μm). The tip of the filopodium, also indicated in A and B (bold black arrow), can be seen in close apposition to vesicle containing structures (arrows). The vesicles seem
to be accumulating in the region of apposition but no membrane den-
sities are discernable. Slightly modified from Ulfhake and
Cullheim (1988a).

formation of new ones.

POSSIBLE MECHANISMS FOR SYNAPTIC REORGANIZATION POSTNATALLY

It has been suggested that the elimination of synapses during development mirrors a process where a presynaptic neuron first makes connections with its target in surplus number to ascertain that contacts are being made. This stage is then followed by a period when surplus or inadequately located connections are eliminated by retraction of terminal axons (see e.g. Purves and Lichtman, 1980; Cowan et al., 1984). This view on the elimination of synapses derives to a large extent from experimental work on the neuromuscular junction. The studies on the α-MN challenge this view in some respects. Thus, it has been demonstrated, that the reduction in number of synaptic terminals on the cell body of cat α-MNs postnatally (Conradi and Ronnevi, 1975) is, at least in part, due to a glial phagocytosis of boutons (Ronnevi, 1977) while no signs of degeneration or phagocytosis of terminals are detected at the neuromuscular junction during the elimination of polyneuronal innervation of muscle fibers (Korneliussen and Jansen, 1976). Boutons can also be engulfed and disintegrated by the MN itself (Ronnevi, 1979). The reason for the developing nervous system to use this type of active process with an apparent waste of membrane material and energy instead of just a retraction of surplus or irrelevant terminal axon branches is not clear. However, the phenomenon indicates a more important role for the postsynaptic neuron and the local micro-environment of the synapse than for the presynaptic neuron in deciding which synaptic connections are to remain through the postnatal development. It may be speculated that synaptic connections with an improper function are disconnected by retraction of preterminal axons, while phagocytosis of synaptic boutons is used to remove functionally intact connections in order to change the composition of synaptic inputs to the MN to a pattern which is relevant for a specific developmental stage (see further below under heading FUNCTIONAL IMPLICATIONS OF SYNAPTIC REORGANIZATION). The central synaptic reorganization of α-MNs should incorporate both types of elimination process.

With regard to the establishment of new synaptic connections with the α-MN, a key role is proposed for the filopodia of dendritic origin seen preferentially in the distal parts of the dendritic tree in young kittens. Electron microscopic observations of such filopodia are suggestive for an active "seeking" behaviour of the filopodia which may not be linked with an outgrowth of new dendritic branches, but instead reflect a search for presynaptic elements which can then be translocated to the dendritic shaft by retraction of the filopodia. The filopodia and other growth-related structures were most frequent in dendrites projecting medially, rostrally and caudally, indicating that these parts of the triceps surae α-MN are the most active ones in producing new dendritic branches and/or establishing new synaptic connections postnatally. Indeed, the

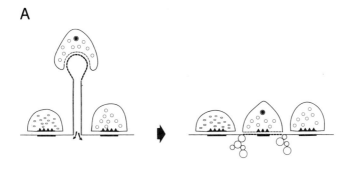

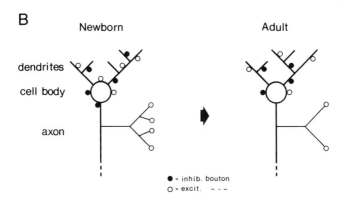

Fig. 2 A. Schematic drawing showing the proposed role for filopodia in establishing new synaptic connections in peripheral α-motoneuron dendrites postnatally. The tip of the filopodium is in contact with an axonal bouton without membrane specializations. The base of the filopodium is surrounded by mature synaptic junctions. Following retraction of the filopodium and translocation of the bouton to the dendritic shaft the synaptic contact is stabilized with membrane specializations. B. Scheme for intramedullary synaptic rearrangements in α-motoneurons postnatally. The number of synaptic terminals of the axon collateral system is reduced by half within a constant terminal field. Half the number of synapses on the cell body and all synapses (predominantly inhibitory) on the initial axon segment are removed. The dendrites are apposed by a constant number of synaptic boutons reflecting a balance between the establishment and removal of synaptic connections. The dendrites are to some degree remodeled during their invasion of new territories, but the total number of dendritic end branches remains constant.

ingrowth of rostrally and caudally oriented dendrites into new
territories of the spinal cord during the first postnatal weeks
should mean that all distal synapses in these directions are
established after birth.

FUNCTIONAL IMPLICATIONS OF SYNAPTIC REORGANIZATION

The differences in the synaptological development between
different parts of the α-MN summarized in Fig. 2B may reflect a
more complicated and "purposeful" development than just a removal
of redundant or inadequately located synaptic terminals, leading to
a diminishing number of innervating axons. Also, the phagocytosis
of synaptic boutons on the cell body of MNs by glial cells or the
MN itself indicates an intricate relationship between individual
presynaptic elements and the MN. The precision of synaptological
changes postnatally is exemplified by the triceps surae γ-MN
(Arvidsson et al., 1987). In the newborn kitten, the cell body of
this neuron is covered predominantly by synaptic boutons of the F
type, containing flat vesicles, which are commonly held to have an
inhibitory function. There is a large reduction in the number of F
type boutons postnatally, while the number of S type boutons (with
spherical vesicles and presumably excitatory in function) remains
fairly constant. The strong inhibitory influence on the immature
γ-MN suggested by these findings is in fact parallelled by a marked
insensitivity of the immature muscle spindle to muscle stretch
(Skoglund, 1960). It should also be noticed that the majority of
synaptic boutons on the initial axon segment (IS) of α-MNs in the
newborn kitten contains flat vesicles (Conradi and Ronnevi, 1977)
with a probable inhibitory function and acts on a part of the MN
which is crucial for the propagation of nerve impulses. It may then
well be that also the α-MN is under an inhibitory influence early
postnatally. Such an inhibition acting on the IS could explain
described difficulties to invade the immature MN cell body with an
antidromically evoked action potential (Kellerth et al., 1971). An
inhibition of those parts of the MN which are most important for
the initiation and propagation of action potentials could be
necessary in order to surpress inadequate activity of the MN
elicited from the synaptic remodeling process in the dendrites. This
remodeling may in turn reflect a changing balance between supraspinal and segmental synaptic inputs on a neuron which is contacted
by a rather fixed number of synaptic boutons throughout the postnatal period. Thus, the gradual development of the supraspinal influence on the spinal cord may force a shift in the pattern of
synaptic connectivity making way for supraspinally derived inputs
at the cost of the segmental connectivity. Such a development could
then explain the postnatal reduction in number of recurrent axon
collateral terminals of the MNs.

ACKNOWLEDGEMENTS

This work was supported by grants from the Swedish Medical Research Council (proj. 6815), Bergwalls stiftelse, Karolinska Institutet, Stiftelsen L. Hiertas minne, I. and L. Ostermans stiftelse and Å. Wibergs stiftelse.

REFERENCES

Arvidsson, U., Svedlund, J., Lagerbäck, P.-Å. and Cullheim, S. (1987). An ultrastructural study of the synaptology of gamma moto-neurons during the postnatal development in the cat. Dev. Brain Res., 37, 303-312.

Bagust, J., Lewis, D.M. and Westerman, R.A. (1973) Polyneuronal innervation of kitten skeletal muscle. J. Physiol. (London), 229, 241-255.

Conradi, S. and Ronnevi, L.-O. (1975) Spontaneous elimination of synapses on cat spinal motoneurons after birth: do half of the synapses on the cell body disappear? Brain Res., 92, 505-510.

Conradi, S. and Ronnevi, L.-O. (1977). Ultrastructure and synaptology of the initial axon segment of cat spinal motoneurons during early postnatal development. J. Neurocytol., 6, 195-210.

Conradi, S. and Skoglund, S. (1969). Observations on the ultrastruc-ture and distribution of neuronal and glial elements on the moto-neuron surface in the lumbosacral spinal cord of the cat during postnatal development. Acta physiol. scand., Suppl. 333, 5-52.

Cowan, W.M., Fawcett, J.W., O'Leary, D.D.M. and Stanfield, B.B. (1984). Regressive events in neurogenesis. Science, 225, 1258-1265.

Cullheim, S. and Kellerth, J.-O. (1976). Combined light and electron microscopic tracing of neurons, including axons and synaptic terminals, after intracellular injection of horseradish peroxidase. Neurosci. Lett., 2, 307-313.

Cullheim, S. and Ulfhake, B. (1982). Evidence for a postnatal elimination of terminal arborizations and synaptic boutons of recurrent motor axon collaterals in the cat. Dev. Brain Res., 5, 234-237.

Cullheim, S. and Ulfhake, B. (1985). Postnatal changes in the termination pattern of recurrent axon collaterals of triceps surae α-motoneurons in the cat. Dev. Brain Res., 17, 63-73.

Eccles, J.C., Fatt, P. and Koketsu, K. (1954). Cholinergic and inhibitory synapses in a pathway from motor-axon collaterals to motoneurones. J. Physiol. (London), 126, 524-562.

Kellerth, J.-O., Mellström, A. and Skoglund, S. (1971). Postnatal excitability changes of kitten motoneurones. Acta physiol. scand., 83, 31-41.

Korneliussen, H. and Jansen, J.K.S. (1976). Morphological aspects of the elimination of polyneuronal innervation of skeletal muscle fibers in newborn rats. J. Neurocytol., 5, 591-604.

Purves, D. and Lichtman, J.W. (1980). Elimination of synapses in the developing nervous system. Science, 210, 153-157.

Remahl, S., Cullheim, S. and Ulfhake, B. (1985) Dimensions and branching patterns of triceps surae alpha motor axons and their recurrent axon collaterals in the spinal cord during the postnatal development in the cat. Dev. Brain Res., 23, 193-200.

Ronnevi, L.-O. (1977). Spontaneous phagocytosis of boutons on spinal motoneurons during early postnatal development. An electron microscopical study in the cat. J. Neurocytol., 6, 487-504.

Ronnevi, L.-O. (1979). Spontaneous phagocytosis of C-type synaptic terminals by spinal α-motoneurons in newborn kittens. An electron microscopic study. Brain Res., 162, 189-199.

Skoglund, S. (1960). The activity of muscle receptors in the kitten. Acta physiol. scand., 50, 203-221.

Ulfhake, B., Cullheim, S. and Franson, P. (1988). Postnatal development of cat hindlimb motoneurons. I. Changes in length, branching structure and spatial distribution of dendrites of cat triceps surae motoneurons. J. comp. Neurol., in press.

Ulfhake, B. and Cullheim, S. (1988a). Postnatal development of cat hindlimb motoneurons. II. In vivo morphology of dendritic growth cones and the maturation of dendrite morphology. J. comp. Neurol., in press.

Ulfhake, B. and Cullheim, S. (1988b). Postnatal development of cat hindlimb motoneurons. III. Changes in size of motoneurons supplying the triceps surae muscle. J. comp. Neurol., in press.

6
Development of Postural Control in Infancy

H. F. R. Prechtl

INTRODUCTION

With the transition from the intrauterine to the extrauterine environment the organism experiences an about threefold increase of the postural load due to the force of gravity. Intuitively one should expect a functional repertoire to be present at birth in order to cope with this change. Actually, infrahuman primates are equipped with postural mechanisms immediately after birth, e.g. they counteract the force of gravity by balancing the head in the horizontal plane even when the trunk is oriented in various directions. In the human neonate such abilities are very limited. This may be due to the surprisingly low muscle power in this species, or to a late postnatal maturation of those neural mechanisms responsible for postural control in relation to space. In order to answer this question polymyographic studies have been carried out in fullterm newborn infants in static conditions (in prone, lateral and supine position) and in situations with acceleration (tilting and rocking). Actually these are all the conditions occurring in the daily life of a neonate. If antigravity movements are absent only because of peripheral factors (i.e. muscle weakness) the contraction patterns should nevertheless appear in the EMG-recordings. If they are also lacking in the contraction patterns of relevant muscle groups it must be concluded that the neural mechanisms are not yet functioning. This raises the question: at what ages do they emerge?

Another source of information on the development of postural mechanisms is the intrauterine position and posture of the fetus which become now available from systematic real-time ultrasound studies. This allows a comparison of postures of the fetus with those of the preterm and fullterm infant.

ACTIVE POSTURE IN FETUS AND NEONATE

Systematic observations of fetal position (supine, lateral and prone) and orientation in the uterus have been provided by De Vries et al. (1982) for the first half of pregnancy. From 20-40 weeks gestation such data are still lacking. The posture of head, trunk and limbs is highly variable but semiflexion of the limbs is common. From about 18 weeks onwards the head is frequently turned to one side. The legs may be extended and an arm lifted with the hand behind the occiput. Retroflexion of the head occurs from time to time. Although there is no recognizable preference posture maintained for most of the time, there can be no doubt that the fetus shows a certain repertoire of repeated active postures. However, they are unrelated to the position in utero.

Similar observations have been made in preterm infants (Prechtl et al., 1979) which were confirmed by Cioni et al. (1988). No age-related preference postures were found between 28 and 40 weeks. Despite this fact the observed postures cannot be considered as random configurations of head and limb positions. The same holds true for fullterm infants, analysed with the same technique (Cioni et al., 1988 in press). Changes of posture are caused by gross movements, but postures are maintained between movements. From these and other observations (Schloon et al., 1976; Casaer, 1979) it can be concluded that the fetus and the young infant have an active, albeit variable, posture which is relatively unrelated to the orientation of the force of gravity.

ELECTROMYOGRAPHIC STUDIES OF NEONATAL POSTURE

In order to distinguish between peripheral and central mechanisms responsible for the poor antigravity function in postural behaviour, we have made polymyographic recordings in 24 healthy fullterm infants on their fifth day in prone and in supine position (3 hours per position) and in 9 infants in left and right lateral position (3 hours per position). The latter study has been described in Schloon et al. (1976).

In addition to the on-line recording we made compressed play-backs of which an example is illustrated in Fig. 1. In this case, the infant was in the supine position for the first three hours and after a feed was put into prone position. The head remained turned to the right from the beginning until min 137, when the infant turned the head to the left and maintained this position

Figure 1 (opposite page). Compressed polymyogram of a five day old fullterm neonate in supine and prone position, respectively. EMG processed with averaging moving window of 200 msec. Logarithmic write out. The cyclic change of state 1 and state 2 epochs is evident in respiratory rate, heart rate and motor activity. For head position see text.

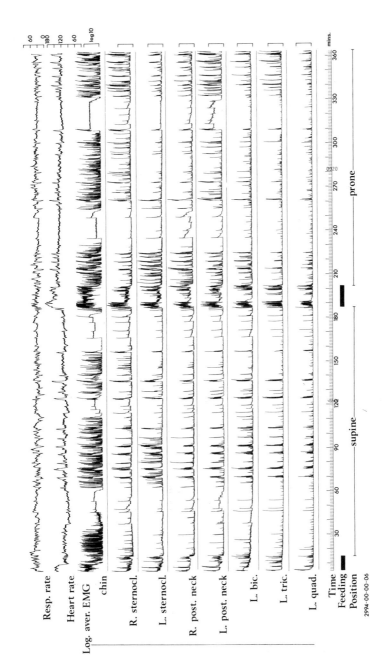

until the feeding. After feeding the infant kept the head to the right but turned spontaneously to the left at minute 262 and kept this position until the end of the recording. Tonic activity was present in large parts of state 1 epoch. During state 2 epochs, general movements occurred periodically every few minutes. When the neck muscles are analysed, an asymmetrical activity is evident in the sterno-cleido muscles with higher and longer tonic activity in the muscles contralateral to the side where the head is turned towards, the phasic activity during state 2 is also asymmetrical. The amplitude of the EMG-activity in the contralateral sterno-cleido muscle exceeds by far the activity in the ipsilateral muscle. During prone position the dorsal neck muscle, ipsilateral to the side the head is turned to, is more active (tonically during state 1 and phasically during state 2) than the contralateral dorsal neck muscle. This means a tendency to turn the head actively to the side and also to lift the head off the ground which is clearly against the force of gravity.

However, when the recording of the supine position is inspected, the muscle activity is the same but the muscle contractions act now in the same direction as the force of gravity. This puzzling result was found to be present in all 24 infants studied. The statistical analysis of the EMG activity in state 1 and state 2 revealed a significant pattern of active head turning to the same side, as the head was already turned towards. This is illustrated in Fig. 2a and b.

State 3 and 4 (wakefulness) were only present in a few percent of the recording time but the EMG activities were identical to those found in the sleep states; but a statistical analysis was not possible because of the small number of observations.

The infants in lateral position had a significantly higher tonic and phasic activity in the upperlying sterno-cleido muscle, turning the head in the direction of the surface the infant is lying on and hence, acting in the same direction as the force of gravity (Schloon et al., 1976).

Analyses of the EMG activity of the limb muscles did also not reveal an activity pattern which would counteract the force of gravity but merely maintains the position actually present which is in full agreement with the assumption of an active posture, especially during state 1 and wakefulness.

RESPONSES TO TILTING

When a newborn infant is picked up from the lying position to be carried in the arms, he or she experiences acceleration in space. During this displacement in space the caretaker feels the active posture of the infant. This becomes particularly evident if the same procedure is carried out with a hypotonic "floppy" infant

tonic emg activity in state 1
median and interquartile range

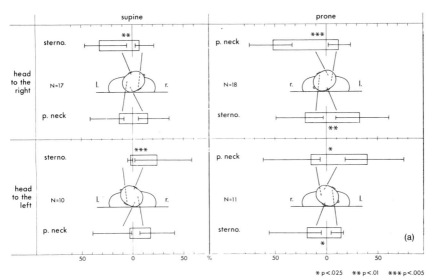

(a)

* p<.025   ** p<.01   *** p<.005

phasic emg activity in state 2
median and interquartile range

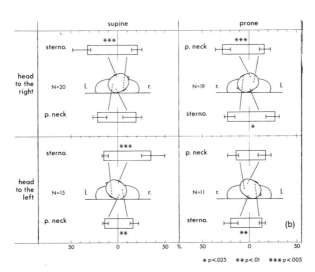

(b)

* p<.025   ** p<.01   *** p<.005

Figures 2a and b. Medians and interquartile ranges of percentage of EMG activity in dorsal neck muscles and sterno-cleido muscles per state 1 and 2. Significance levels between pairs of muscles from t-test (two-tailed).

who gives the impression of "slipping through the fingers". It
remains to be seen, however, as to whether this posture is in the
normal infant an "en bloc" response or is acting in relation to
gravity.

To this end we carried out tilting experiments with a rocking
table on which the infant was lying in prone or supine. The
tilting was through the transverse axis at the height of the
diaphragm and had a range of 30 degrees, i.e. ± 15 degrees from
the horizontal plane. Speed of the tilts could be varied. A total
of 32 infants between the age of 4 days to 25 weeks were examined.
Simultaneous EMG recordings of various neck, trunk and limb
muscles, together with time-coded videorecordings were obtained.
Newborns and infants up to the age of 8 to 10 weeks did not
respond, neither to head downwards nor head upwards tilts. Not
only were there no responses during sleep states but also none
during quiet wakefulness (Fig. 3). If the infant moved at all
within a reasonable latency, the EMG pattern and the video image
were indistinguishable from those of spontaneously occurring
movements without tilting. This picture changed when spontaneous

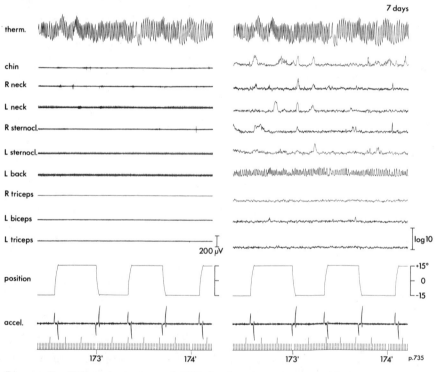

Figure 3. EMG and processed EMG during transverse tilting.
          No response during wakefulness.

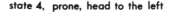

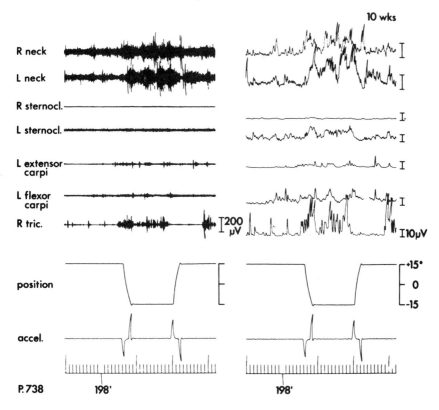

Figure 4. Response to tilt in a 10 weeks old awake infant. Note
activity in dorsal neck muscles and triceps muscle
during downward tilt which disappears during upward
tilt.

head control in vertical suspension and prone position was
observed. Infants of about 10 weeks of age showed a clear head
retroflexion and extension of the arms, when tilted with the head
downwards. This was also evident in the EMG patterns (Fig. 4).
When tilted in the upward direction, the head became anteflexed
and kept in the horizontal plane. From about the beginning of the
third month of age (with some interindividual variation) this
antigravity response to tilting became consistent.

DISCUSSION

In contrast to the naive expectation, the newborn and young infant seems poorly adapted to counteract the force of gravity. On the other hand, the fetus, the neonate and the young infant have a variable but limited repertoire of active postures. These postures are unrelated to space as they lack systematic responses to the orientation in space. It is most likely that they are proprioceptively controled while the vestibulum seems to play no important role. The mechanisms providing the postures at these early ages may be considered to be "body-oriented".

At about the beginning of the third month, a major transformation of many neural functions (see Prechtl, 1984) can be observed. The muscle power increases, the head becomes centered in the midline, when the awake infant is lying in supine position. When sitting reclined in a baby chair, the posture is no longer slumped but counteracts the force of gravity (Wulfften Palthe and Hopkins, 1984). At the same age the quality of the general movements changes from a writhing character to a fidgety like activity (Hopkins and Prechtl, 1984; Prechtl and Hopkins, 1986). Social vocalisation starts and social interaction expands rapidly.

It is at this transformation that postural adjustment to tilting develops. These responses are clearly antigravity and make the posture now "space-oriented". Preliminary observations indicate that the visual system plays a neglishable role for the stabilisation of head and trunk at this age. It can be concluded that with the transition from body-oriented to space-oriented postural control a new adaptation to the extrauterine environment is reached.

ACKNOWLEDGEMENTS

The cooperation of Drs. M.John O'Brien, H.H. Bakker and E. Buiten is greatly acknowledged. This paper is part of the research program on Pregnancy and Early Development at the University of Groningen.

REFERENCES

Casaer, P. (1979). Postural Behaviour in Newborn Infants. Clinics in Developmental Medicine, no. 72. Heinemann, London, pp. 112.

Cioni, C., Ferrari, F. and Prechtl, H.F.R. (1988). Posture and spontaneous motility in fullterm infants. Early Hum. Dev., in press.

Cioni, G. and Prechtl, H.F.R. This volume.

Hopkins, B. and Prechtl, H.F.R. (1984). A qualitative approach to the development of movements during early infancy. In <u>Continuity of Neural Functions from Prenatal to Postnatal Life</u>. (ed. H.F.R. Prechtl). Blackwell, Oxford, Clinics in Developmental Medicine, no. 94, 179-197.

Prechtl, H.F.R. (ed.) (1984). <u>Continuity of Neural Functions from Prenatal to Postnatal Life</u>. Blackwell, Oxford, Clinics in Developmental Medicine, no. 94, pp. 255.

Prechtl, H.F.R., Fargel, J.W., Weinmann, H.M. and Bakker, H.H. (1979). Posture, motility and respiration in low-risk preterm infants. Develop. Med. Child Neurol. <u>21</u>, 3-27.

Prechtl, H.F.R. and Hopkins, B. (1986). Developmental transformations of spontaneous movements in early infancy. Early Hum. Dev., <u>14</u>, 233-238.

Schloon, H., O'Brien, M.J., Scholten, C.A. and Prechtl, H.F.R. (1976). Muscle activity and postural behaviour in newborn infants. Neuropädiatrie, <u>7</u>, 384-415.

Vries, J.I.P. de, Visser, G.H.A. and Prechtl, H.F.R. (1982). The emergence of fetal behaviour. I. Qualitative aspects. Early Hum. Dev., <u>7</u>, 301-322.

Wulfften Palthe, T. van and Hopkins, B. (1984). Development of the infant's social competence during early face-to-face interaction: a longitudinal study. In <u>Continuity of Neural Functions from Prenatal to Postnatal Life</u>. (ed. H.F.R. Prechtl). Blackwell, Oxford, Clinics in Developmental Medicine, no. 94, 179-197.

7

Development of Posture and Motility in Preterm Infants

Giovanni Cioni and Heinz F. R. Prechtl

Low-risk preterm infants provide a unique opportunity for studying the development ex utero of neural functions which usually develop in the maternal womb. Despite all attempts to simulate intrauterine conditions in the incubator, there are still enormous differences between the environment of the preterm infants and the fetus. In this regard preterm birth could throw light on the major questions relating to the role of the environment on the development of the nervous system. If particular behaviours in the preterm infant and the fetus do not differ, an influence of the environment on early development must be minimal.

SELECTION OF THE OBSERVATIONS

Motor and postural behaviour was studied longitudinally in 14 carefully selected low-risk preterm infants. They were born at a gestational age (G.A.) of 27 to 35 weeks (mean 31) and with a birth weight of between 850 and 2490 g (mean 1625). They were judged to be low-risk on the basis of a birthweight appropriate to G.A., good condition at birth, the absence of serious complications during the neonatal period, no pathological images on the ultrasound scan, and normal neurological examinations at 38-40 wks of conceptional age (C.A.). Their neurodevelopmental outcome at 18 months of corrected age was also normal. The data were abstracted from weekly one-hour videorecordings of undisturbed infants. Analysis of the movements was carried out from replay of the videotapes by using Prechtl's classifications of fetal and neonatal spontaneous movement patterns (Prechtl,1985; Prechtl et al., 1979). After classifying the different movement patterns, an actogram was produced, on which rest-activity cycles were identified with the aid of a three min moving window. Rate of occurrence per 10 mins and, where applicable, duration of the events, were computed for activity and rest periods respectively.

DEVELOPMENTAL COURSE OF MOTILITY

With the exception of startles (ST), almost equally represented in rest and activity periods, all other spontaneously generated movement patterns rarely occurred in rest periods in the age range under consideration.

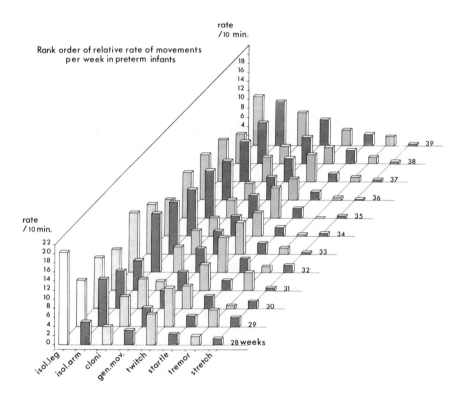

Fig.1. Rank order of rates (median values) of movement patterns in activity periods in preterm infants from 28 to 39 wks of C.A.

When the most frequently occurring movement patterns were rank ordered according to their relative rate in activity periods, the following sequence was found at 39 wks: isolated leg movement (IL), isolated arm movement (IA), general movement (GM), twitch (TW), cloni (CL), ST, stretch (SR), tremulous movement (TM). A similar sequence was obtained in 10 fullterm infants on their 1st and 4th days of life (Cioni et al., 1988).

From 28 to 39 wks fluctuations in the median rates of all movement patterns were observed (Fig.1). In the same period none of the infants showed a marked increase or decrease in the absolute rate of the different movement patterns, either in activity or in rest periods. In activity periods we found a significant decrease in the incidence of TW and SR only (Fig.2),

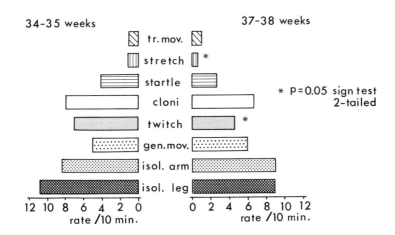

Fig. 2. Averaged rates (mean values) of movement patterns at 34-35 and 37-38 wks for 12 preterm infants.

when the averaged rates from 34 and 35 wks were compared with the averaged rates from 37 and 38 wks (p = 0.05, sign-test 2-tailed).

Although a decrease in the total number of movements during the last weeks of pregnancy has been reported both in the fetus (de Vries et al.,1987) and in preterm infants (Prechtl et al.,1979), this is probably due to the relative increase of quiescence or state 1 approaching term age (Nijhuis et al.,1982; Nolte & Haas,1978).

The median rates of movement patterns in the preterm infants at term age were similar to those previously found in fullterm infants (Cioni et al., 1988). Only TW and CL occur more often in preterm infants (Fig.3).

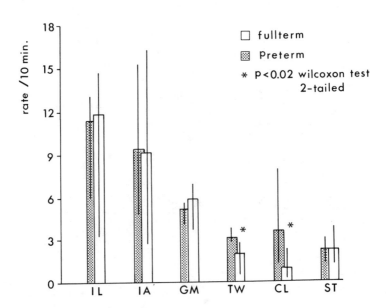

MOVEMENT PATTERNS

Fig. 3. Rate of movement patterns (medians and interquartile ranges) in state 2 of 10 fullterm infants on day 4 and 10 preterm infants at term age.

There is a strong indication that the various spontaneously generated movement patterns are produced independently of each other. No correlation between the incidences of movement could be found when correlation matrices were produced for each of the weeks from 35 to 38. Similar results have already been reported in the fetus (de Vries et al.,1987) and fullterm infants (Cioni et al.,1988).

The data of our longitudinal observation, compared with the results of similar studies on the fetus and fullterm infants, indicate a considerable stability in human motor behaviour in the last months of gestation, irrespective of the intra- or extrauterine environment and of the time of delivery.

In order to study the post-natal development of motor activity, 10 of the preterm infants were observed at 3 wk intervals, from 3 to 18 wks of post-term age, in the "home" situation (for more details on the observation procedure see Hopkins & Prechtl, 1984).

Prechtl and Hopkins have recently (1986) described details of the change in appearance of GMs at the end of the second post-natal month. They lose their writhing character which is replaced by a qualitatively different, transient character, described as "fidgety". The authors have speculated that "fidgety" movements may be related to a postnatal "recalibration" of the proprioceptive system. In our study special attention was paid to the change from the writhing to the fidgety character in GM, and to the onset of manipulation and reaching. For comparison the same procedure was applied to 10 healthy fullterm infants. The results are shown in Fig.4.

The onset of fidgety movements occurred at 6 wks in 9 preterm infants, whereas of the fullterm infants 5 started at 6 wks, 3 at 9 wks and 2 at 12 wks. In both groups this movement pattern was transient, never lasting longer than 6 to 9 wks. In contrast with the earlier onset of fidgety movements in the preterm group, no difference was found in the onset of manipulation, reaching, head control, and in the disappearance of athetoid-like movements.

These observations provide another strong argument in favour of a high degree of independence in the maturation of the neural functions studied.

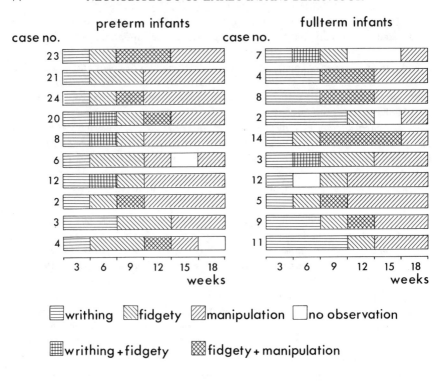

Fig. 4. Developmental course of writhing, fidgety and manipulating movements in 10 preterm and 10 fullterm infants followed at 3 wk intervals. .

POSTURE

In addition to the motor development, systematic observations of all postures occurring during the recording time were carried out. Preference posture was defined as the position of head, trunk and limbs assumed by the infant for the largest percentage of observation time. In the preterm period a large variability in the postural repertoire of the infants was observed. Fully confirming

Prechtl's previous report (Prechtl et al.,1979), we could not find any age-dependent characteristic posture. There was more intra-individual consistency of the preferred posture than similarities between babies at the same C.A.. When approaching term age there appear to be minimal differences between the preferred postures of preterm infants and those of full-term babies (Cioni et al.,1988), despite the spatial restriction in the uterus and the lack of restriction in the incubator. As reported by other authors (Palmer et al.,1982), extended postures of the legs are assumed slightly more frequently by the preterm infants, but this difference is already reduced when fullterm infants are observed in their fourth day of life (compared with the first), and almost disappears after 3-6 wks.

At term age postures assumed by the preterm infants in state 1 contributed more to the preference posture than postures in state 2. The infants studied did not show one particular posture characteristic of state 1, nor another characteristic of state 2. Again, similar findings have previously been obtained in fullterm infants (Cioni et al.,1988).

Still more similarities between preterm and fullterm infants were observed in the postural behaviour of the post-term period. Both showed a rapid increase of the midline position of the head in supine from 9 to 12 wks.

A parallel developmental course was also observed for the influence of head position and change of head position upon limbs posture. Asymmetrical tonic neck response (A.T.N.R.) was scored positive when one or both limbs on the chin side extended and the corresponding limbs flexed on the opposite side within 3 secs of each head turn. While present in both groups at 3 and 6 wks, A.T.N.R. decreased rapidly in frequency and intensity from 9 to 12 wks and disappeared at 15-18 wks.

CONCLUSIONS

The results of our longitudinal observations on posture and spontaneously generated movement patterns in preterm infants have confirmed the strict continuity between prenatal and postnatal life. Fetal motor patterns continue to be present up to and beyond term age. A major transformation of neural functions was observed only after the first month of life. That holds true for several postural and motor characteristics of the infants, as well as for many other aspects of their behaviour.

When data from the preterm infants were compared with those of the fetus and fullterm infants, we found striking similarities in motility and posture and also in their age-related transformations. Environmental conditions, provided they are not adverse, seem to have a very limited influence on the maturation of these neural functions in the healthy human fetus born before term.

REFERENCES

Cioni, G., Ferrari, F., Prechtl, H.F.R. (1988). Posture and spontaneous motility in fullterm infants. Early Hum. Develop., (in press).

Hopkins, B.,Prechtl, H.F.R. (1984). A qualitative approach to the development of movements during early infancy. In: H.F.R. Prechtl (Ed.), Continuity of Neural Functions from Prenatal to Postnatal Life. CDM 94. pp.179-197. London: Blackwell.

Nijhuis, J.G., Prechtl, H.F.R., Martin, C.B. Jr., Bots, R.S.G.M. (1982). Are there behavioural states in the human fetus ?. Early Hum. Develop. 6, 177-195.

Nolte, R., Haas, G.A (1978). Polygraphic study of bioelectrical brain maturation in preterm infants. Develop. Med. Child. Neurol., 20, 167-182.

Palmer, P.G., Dubowitz, L.M.S., Verghote, M., Dubowitz, V. (1982). Neurological and neurobehavioural differences between preterm infants and full-term newborn infants. Neuropediatrics, 13, 183-189.

Prechtl, H.F.R. (1985). Prenatal motor development. In: M.G. Wade and H.T.A. Whiting (Eds.), Motor Development in Children: Aspects of Coordination and Control. pp.53-64. Dordrech: Martinus Nijhoff Publishers.

Prechtl, H.F.R., Fargel, J.W., Weinmann, H.M., Bakker, H.H. (1979). Postures, motility and respiration of low-risk preterm infants. Develop. Med. Child. Neurol., 21, 3-27.

Prechtl, H.F.R., Hopkins, B. (1986) Developmental transformations of spontaneous movements in early infancy. Early Hum. Develop. 14, 233-238.

Vries, J.I.P. de, Visser, G.H.Å., Prechtl, H.F.R (1987). The emergence of fetal behaviour. III. Individual differences and consistences. Early Hum. Develop., 15, 333-349

III. Motor Control

8
Continuity of Pattern Generating Mechanisms in Embryonic and Posthatching Chicks

Anne Bekoff

The motor behavior that is seen at early embryonic stages in birds and mammals consists of Type I embryonic motility. This is a unique form of behavior, strikingly different in appearance from postnatal behaviors. While most postnatal behaviors, such as walking or grasping, appear smooth, goal-directed and coordinated, embryonic motility is typically characterized as jerky, random and uncoordinated (Hamburger, 1963; Hamburger and Oppenheim, 1967). Even in mammals, in which the embryonic movements are often less jerky than in birds, the behavior typically looks unorganized in that various body parts appear to move independently of one another (Hamburger, 1975; Smotherman et al., 1984). Nevertheless, despite the apparent discontinuity in appearance, it has often been suggested that embryonic behavior may serve as an antecedent or precursor of postnatal behaviors (Oppenheim, 1982; Bekoff, 1978; 1986).

Domestic chickens are ideal organisms in which to examine the issue of continuity between embryonic and postnatal motor behaviors for several reasons. First, fertile chicken eggs are available throughout the year. Second, the embryos are easily accessible once a hole is made in the eggshell. This means that early developmental stages can be readily studied. The third advantage to studying chicks is that they produce a wide repertoire of different behaviors, including embryonic motility, which involve leg movements. This means that it is possible to narrow our focus to consider continuity in the mechanisms involved in generating leg movements without compromising our ability to examine a variety of behaviors.

The purpose of this chapter is first to examine the characteristics of embryonic motility in chicks in order to obtain some insights into the nature of the underlying pattern generating circuitry. Second, the possibility that the circuit used for generating leg movements in the embryo is a basic circuit which is used and re-used throughout ontogeny to produce many different behaviors will be explored.

KINEMATIC ANALYSES

Early studies focussed on real-time visual observations of embryonic motility. This technique is useful for counting the number of movements per time interval and for making general qualitative observations of the movements (Bekoff, in press). However, because the movements appear jerky and uncoordinated, it has been difficult to characterize the movements in a way that facilitates comparison with other behaviors.

A recent study of the kinematics of embryonic motility in 9- and 10-day old chick embryos has provided some important new insights into the nature of this unique behavior (Watson and Bekoff, 1987; in preparation). Detailed analyses have been carried out on the movements of the right leg. To accomplish this, the hip, knee and ankle joints were marked as indicated in Figure 1. For each embryo normal, spontaneous, episodes of embryonic motility were videotaped at 60 frames per second for at least 20 minutes. Within each episode several leg movements occurred. To analyze a particular movement, the joint markers were digitized in each frame of the videotape records throughout the duration of the movement and computer programs were used to calculate joint angles. From these data, the duration of the movements, the direction of joint movement (extension or flexion), interjoint coordination patterns and the amplitude of joint excursions could all be determined.

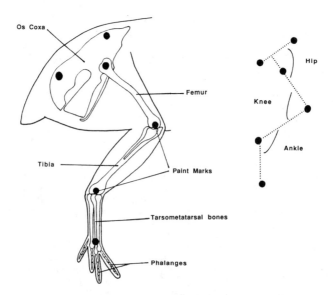

Figure 1. On the left is a schematic diagram of the right leg of a 10-day old chick embryo showing the placement of the paint spots used to mark the joints. The way in which hip, knee and ankle joint angles were determined from the digitized marks is indicated on the right.

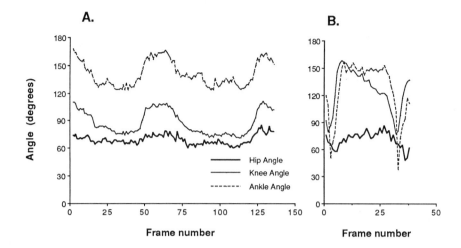

Figure 2. Graphs of joint angles for hip, knee and ankle plotted
against frame number. One frame = 16.7 msec. (A) Embryonic
motility. (B) Walking. Note different time scales on graphs. The
hip shows the smallest excursions in both behaviors while the
ankle shows the largest excursions.

These analyses demonstrate that a wide variety of leg
movement patterns is produced in the 9- to 10-day old embryo. That
is, any one, all three, or any combination of two, leg joints can
participate in a given movement. The amplitude of joint excursion
is typically quite small, but is also variable. The movement
duration can be anywhere from very short (300 ms) to very long
(3000 ms). Furthermore, a movement can occur individually, with a
pause before its onset and after its termination, or as part of a
rhythmic sequence of movements, as shown in Figure 2A. This
variability appears to account for the earlier characterizations
of embryonic motility as jerky and disorganized (Hamburger, 1963;
Hamburger and Oppenheim, 1967).

While there is a great deal of variability, some patterns
also emerge from the data. For example, the shortest movements are
all individual movements, usually consisting of a brief extension
from the rest position, followed by a flexion back to the rest
position. The longest movements are all part of rhythmic
sequences. Both the knee and the ankle participate in the majority
of movements. Motion in both knee and ankle almost always begins
synchronously and the joints usually move in the same direction.
Thus, although there are exceptions to these general rules, the
typical pattern is for knee and ankle, or in many cases hip, knee
and ankle, to. show a synchronous pattern of interjoint
coordination in which all three joints extend and flex together.
The pattern of synchronous interjoint coordination seen in the
kinematic analyses of embryonic leg movments is particularly
characteristic of the longer duration, rhythmic, movements.

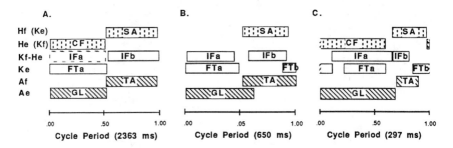

Figure 3. Bar graphs showing normalized EMG data for (A) Embryonic motility in 9- and 10-day old chick embryos, (B) Walking in cervical spinal and deafferented posthatching chicks and (C) Walking in normal posthatching chicks. H = hip, K = knee, A = ankle, e = extensor, f = flexor. Mean cycle period is in parentheses.

EMG ANALYSES

     EMG studies of embryonic motility have typically focussed on rhythmic activity (Bekoff, 1976; O'Donovan and Landmesser, 1984; Bradley and Bekoff, 1987). Similarities in cycle periods suggests that the EMGs that have typically been analyzed are from the longer, rhythmic embryonic movements. Analysis of these EMG records shows consistent muscle synergies: hip, knee and ankle extensors are active synchronously and their activity alternates with hip, knee and ankle flexors (Figure 3A).

     A recent study involving more detailed examination of the synergies has shown that these synergies are maintained even when only a subset of the muscles are active (Bradley and Bekoff, 1987). That is, any one or any combination of muscles can be active during rhythmic activity. However, whenever two or more muscles are active, they are active in the predicted pattern, independent of whether the active muscles include an ankle extensor and flexor, a hip and a knee extensor, or a hip flexor and an ankle extensor. Analyses of these data also show that the extensor and flexor bursts are similar in duration. Furthermore, the burst durations for flexors and extensors increase to a moderate and similar extent with increasing cycle period (Figure 4A).

Therefore, the kinematic and EMG data for rhythmic movements during embryonic motility in 9- to 10-day old chick embryos correspond well. Both kinds of data point to a relatively simple, basic, pattern of motor output. The movements of the right leg consist of alternation of extension and flexion at all of the active joints. These movements are produced when the leg muscles are active in a simple, symmetrical pattern in which extensors and flexors alternate. These data, then, suggest that a basic pattern generating circuit is assembled to produce leg movements in the early embryo.

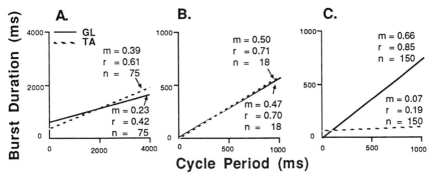

Figure 4. Burst durations for the ankle extensor, GL, and the ankle flexor, TA, have been plotted against cycle period for (A) Embryonic motility in 9- to 10-day old chick embryos, (B) Walking in cervical spinal and deafferented posthatching chicks and (C) Normal walking in posthatching chicks.

CONTINUITY?

The next question, then, is whether there is any evidence to suggest that this basic circuit is used in posthatching chicks in the production of other behaviors. Neither kinematic nor EMG studies have found evidence for the presence of the unaltered embryonic motor pattern in posthatching chicks despite examination of a variety of different behaviors, including, hatching, walking, swimming, airstepping and scratching (Jacobson and Hollyday, 1982; Bekoff, 1986; Bekoff et al., 1987a,b; Johnston and Bekoff, 1987; in press; Smith, Bradley and Bekoff, 1987; Smith and Bekoff, in press). For example, walking is a distinctive behavior that differs in several ways from embryonic motility. Kinematic data show that the step cycle during walking in chicks is similar to that seen in many animals in that it is divided into two distinct phases (Figure 2B). During a prolonged *stance phase* the leg joints are in a relatively extended position and the toes are in contact with the ground. During a shorter *swing phase* the leg joints first flex rapidly to lift the toes off the ground and then extend rapidly to prepare for the next toe touch. During embryonic motility, there is no contact with a substrate and the extension and flexion phases of the leg movement cycle are more symmetrical.

A second characteristic of walking that can be seen in the joint angle versus frame graph is the phase lag in onset of extension at the three leg joints. While flexion typically begins almost synchronously in hip, knee and ankle, extension consistently begins first at the knee, followed by ankle and then hip (Jacobson and Hollyday, 1982; Johnston and Bekoff, 1987; in preparation). In embryonic motility, extension and flexion of the three joint typically begins synchronously (Figure 2A).

A third characteristic feature of walking, which has been seen in EMG recordings from a wide range of animals, including chicks, is an asymmetry between extensor and flexor muscle activity (Grillner, 1981; Jacobson and Hollyday, 1982; Bekoff et al., 1987). Extensor burst durations are longer than flexor burst durations (Figure 3C) and they increase dramatically with increasing cycle period, while flexor burst durations increase relatively little (Figure 4C). This contrasts with the situation seen in embryonic motility, in which the pattern of flexor and extensor alternation is more symmetrical (Figures 3A,4A).

If the basic circuit used to produce the leg movements of embryonic motility were also used in the production of walking, then it would have to be modified or modulated to produce the different motor patterns. If the circuitry is permanently modified, then it should not be possible to elicit a motor pattern similar to embryonic motility from posthatching chicks. On the other hand, if the circuit is temporarily modulated so as to produce the walking motor pattern, then removal of the modulatory input should allow the circuit to produce the embryonic pattern.

We have therefore carried out an experiment in which two major potential sources of modulatory input were removed from several posthatching chicks (Bekoff et al., in press). Brain input was eliminated by carrying out a cervical spinal transection and leg-related sensory feedback was removed by carrying out a bilateral lumbosacral deafferentation. The effect of this experimental manipulation on the EMG pattern when these spinal, deafferented chicks were placed on a moving treadmill to elicit walking, were then examined. One major change is that the relative durations of extensors and flexors become more similar (Figure 3B). In addition, the asymmetry seen in the duration versus period relationships for extensors and flexors during normal walking is no longer present in these animals (Figure 4B).

Thus several characteristic features of walking are lost after brain and leg-related sensory inputs are removed. Furthermore, the pattern is similar, though not identical, to the pattern seen during embryonic motility. It is possible that the remaining differences between the motor pattern seen in the spinal, deafferented animals and the 9- and 10-day old embryos is due to remaining sensory and propriospinal inputs to the lumbosacral spinal cord. Because the transection was at C3, input was still available from the neck and thoracic region. To eliminate these inputs, future experiments are planned in which thoracic spinal cord transections will be performed.

ACKNOWLEDGEMENTS

        I would like to thank M. Bekoff for useful comments on the manuscript. N. S. Bradley, R. M. Johnston and S. J. Watson contibuted to the development of the ideas presented here by providing data and many stimulating conversations. The research reported here has been supported by NSF grant BNS 79-13826 and NIH grant NS20310.

REFERENCES

Bekoff, A. (1976). Ontogeny of leg motor output in the chick embryo: a neural analysis. Brain Res., 106, 271-291.

Bekoff, A. (1986). Ontogeny of chicken motor behaviours: evidence for multi-use limb pattern generating circuitry. In Neurobiology of Vertebrate Locomotion. (eds. S. Grillner, P.S.G. Stein, D.G. Stuart, H. Forssberg, R.M. Herman and P. Wallen). Macmillan Press, Hampshire, England. pp. 433-453.

Bekoff, A. (1978). A neuroethological approach to the study of the ontogeny of coordinated behavior. In The Development of Behavior. (eds. G.M. Burghhardt and M. Bekoff). Garland, NY. pp. 19-41.

Bekoff, A. (1986). Is the basic output of the locomotor CPG to flexor and extensor muscles symmetrical? Evidence from walking, swimming and embryonic motility in chicks. Soc. Neurosci. Abstr. 12, 880.

Bekoff, A. (in press). Embryonic motor output and movement patterns: relationship to postnatal behavior. In Behavior of the Fetus. (eds. W.P. Smotherman and S.R. Robinson). Telford Press, New Caldwell, NJ.

Bekoff, A., Feucht, P., Johnston, R.M. and H.E.Settles. (1987a) Comparison of forward and backward walking in chicks. Soc. Neurosci. Abstr., 13, 1541.

Bekoff, A., M.P. Nusbaum, Sabichi, A.L. and Clifford, M. (1987b). Neural control of limb coordination in chicks. I. Comparison of hatching and walking motor output patterns in normal and deafferented chicks. J. Neurosci., 7, 2320-2330.

Bekoff, A., Kauer, J.A., Fulstone, A. and Summers, T.R. (in press). Neural control of limb coordination. II. Hatching and walking motor output patterns in the absence of input from the brain. Exp. Brain Res.

Bradley, N.S. and Bekoff, A. (1987). Emergence of flexion and extension muscle synergies in the hindlimb of chick embryos. Soc. Neurosci. Abstr., 13, 1504.

Hamburger, V. (1963). Some aspects of the embryology of behavior. Quart. Rev. Biol., 38, 342-365.

Hamburger, V. (1975). Fetal behavior. In The Mammalian Fetus. (ed. E.S.E. Hafez). Charles C. Thomas, Springfield, Illinois. pp. 68-81.

Hamburger, V. and Oppenheim, R.W. (1967). Prehatching motility and hatching behavior in the chick. J. Exp. Zool., 166, 171-204.

Jacobson, R.D. and Hollyday, M.   (1982). A behavioral and
electromyographic study of walking in the chick.   J.
Neurophysiol., _48_, 238-256.

Johnston, R.M. and Bekoff, A. (1987).   Kinematic analysis of
walking, swimming and airstepping in chicks.   Soc. Neurosci.
Abstr., _13_, 356.

Johnston, R.M. and Bekoff, A. (in press). What are the
relationships between walking and airstepping in chicks?   Soc.
Neurosci. Abstr., _14_.

Landmesser, L.T. and O'Donovan, M.J.   (1984).   Activation patterns
of embryonic chick hind limb muscles recorded _in ovo_ and in an
isolated spinal cord preparation.   J. Physiol., Lond., _347_, 189-
204.

Oppenheim, R.W.   (1982).   The neuroembryological study of
behavior: progress, problems, perspectives.   In _Neural
Development, Part III_.   (ed. R.K. Hunt).   Academic Press, NY.   pp.
257-309.

Smith, M.B., Bradley, N.S. and Bekoff, A. (1987).   An EMG study of
scratching in chicks.   Soc. Neurosci. Abstr., _13_, 355.

Smith, M.B. and Bekoff, A. (in press).   Kinematic analysis of
scratching in chicks.   Soc. Neurosci. Abstr., _14_.

Smotherman, W.P., Richards, L.S. and Robinson, S.R.   (1984).
Techniques for observing fetal behavior in utero: a comparison of
chemomyelotomy and spinal transection.   Devel. Psychobiol., _17_,
661-674.

Watson, S.J. and Bekoff, A. (1987).   A kinematic study of chick
embryonic motility.   Soc. Neurosci. Abstr., _13_, 1504.

9

Continuity and Consequences of Behavior in Preterm Infants

Heidelise Als

INTRODUCTION

The development of the preterm infant presents an experiment of nature from which one might infer the importance of the specificity of sensory input for the normal unfolding and differentiation of early human functioning. Many more preterms survive now due to advances in neonatal medical technology than has ever been the case before. Twenty-four to 25 weeks gestation is the current lower limit of extrauterine viability. Longitudinal outcome studies, especially of the <32 weeks preterm, show a high incidence of motor problems, learning disabilities, behavior problems, attentional deficit disorder and emotional problems (see, for example, Kitchen et al., 1980; Catto-Smith et al., 1985; Hack & Breslau, 1986; and Minde et al., in press). There is some suggestion that these problems diminish only to some degree by exclusion of infants with such morbidities as fetal brain insults (Larroche, 1986), intraventricular hemorrhage and bronchopulmonary dysplasia (e.g., Sostek et al., 1987). Developmental impairment or difference appears due not only to focal insult by hemorrhage or anoxic event, but possibly also to a difference in sensory experience *ex utero*, including cutaneous tactile, somasthetic kinesthetic as well as visual, auditory, gustatory and olfactory experiences. Since species appropriate sensory information is thought to potentiate species appropriate ontogenetic differentiation and modulation patterns, it would not be surprising that difference in sensory information input would lead to difference in development, especially given the rapid development of the brain from the 24th to the 40th week of fetal life, and especially the rapid emergence of association cortical areas. Animal models, such as in the work of Duffy and colleagues (Duffy et al., 1985, 1978-a,b, 1976; Mower et al., 1981, 1985, 1984; Mower & Duffy, 1983), Spinelli (Spinelli & Jensen, 1979; Spinelli et al., 1980) and others (for a review, see Duffy et al., 1984) investigating the effects of developmentally inappropriate inputs during periods of rapid brain development, have largely implicated active suppression and inhibition of pathways through overactivation of already functional pathways, thus leading to less differentiated and less modulated overall functioning. We have examined this hypothesis in two research projects, the longitudinal investigation of the behavioral functioning of medically healthy preterm infants of various gestational ages in comparison to fullterm infants and the study of environmental restructuring of the early extrauterine environment in which the very early preterm infant finds him or herself.

QUESTION 1: DO MEDICALLY HEALTHY PRETERMS SHOW BEHAVIORAL MODULATION DIFFERENCES WHEN COMPARED TO FULLTERMS?

1. Behavioral Assessment

We have developed two behavioral assessment methodologies specifically designed to assess the behavioral regulation and organizational differences between preterm and fullterm infants. The first is an assessment of newborn behavioral organization called the APIB (Assessment of Preterm Infants' Behavior) (Als et al., 1982-a,b); the second is an experimental play paradigm called the Kangaroo-Box Paradigm (Als & Berger, 1986). Both were developed in a synactive formulation of development (Als, 1982) assessing the degree of flexibility and modulation of behaviorally identified subsystems of functioning in their interplay with each other and, in turn, in their joint interplay with the environment. Figure 1 shows the schematic presentation of this formulation (reprinted with permission). The subsystems observed include the autonomic, motor, state regulatory and the attentional interactive systems. These are assessed when the organism is brought through a systematic sequence of manipulations or is observed in a standard paradigm designed to bring out the infant's current level of regulation.

The *APIB* was developed in an effort to extend the Brazelton Neonatal Behavioral Assessment Scale (BNBAS) (Brazelton, 1984) to specifically assess the behavior of prematurely born infants and, furthermore, to allow for the assessment of the level differentiation and modulation of functioning. The APIB casts the maneuvers of the BNBAS into a graded sequence of increasingly vigorous environmental inputs in order to systematically assess the infant's threshold from organization to disorganization. The differential cost to the infant in handling and responding to the maneuvers of the examination becomes a key feature of analysis. For instance, one newborn may move from sleep state to alert state only with accompanying respiratory irregularity consisting of respiratory pauses, alternating with tachypneic episodes, accompanied by visceral upheaval, color changes, and motoric hyperextension oscillating with flaccidity. Once he brings about an alert state, he appears facially bland or even strained, with acrocyanosis and poor respiratory stability, unable to consistently focus on a stimulus and process the sensory input. After a fleeting episode of strained alerting, he moves quickly to a motorically hyperaroused state accompanied by tachypnea, from which he can be brought to a more balanced level of modulated flexor tone with regular respirations only with great difficulty. Yet he will visually track and follow a target through a 60 degree angle. Another newborn, in contrast, will move easily from sleep to alert state without autonomic instability or motoric disorganization. Once in alertness, he maintains himself there readily and focuses on various stimuli with ease and alacrity while his angle of visual excursion is also 60 degrees. Despite the same visual orientation angle, this second infant would be considered more well organized than the first infant along the differentiation and modulation continuum of subsystems, and his scores on the autonomic, motor, state, attentional, and self-regulatory systems as well as on examiner facilitation would be lower, reflecting better behavioral organization and, therewith, a difference in regulation as defined here.

MODEL OF THE SYNACTIVE
ORGANIZATION OF BEHAVIORAL DEVELOPMENT

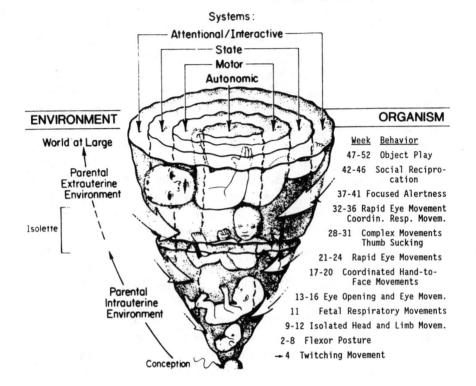

*Figure 1. Model of the synactive organization of behavioral develop-
ment [from Als H, 1982; with permission]. Note: Approximate time
of appearance of selected fetal behaviors is listed on the right.*

The ***Kangaroo-Box Paradigm*** was developed to assess the strategies and the degree of overall subsystem modulation and differentiation exhibited by infants at 9, 18 and 36 months, with a version available for the 5-8 year range. By 9 months post term, the infants' world
has expanded considerably. Their mobility allows them to approach
and leave situations, objects, and persons in a very different way than

they did earlier. They initiate interactions and explorations beyond their immediate reach space, pursue objects and persons locomotively and structure situations by incorporation of much larger space frames and with more temporal flexibility than before. In order to assess competence along comparable dimensions of subsystem differentiation and modulation in analogy to the newborn period via the APIB, we constructed a paradigm which involves a toy task consisting of a transparent plexiglass box accessible through a transparent mobile porthole latch door and containing a hopping, wind-up kangaroo. The box is placed on the floor of a playroom. During the observation, all other distractions (pictures, chair, etc.) are removed, and mother and infant are asked to go into the room and play with the toy in whatever way so that "they both have a good time." They are observed and videotaped with a two-camera split-screen system through one-way mirror walls for six minutes. Then the kangaroo is placed back into the box, the latch door closed, and the mother is asked to sit against the wall of the room looking at the infant, but not interacting or reacting. The infant is observed in this stillface situation for six minutes. Then a three-minute reunion is observed when the mother is again allowed to play with the infant. The Kangaroo-Box Paradigm (K-Box) challenges the infant's cognitive, gross and fine motor, social and affective capacities and, for some more stressed infants, even physiological regulation, as the infant attempts to retrieve the kangaroo from the box. It, furthermore, provides an opportunity to observe the mother's strategies in facilitating and expanding the infant's competence.

We have developed a scoring manual (Als & Berger, 1986) to score the infant's capacities during the play and stillface episodes along 12 dimensions on a scale from 1 (minimum) to 5 (optimal). These include autonomic organization, gross and fine motor organization, symmetry of tonus, movement and posture, apparent cognitive functioning, language and vocal organization, affective organization, social-interactive organization, competence in play with the object, competence in combining object play and social interaction, degree of self-regulation, degree of facilitation and structure necessary, and degree of pleasure and pride displayed by the infant. Attention is paid to autonomic reactions, movements, tone, vocalizations, and facial expressions in their interplay. And, as in the APIB, the degree of

flexibility, differentiation and modulation of each subsystem is measured as an index of competence and regulation. The mother is also
scored on parallel scales.

The Kangaroo-Box Paradigm for the older children consists of a
large plexiglass tower with three tiers and varying degrees of difficulty
of access to the wind-up toy inside two of the plexiglass cubes making up the tower. As an aid to reaching the top level, a footstool and
various raking tools are provided. The kangaroo can either be taken
out or can be dropped through a latch door in the floor of the top cube
to the second level. Once on the second level, it needs to be pushed
via one of the several raking tools provided at the second level opening to fall to the ground level, from where it can be obtained via the
door, openable by a key. The second kangaroo sitting in the ground
level cube can be obtained independently of the first. Both can be
obtained and incorporated into exploration of the various possibilities
of this apparatus.

The K-Box apparatus of the different age levels is designed to
have built-in, immediate demand characteristics, yet to allow for individual differences in the order, sophistication and complexity of its
manipulation and use. The total child is directly involved in the
Kangaroo-Box Paradigm rather than only selected facets of the child's
functioning. It, therefore, is expected to yield useful and systematic
information in the integration and modulation of overall behavioral
functioning.

2. Results

We have studied 160 healthy preterm and fullterm infants who
spanned the gestational age continuum in relatively equal numbers
from the 26-32 week preterm, the 33 to 37 week preterm, and the 38
to 41 week fullterm. All infants were selected to be free of known
neurological insult including perinatal asphyxia, neonatal seizures,
bronchopulmonary dysplasia, and intraventricular hemorrhage as well
as free of necrotizing enterocolitis and sepsis. All infants were
appropriate for age in weight at birth; all were singletons and free of
any congenital abnormalities and infections. There were 48 fullterms
(FT), 48 preterms (PT), and 64 pre-preterms (PPT). All infants were

studied with the APIB at 2 weeks after due date. The results indicate that the six system variables (autonomic, motor, state and attentional organization, self-regulation and examiner facilitation) show strong differences between FTs, PTs and PPTs, with the strongest differences between FTs and the two PT groups together, and fewer yet significant differences also between the PTs and PPTs. The PPTs are consistently the most reactive, hypersensitive and disorganized, the PTs take a middle position, and the FTs are the most well modulated and well differentiated. Thus, the APIB appears very sensitive in identifying gestational age effects (Als et al., 1988-a,b). The robustness of the APIB in identifying gestational age [GA] group membership was also shown by successful prospective classification of an earlier sample of 20 FTs and 20 PTs. Ninety-five percent (38/40) of the infants were correctly classified as to GA status on the basis of their APIB scores (Als et al., 1988-a). Furthermore, three reliable (tested on two independent split-half samples), behaviorally defined clusters of infants were identified (Als et al., in press-a,1988-b), with a preponderance of PPTs in the most reactive group and a preponderance of FTs in the most well organized group. Brain electrical activity mapping (BEAM) data (for methodology, see chapter by Duffy in this volume) implicated primarily right hemispheric and frontal lobe function differences between the behaviorally defined clusters (Als et al., in press-b).

One-hundred forty-eight infants were restudied at 9 months post-EDC (expected date of confinement) with the Bayley Scales (Bayley, 1969) and in the Kangaroo-Box Paradigm; 73 of the infants were restudied at 3 years post EDC with a comprehensive neuropsychological battery as well as the Kangaroo-Box Paradigm. While the Bayley Scale Scores (MDI and PDI) did not show gestational age differences, the Kangaroo-Box Paradigm elicited consistent differences in autonomic, gross and fine motor regulation, social interactive, affective, and spatial regulation. Preliminary analyses of the data at age 3 years showed, again, on the standardized psychological assessments few differences, yet the Kangaroo-Box Paradigm showed many highly significant gestational-age group effects (autonomic regulation, gross and fine motor modulation, social interactive and affective regulation, and language functioning). Furthermore, again three clusters of neurobehavioral functioning emerged on the basis of the K-Box data at each of the age points. Cluster concordance from the newborn period to the later age points was very good.

Aside from these findings, K-Box data on 14 healthy preterm (<34 weeks) and 14 healthy fullterm children from the earlier sample of 20 and 20 have been collected and analyzed at age 5 years. The results showed striking group differences in this paradigm in the face of only very small differences on standardized cognitive assessments, and BEAM again implicates frontal and right hemispheric functioning (Als et al., in press-b; Duffy & Als, 1988).

Thus, it appears that there is a profile of regulatory difficulties characteristic of preterm infants and increasing with lower gestational age at birth which can be documented from the newborn period on and which shows consistency to age 3 years and perhaps to age 5 years. It appears to encompass not only greater autonomic reactivity, but also poorer modulation of gross and fine motor functioning, poorer affective and attentional regulation, with more static facial expression, narrowed affective range, higher distractibility and perseveration, poorer modulation of transition from one task aspect to another, and poorer articulation and expressive language use, in the face of normal overall intellectual capacity. These differences were found in the absence of documented brain injury. They, thus, speak to a difference in neurobehavioral organization due possibly to difference in sensory experience and consequent brain maturation in the trimester preceding term.

QUESTION 2: WILL THE COMPREHENSIVE MODIFICATION OF SENSORY INPUT TO THE VERY EARLY BORN PRETERM INFANT (< 32 WEEKS) REDUCE DEVELOPMENTAL COMPROMISE?

On the basis of the synactive theoretical model, we developed an intervention approach which focusses on reduction of purported stress behaviors and increase of self-regulatory behaviors of the preterm infant by modification of the physical environment in the neonatal intensive care unit [NICU] (e.g., shielding from overhead lighting and from noise) and the caregiving practices by nurses and other professionals as well as the parents interacting with the infant (e.g., provision of prone or sidelying flexor position support by specially constructed buntings; of nonnutritive sucking; containment during medical procedures; sleep state regulation protection, etc.) (Als, 1986; Als et al., 1986). A training program in the individualized caregiving approach is now available at our hospital with focus on the behavioral observation of the infant, on designing an individualized care plan, and on comprehensive implementation with appropriate modification as the baby's behavior matures and changes. Figures 2 through 4 show examples of caregiving modifications.

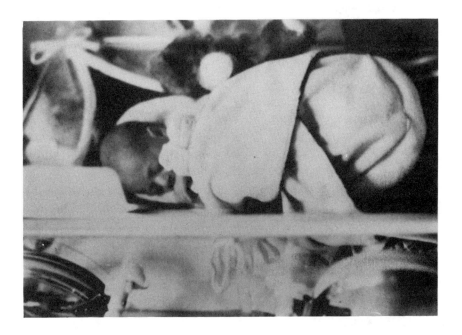

Figure 2. Very sensitive former 26-week preterm, now 29 weeks, in bunting on hammock in isolette, sidelying with arms in flexion, in relaxed sleep

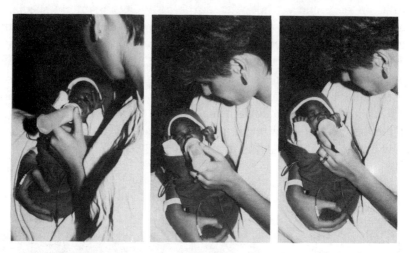

Figure 3a. 27-week preterm, now 35 weeks post-conception; bottle feeding in bunting to facilitate shoulder, arm, and leg flexor position and, therewith, sucking and relaxation [Figures 3-4 from Als H, 1986; with permission]

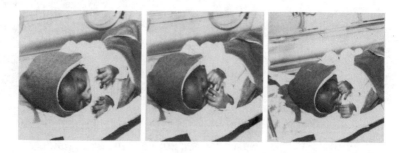

Figure 3b. Increasingly competent use of special "suckel" without help by caregiver; gradual relaxation into sleep

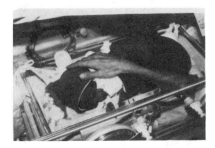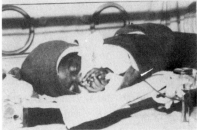

Figure 3c. After a taxing caregiving procedure, in isolette on hammock supported by special frame; facilitation by containment in bunting, sidelying position, aided by caregiver's encasing arm and hand, and by opportunity to suck on special "suckel" (nipple in soft cloth strip)

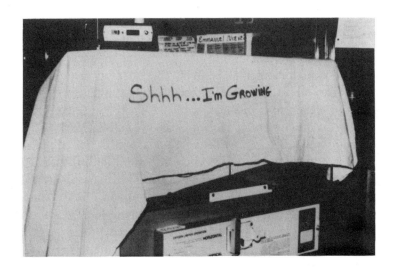

Figure 4. Shielding of isolette with blanket

We have tested this approach in two studies with encouraging results:

1. Initial Study

We studied eight control infants in the course of one year, conducting detailed behavioral observations (Als et al., 1986) on the infants every 10th day. In the second year of the study, intervention infants received the same observations and, in addition, carefully designed individualized caregiving modifications implemented by the primary nursing team of the baby. All infants were initially respirator-dependent and met stringent selection criteria which put them at high risk for the development of bronchopulmonary dysplasia (birthweight <1250g; mechanical ventilation within 48 hours of delivery; mechanical ventilation >24 hours in the first 48 hours at > .40 FiO2 for >4 hours (Cohen & Taeusch, 1983); no chromosomal or other genetic anomalies; no major congenital infections; no major maternal illness including intrauterine infections; no twins; etc.). The control and intervention groups did not differ on any other medical variables up to day 10, when intervention started, nor did they differ on any demographic variables. The results of the study showed the intervention group with a significantly decreased number of days on the respirator, on supplemental oxygen, and on tube feeding (Als et al., 1986). The children were subsequently studied after NICU discharge at 4 weeks post due date with the APIB; at 3, 6, 9 and 18 months post due date with the Bayley Scales (Bayley, 1969); at 9, 18 and 36 months post due date with the Kangaroo-Box Paradigm (Als, 1984); and at 36 months post due date with the McCarthy Scales of Children's Abilities (McCarthy, 1972), the Kaufman Assessment Battery for Children (K-ABC) (Kaufman & Kaufman, 1983), and the Psychomotor Scale of the Bayley Scales (Bayley, 1969). The intervention infants were better modulated, as measured by the APIB systems scores, in terms of motor system and self-regulation ability. Of the five body signal parameters measured, the intervention group showed a significantly lower incidence of motoric extension behavior such as grimacing, arching, etc., considered indicators of stress. They also showed a higher number of normal reflexes. Further, the Mental Developmental Index (MDI) scores and the Psychomotor Developmental Index (PDI) scores for the control and intervention groups at 3,

6 and 9 months consistently showed the intervention infants significantly above the control infants. Thus the intervention appears to have had a substantial impact on both the mental development of these infants and the motor development (Als et al., 1986; Als et al., 1988-c). Preliminary analyses (ANOVA) on results of the Kangaroo-Box Paradigm at 9, 18 and 36 months (Als et al., 1986; Als et al., 1988-c,d) showed that the intervention children performed significantly better than the control infants. Furthermore, the initial advantage of the intervention children was well maintained, while the control children deteriorated over time on many of the parameters. All parent-child interaction parameters favor the intervention children significantly. This advantage was also demonstrated on the McCarthy Scales at age 3 years, the Bayley Psychomotor Scale raw score, and K-ABC performance (Kaufman & Kaufman, 1983). We feel that these results demonstrate that behavioral modulation, implemented in the early preterm phase by modification of sensory input, shows striking continuity in behavioral improvement over time, at least to age 3 years.

2. Replication Study

We have very recently replicated and extended this study on a larger sample (18 control and 20 intervention infants) using similar selection criteria. This time, we randomly assigned the preterms to the control and intervention groups, with intervention starting in the first 48 hours after delivery, i.e., as soon as selection criteria were met. The results again showed striking medical course improvement of the intervention infants, with significantly reduced respirator stay, oxygen need, tube feeding, bronchopulmonary dysplasia, and marked reduction in the incidence of intraventricular hemorrhage (10 out of 18 controls; 1 out of 20 intervention infants). Furthermore, length of hospital stay was significantly reduced, as was hospital cost. APIB scores at 2 weeks after due date and electrophysiological functioning at the same data point, as assessed with BEAM, show again highly significant group differences favoring the intervention infants (Als et al., 1988c]. We fully expect that the functional advantage of the intervention infants will be lasting over time, as was seen in the initial intervention study reported above.

SUMMARY

Understanding and documentation of the continuity and consequences of preterm infant behavior is a constant challenge to the researcher and the clinician. We have formulated a functional model which attempts to specify the behavioral subsystems of functioning, which, in their respective interplay, in the manner in which they move from stable to disorganized functioning, and in the flexibility with which they maintain organized functioning in the face of varied exogenous and endogenous events, may exemplify an infant's individuality of behavioral functioning. Based on this model, we have attempted to develop systematic assessments, the APIB and the Kangaroo-Box Paradigm, to quantify the degree of differentiation and modulation of these behaviorally defined subsystems of functioning. We hypothesize that the differences documented via these assessments are brain-based, i.e., part of the child's biological make-up, which is influenced by the environment and which shows a recognizable pattern along a defineable trajectory.

The studies reported in this chapter show the following:

Medically healthy preterm infants show a gradient of modulation differences by gestational age group, with the earlier born babies showing much greater sensitivity, reactivity and lower threshold to disorganization. Brain electrical activity mapping studies appear to implicate primarily the right hemisphere and frontal lobes.

Behavioral organizational group membership in the newborn period predicts to neuropsychological functioning at later ages, with the low threshold reactive newborns showing much greater difficulties in motor and spatial planning, social interactive modulation capacity, and attentional regulation.

Behavioral organizational functioning of the very early-born preterm infant appears to be modifiable and supportable by individualized caregiving based on the infant's own behavioral cues indicating his sensory thresholds to disorganization.

The brain of the immature fetal infant is the organ which orchestrates and influences all aspects of functioning. The synactive model of development outlines access avenues for the observation of that brain's function via the behavior displayed by the infant. Autonomic, motoric, state organizational, attentional, and self-regulatory capacities of the infant can be observed in order to identify succinctly and specifically where an individual infant's thresholds to sensory input and ability not only for self-maintenance, but for increasing differentiation lie. In order to take the next step in differentiation, previously integrated and synchronized connections open up, necessitating the temporary disorganization and dyssynchronization of subsystems in their interplay. Yet, then the subsystems realign and support each other again at a more differentiated level of functioning. In this model, if stress is too massive, more differentiated new alignment of subsystems is not possible, and maladaptive, costly realignment occurs at a more rigid, canalized level of functioning. Detailed observation of the behavior of the fetus displaced from the womb into the NICU environment and reacting to the onslaught of sensory experiences can be our opportunity to estimate and infer from the infant's behavior how an appropriate comprehensive physical and caregiving environment can be provided sufficiently astutely in order to support the highly sensitive and rapid brain and behavioral development of this infant.

It appears such strenuous medical management and even programs of environmental enrichment not geared to the individual infant's sensory thresholds may force the organism to reject such stimulation with consequences akin to deprivation and subsequent active neuronal suppression (Duffy et al., 1984). Only careful environmental manipulation in controlled studies with sensitive outcome measures will provide us with the answers.

ACKNOWLEDGEMENTS

The work reported here was supported by grant 1RO1HD15482 from NICHD, grant GO-08435063 from NIDRR, MR Center Grant P30-HD18655 from NICHD, a grant from the H. P. Hood Foundation and the Merck Family Fund. Special thanks go to all our research assistants over the years and to my secretary Christine Murray whose unflagging support makes it all possible. Further thanks go to the nurses and medical staff in our NICU, and, foremost, to our study parents and their infants, who are helping us become more astute in understanding the amazing complexity of early development.

REFERENCES

Als, H. (1982). Towards a synactive theory of development: Promise for the assessment of infant individuality. *Infant Mental Health J.*, *3*, 229-243.

Als, H. (1984). *Manual and scoring system for the assessment of children's behavior: Kangaroo-box paradigm* Unpublished manuscript, The Children's Hospital, Boston.

Als, H. (1986). Synactive model of neonatal behavioral organization: Framework for the assessment and support of the neurobehavioral development of the premature infant and his parents in the environment of the neonatal intensive care unit. In J. K. Sweeney (Ed.), *The High-Risk Neonate: Developmental Therapy Perspectives* (pp. 3-55). The Haworth Press.

Als, H., & Berger, A. (1986). Manual and Scoring System for the Assessment of Infants' Behavior: Kangaroo - Box Paradigm Unpublished manuscript, Children's Hospital, Boston.

Als, H., Lawhon, G., Brown, E., Gibes, R., Duffy, F. H., McAnulty, G., & Blickman, J. G. (1986). Individualized behavioral and environmental care for the very low birth weight preterm infant at high risk for bronchopulmonary dysplasia: Neonatal intensive care unit and developmental outcome. *Pediatr.*, *78*, 1123-1132.

Als, H., Duffy, F. H., & McAnulty, G. B. (in press-a). Neurobehavioral competence in healthy preterm and fullterm infants: Newborn period to 9 months. *Dev. Psychol.*

Als, H., Duffy, F. H., McAnulty, G., & Badian, N. (in press-b). Assessment of neurobehavioral functioning in preterm and fullterm newborns and the question of predictability of later development. In N. Krasnegor and M. Bornstein (Eds.), *Continuity in Development*. Hillsdale, NJ: Lawrence Erlbaum.

Als, H., Duffy, F. H., & McAnulty, G. B. (1988-a). Behavioral differences between preterm and fullterm newborns as measured with the APIB system scores: I. *Infant Behav. Dev, 11*, 305-318.

Als, H., Duffy, F. H., & McAnulty, G. B. (1988-b). The APIB, an assessment of functional competence in preterm and fullterm newborns regardless of gestational age at birth: II. *Infant Behav. Dev., 11*, 319-331.

Als, H., Lawhon, G., Gibes, R., Duffy, F. H., McAnulty, G. B., & Blickman, J. G. (1988-c). *Individualized behavioral and developmental care for the VLBW preterm infant at high risk for bronchopulmonary dysplasia and intraventricular hemorrhage. Study II NICU outcome.* New England Perinatal Association Annual Meeting, Woodstock, VT.

Als, H., Lawhon, G., McAnulty, G., Duffy, F. H., & Gibes, R. (1988-d). Developmental outcomes to age 3 years of early behaviorally based care in the NICU. *in preparation.*

Als, H., Lester, B. M., Tronick, E., & Brazelton, T. B. (1982-a). Towards a research instrument for the assessment of preterm infants' behavior. In H. E. Fitzgerald, B. M. Lester and M. W. Yogman (Eds.), *Theory and Research in Behavioral Pediatrics* (pp. 35-63). New York: Plenum Press.

Als, H., Lester, B. M., Tronick, E. C., & Brazelton, T. B. (1982-b). Manual for the assessment of preterm infants' behavior (APIB). In H. E. Fitzgerald, B. M. Lester and M. W. Yogman (Eds.), *Theory and Research in Behavioral Pediatrics. Vol. I* (pp. 65-132). New York: Plenum Press.

Bayley, N. (1969). *Manual for the Bayley Scales of Infant Development.* New York: The Psychological Corporation.

Brazelton, T. B. (1984). *Neonatal Behavioral Assessment Scale. Clinics in Developmental Medicine, No. 88 (rev. ed.).* Philadelphia: Lippincott.

Catto-Smith, A. G., Yu, V. Y. H., Bajuk, B., Orgill, A. A., & Astbury, J. (1985). Effect of Neonatal Periventricular Hemorrhage on neurodevelopmental outcome. *Archives of Disease, 60,*

8-11.

Cohen, A., & Taeusch, H. W. (1983). Prediction of risk for bronchpul-monary dysplasia. *Am. J. Perinatology, 1*, 21-22.

Duffy, F. H. (this volume) Electrophysiological evidence for gesta-tional age effects in infant studied at term: a Beam study. In C. von Euler, H. Forssberg, & H. Lagercrantz (Eds.), *Neurobiology of Early Infant Behavior. Wenner-Gren Center International Symposium Series.* Hampshire, England: Macmillan Press.

Duffy, F. H., & Als, H. (1988). Neural plasticity and the effect of a supportive hospital environment on premature newborns. In J. F. Kavanagh (Ed.), *Understanding mental retarda-tion. Research accomplishments and new frontiers* (pp. 179-206). Baltimore: Paul H. Brookes Publishing Co.

Duffy, F. H., Burchfiel, J. L., Mower, G. D., Joy, R. M., & Snodgrass, S. R. (1985). Comparative pharmacological effects on visual cortical neurons in monocularly deprived cats. *Brain Res., 339*, 257-264.

Duffy, F. H., Burchfiel, J. L., & Snodgrass, S. R. (1978-a). The phar-macology of amblyopia. *Arch. Ophthal., 85*, 489-495.

Duffy, F. H., Mower, G. D., & Burchfiel, J. L. (1978-b). Experimental amblyopia production by random monocular shifts of visual inputs. *Soc. Neurosci. Abstracts, 4*, 625.

Duffy, F. H., Mower, G. D., Jensen, F., & Als, H. (1984). Neural plasticity: A new frontier for infant development. In H. E. Fitzgerald, B. M. Lester and M. W. Yogman (Eds.), *Theory and Research in Behavioral Pediatrics II* (pp. 67-96). New York: Plenum.

Duffy, F. H., Snodgrass, R., Burchfiel, J. L., & Conway, J. (1976). Bicuculline reversal of deprivation amblyopia in the cat. *Nature, 260*, 256-257.

Hack, M., & Breslau, N. (1986). Very Low Birth Weight Infants: Effects of Brain Growth During Infancy on Intelligence Quotient at 3 years of age. *Pediat., 77(2)*.

Kaufman, A. S., & Kaufman, N. L. (1983). *Kaufman Assessment Battery for Children, K-ABC.*. Circle Pines, Minn.: American Guidance Service.

Kitchen, W. H., Ryan, M. M., Richards, A., McDougall, A. B., Billson, F. A., Keir, E. H., & Naylor, F. D. (1980). A longitudinal study of very low-birthweight infants IV. An overview of performance at eight years of age. *Dev. Med. Child Neurol.*, *22*, 172-188.

Larroche, J. (1986). Fetal encephalopathies of circulatory origin. *Biol. Neonate*, *50*, 61-74.

McCarthy, D. (1972). *Manual for the McCarthy Scales of Children's Abilities*. New York: The Psychological Corporation.

Minde, K., Goldberg, S., Perrotta, M., Washington, J., Lojsak, M., Corter, C., & Parker, K. (in press), Continuities and discontinuities in the development of 64 very small premature infants to four years of age. *J. Child Psychol. Psychiatry*.

Mower, G. D., Berry, D., Burchfiel, J. L., & Duffy, F. H. (1981). Comparison of the effects of dark rearing and binocular suture on development and plasticity of cat visual cortex. *Brain Res.*, *220*, 255-267.

Mower, G. D., Caplan, C. J., Christen, W. G., & Duffy, F. H. (1985). Dark rearing prolongs physiological but not anatomical plasticity in the cat visual cortex. *J. Comp. Neurol.*, *235*, 448-466.

Mower, G. D., Christen, W. G., Burchfiel, J. L., & Duffy, F. H. (1984). Microiontophoretic bicuculline restores binocular responses to visual cortical neurons in strabismic cats. *Brain Res.*, *309*, 168-172.

Mower, G. D., & Duffy, F. H. (1983). Animal models of strabismic amblyopia: comparative behavioral studies. *Behav. Brain Res.*, *7*, 239-251.

Sostek, A. M., Smith, Y. F., Katz, K. S., & Grant, E. G. (1987). Developmental outcome of preterm infants with intraventricular hemorrhage at one and two years of age. *Child Dev.*, *58*, 779-786.

Spinelli, D. N., & Jensen, F. E. (1979). Plasticity: The mirror of experience. *Science*, *203*, 75-78.

Spinelli, D. N., Jensen, F. E., & DePrisco, G. V. (1980). Early experience effect on dendritic branchings in normally reared kittens. *Exper. Neurol*, *68*, 1-11.

10

An 'Outside-in' Approach to the Development of Leg Movement Patterns

Esther Thelen, Beverly D. Ulrich and Jody L. Jensen

INTRODUCTION

During the first year, the developmental course of coordination and control of leg movements is complex and nonlinear. Movement patterns undergo cycles of stability and change, symmetry and asymmetry, and spurts and regressions. At every age, motor coordination is a function not only of infants' maturational status but also of their immediate internal state and the context in which the action is performed. The thesis of this chapter is that these developmental events can best be interpreted from a dynamical framework. First, at any age movements emerge from the "soft-assembly" of a multicomponent neuromuscular system operating in a specific environmental or task context. And second, new motor forms arise in ontogeny as a result of a continual "dialogue" between the central nervous system and the periphery.

In the first section, we illustrate the context-dependency of leg actions by tracing the ontogenetic course of various kicking and stepping movements in the first year. In the second section, we report experiments that show that infants are sensitive to their own self-movement through proprioception and other modalities. Then, we argue that spontaneous and elicited movements allow infants to explore a wide universe of movement possibilities and their multimodal perceptual correlates. Finally, we suggest that certain movement configurations become preferred and stable as a result of this dialogue with the periphery. In this view, central nervous system (CNS) maturation sets only the broad outlines for motor development; the details are filled in by continual experience in the real world.

THE CONTEXT ASSEMBLES MOTOR PATTERNS

With the rediscovery of the work of N. Bernstein (1967; Whiting, 1984), there has been increasing recognition that in order to coordinate and control movement, the CNS must deal with the biomechanical properties of the body. Limbs and body segments have mass, viscoelastic properties; they are linked together and subject to gravity. When a person moves, the movement trajectory is determined not only by active muscle contractions, but also by these nonmuscle forces, which change in a complex and nonlinear way during the movement.

A central question for understanding movement is how the nervous system turns on and off the muscles to account for the biomechanics of the body and to produce the adaptive and flexible actions needed for everyday tasks. It is highly unlikely that the CNS could store and read out a muscle-specific code for each and every action in each and every situation. In the absence of a "motor program," how are stable, yet flexible actions produced?

Evidence is rapidly accumulating to show that patterns of coordination are not "hard-wired" anywhere in the nervous system, but "softly-assembled" specifically in response to the total task context (e.g. Schoner & Kelso, 1988). According to Kugler and Turvey (1987), temporally ordered rhythmic behavior such as locomotion can arise from a biokinematic system "assembled temporarily and for a particular purpose from whatever neural and skeletomuscular elements are available and befitting the task" (p.3). Such a system exhibits stability of form under uniform conditions, but retains flexibility to adjust to changing conditions within the organism and in the environment.

The patterns of leg coordinations seen in infants, which culminate in independent upright locomotion, can best be understood from this context-specific perspective. During their first year infants move their legs rhythmically in a number of configurations and from a variety of postures. They "step" while upright. They kick while supine, prone, and sitting. They propel forward on their knees, and they "walk" on a treadmill.

Each of these movement topographies follows a different developmental course (Figure 1). Stepping movements while supported upright decline dramatically within the first 2 months. At the same time kicking movements in supine and prone increase, and continue to do so. Stepping on the treadmill is also increasingly easy to elicit after about 3 months, although a few infants respond to the treadmill earlier. Much later in the first

year, infants creep, crawl, step with support, and walk
alone (see Thelen, in press, for review).

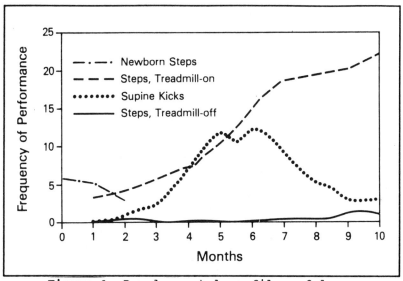

Figure 1 Developmental profiles of leg
movement types during the first year
(arbitrary units). Data are redrawn from
Thelen (1979), Thelen & Ulrich (1988), and
Zelazo, (1983).

Are, then, kicking, stepping, treadmill stepping, crawling
and walking different behaviors controlled by specific and
dedicated <u>a priori</u> neural codes, each with its own
maturational profile? The difficulty with this hypothesis
is the ease by which very simple physical manipulations
shift the infant from one behavior to another. An infant
of 5 months, for example, will not step at all when simply
supported upright. The same infant, however, will kick
frequently in both in-phase and out-of-phase
configurations when placed supine or prone, and will
perform well-coordinated and mature-looking alternating
steps as soon as the treadmill is turned on. Simply
submerging the infant in torso-deep warm water elicits
stepping movements, and some babies respond to walkers and
jumpers with appropriately organized movements (Thelen,
1988). It seems unlikely that special purpose generators
would be built into the CNS to await treadmills, tanks of
water, or mechanical devices such as walkers or jumping
harnesses.

It is more satisfactory to postulate that each of these rhythmical behaviors is assembled from the available neurological and anatomical components strictly in response to the context. Recent theorists have shown that under certain thermodynamic constraints, complex, open systems (most notably, biological systems) self-organize to produce ordered behavior, without prescriptions for those behaviors existing beforehand. Nonetheless, these systems will naturally prefer certain pattern configurations under specific circumstances (Schoner & Kelso, 1988). We suggest here that infant leg movements are such self-organizing phenomena: preferred, but not obligatory, coordinated and rhythmical patterns sensitive to the entire organismic and environmental influences on the baby. This means that movement outcome is determined not by the maturational status of the CNS alone, but also by more general variables. These may include, but not be limited to, infants' level of behavioral activation (the energy pumped into the system), their postural set and therefore their relation to the gravitational field, the biomechanical constraints of the body, and the nature of the task at hand (Thelen, Kelso, & Fogel, 1987).

If it is true that these rhythmicities are emergent rather than prescribed, then we must show that infants are indeed both sensitive to the general situational variables that change movement topography, and that they are responsive to these variables. This evidence is presented in the next section.

INFANTS ARE SENSITIVE TO THE DYNAMICS OF THEIR MOVING LIMBS

For movement topographies to be dynamically assembled, there must be a continual dialogue between the CNS and the changing conditions of the limbs and body segments- an "outside-in" as well as an "inside-out" flow of information. From several lines of experimental evidence, we believe that this proprioceptive sense is used in a functional manner very early in ontogeny. Please note that this "motor sense" need not in any way be conscious.

We consider first the coupling of the movements between the legs. Infants between 1 and 4 months of age often kick asymmetrically, that is, a single leg at a time. Because in any infant, this lateral preference for kicking was highly unstable, it seemed unlikely that this asymmetry reflected a fundamental CNS laterality. Rather, we suggested more peripheral influences such as subtle postural or tonus asymmetries or asymmetrical growth patterns affected the moment-to-moment choice of kicking leg (Thelen, Ridley-Johnson, & Fisher, 1983).

In fact, Thelen, Skala & Kelso (1987) experimentally shifted the laterality of spontaneous kicking in 6-week old infants by adding small weights to one leg. Weighting caused infants to decrease the kick rate in the weighted leg and <u>increase</u> the kick rate in the unweighted leg so that an overall rate was preserved. Likewise, movement amplitude and velocity were maintained in the weighted leg, but dramatically increased in the unweighted leg. Infants must have <u>sensed</u> the load perturbation and <u>responded</u> by increasing the activation levels to the two-leg <u>system as a whole</u>. This adjustment was then manifested as a higher amplitude and velocity of the unweighted leg. The kinematics of the unperturbed leg reflected the dynamic manipulations to the other limbs.

Infants' performance on a <u>split-belt</u> treadmill constituted a second demonstration of the responsiveness of a two-leg synergy to biodynamic manipulations. Thelen, Ulrich, & Niles (1987) supported 7-month old infants so that their feet rested on each of two parallel treadmill belts whose speed could be independently controlled. Infants maintained alternating stepping even when one belt was driven at twice the speed of the other belt. Like mesencephalic and spinal cats (Kulagin & Shik, 1970; Forssberg, Grillner, Halbertsma, & Rossignol, 1980) infants compensated for the speed discrepancy by precisely shortening the stance phase of the step on the slow belt and increasing the stance on the fast belt to maintain precise alternation at a step rate intermediate between the slow and fast belts. Recently, Thelen & Ulrich (1988) have found adjustments to the split-belt in infants as young as 5 months.

Infants must again have <u>detected</u> the dynamical course of the stretch of one leg and <u>adjusted</u> the temporal phasing of the second leg, even in this asymmetric condition. This cooperativity was entirely context-specific. Alternation is a strongly attractive (and functional) configuration for the two legs when the legs are pulled backward, either mechanically by the treadmill, or in natural locomotion when the weight is shifted forward on the stance leg. Nonetheless, the flexibility of the individual phases in the cycle make it unlikely that the rhythmicity is embedded in a predetermined code. The cycles could only have been initiated and terminated by information about the status of other moving leg.

Infants generate and use this information long in advance of voluntary control of these movements.

Finally, we present evidence from the dynamic control of forces within a single limb that infants "know" about their own movement status. When a limb is moved through space, its trajectory is determined by forces originating from several sources. First, torques are created by active muscle contraction and by the viscoelastic properties of the muscle. But because the body is a mechanically linked system, a limb segment is also affected by the inertial forces generated by the other moving segments coupled to it -- the intersegmental dynamics. (Imagine, if you will, a jointed marionette, and the effect of pulling on just one string.) Thirdly, all movements are affected by the pull of gravity, which helps or hinders a movement, depending on that movement's orientation in respect to the gravity vector.

In natural movements, people adjust their active muscle contractions to control the inevitable passive forces from the other segments and from gravity. This means that they must stabilize some joints from movement-related forces impinging upon them and counteract gravity when necessary. Recent observations have shown that people do more than just control these changing nonmuscular forces, however. They actually use them to their advantage. That is, by turning on and off the muscle contractions at precisely the right times in a movement trajectory, people can allow these passive forces to do some of the work. For example, it is well known that gravitational and inertial forces are significant determinants of the swing phase trajectory in upright locomotion. These dynamical interactions require continual adjustments between the ongoing movement and the neuromotor commands.

Using new techniques of inverse dynamics combined with mathematical models of body segment parameters, we are currently investigating how infants manage the forces underlying their natural movements. These techniques allow us to partition the torques acting at each joint into those generated by gravity, those resulting from the movement of other segments, and those produced by muscle components. The question is whether and when infants can detect the changing array of forces as they move and compensate for them with active muscle participation (see Schneider, Zernicke, Ulrich, Jensen, & Thelen, 1988).

Figure 2 reports such an analysis for two kicks in a single 2-month-old infant who was reclining (45 deg.) in an infant seat. Each kick is a single flexion and extension of the leg, with nearly simultaneous rotations of the hip, knee, and ankle joint. We characterized the kick in the left panel as a low-intensity kick; it was of relatively long duration and low velocity. In contrast, the kick on the right was stronger and more vigorous, of shorter duration and higher velocity. The plots show the partitioning of forces around the hip joint. What is noteworthy about these plots is that infants, even at 2 months, <u>detect</u> and <u>manage</u> passive forces by the precise use of active muscle contraction. In the low-intensity kick, the infant used active muscle contraction primarily to counteract gravity as the leg was slowly and smoothly lifted into the air. In contrast, in the rapid kick, there was a significant effect of the inertial forces from the leg and foot segments on the hip joint. Thus, in addition to contracting the muscles around the hip to counteract gravity, muscle action was precisely modulated to stabilize the hip against the forces generated by the other segments.

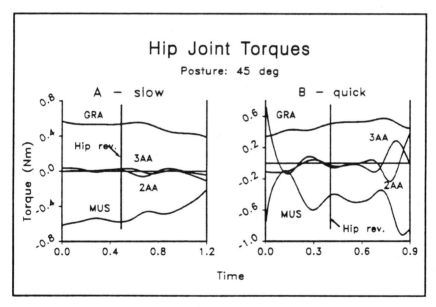

Figure 2 Selected hip joint torques during a slow (A) and quick (B) kick. MUS = generalized muscle torque, GRA = gravity torque, 3AA = torque due to thigh angular acceleration, 2AA = torque due to leg angular acceleration.

It is remarkable that even at two months, the neuromuscular system is continually monitoring the torques acting on the moving limb, and immediately using muscle contraction appropriately to balance those forces. In the slowly moving limb, the reactive forces from other segments were minimal, and the muscles assumed the primary task of counteracting gravity to keep the leg in the air. During a kick of greater vigor, the other segments generated considerable inertial moments on the hip, which were precisely counteracted by the muscle components.

INFANT MOVEMENTS HAVE MULTIMODAL CONSEQUENCES

In infant kicking and stepping, the neuromotor system must be monitoring the changes of forces generated by the limbs' movements. The proprioceptive mechanisms by which this is accomplished are not yet known (Hasan & Stuart, 1988). However, it is clear from the above results that as infants move their legs spontaneously as a result of generalized excitation, or to accomplish a task such as support or locomotion, proprioceptive and tactile information must be received and used by the CNS. In addition, certain leg actions result in visual, vestibular, and auditory feedback, and occasionally sensations of taste and smell as well!

Self-generated movements, therefore, provide continual information to infants on the status of their own bodies, and at the same time, on their interactions with the physical environment. That is, each preferred motor synergy in a particular postural or contextual set has immediate and simultaneous multimodal efferent consequences. In this sense, infants, with their movements, are exploring a universe of motor and sensory spaces.

MOVEMENT CATEGORIES BECOME STABLE AND EFFICIENT THROUGH DIALOGUE WITH THE PERIPHERY

We earlier stated that the complex and asynchronous course of the development of leg coordination could best be understood as the interaction of many developing subsystems assembled within a specific task context. How does it happen, then, that infants universally develop species-typical action patterns such as reaching, walking, jumping, feeding themselves, and so on, as well as culture-specific coordinations such as tool-use, dancing, and riding a bicycle?

Here we enter a more speculative realm. Specifically, we invoke the <u>neuronal group selection</u> theory of Edelman (1987). Very briefly, Edelman proposed that the anatomical structure of the CNS allows for both the afferent and efferent consequences of all actions to be captured in the form of local network maps. These maps are highly overlapping with each other, which allows the input-output array to be continuously and multiply correlated to produce more global mappings of the motor gesture and its sensory consequences. As the infant explores its motor universe, each variant of the movement combination is generated in presumably slightly different contextual conditions, which are associated with their sensory consequences. Current models show that this process of feature correlation can produce stable categories of action in response to repetition alone. Thus, action categories are self-organizing by this dynamic interplay of motor and sensory components and do not require an explicit schema existing beforehand. As Edelman put it, "Selection 'carves' out effective motions from the large set of postural and gestural components, ranging from the mechanical and muscular components of the motor ensemble to the complex neuronal adaptations that are the components of reentrant maps" (p.230).

By this scheme, therefore, stable, functional, and efficient topologies of movement are established in the CNS by continual motor activity and its sensory consequences. Because the contexts in which infants move change dramatically during the first year, development itself sets new challenges for the nervous system (Bernstein, 1967).

We suggest several major reorganizing contextual events for coordinative categories of leg movements. First is the transition from the fluid, confined environment of the uterus to a gravity-dominated world. The loss of perinatal coordinative patterns- hyperflexion, alternation, synchronous joint actions-- may result more from this confrontation with gravity and an expanded movement space than with intrinsically driven neural reorganization. Secondly, bearing the weight on the feet opens up yet another movement space with profoundly different proprioceptive consequences. Effective muscle synergies used for static balance may then be carved out of the infant's continual exploration of this space. A third challenge for the nervous system is dynamic balance while walking. As infants gain stability in static balance, they can begin to explore the coordinative spaces for shifting and bearing weight on one leg while swinging the other leg forward. Once the dynamic condition is established where the center of mass is over the stiff stance leg and the opposite leg is stretched back, the normal biomechanics of the system allow the leg to swing forward, as it did in the treadmill. Maturational refinements in gait, such as the heel strike during swing and the increasing use of reciprocally alternating muscle patterns emerge as "optimization" strategies as new walkers continually explore and select functional patterns of coordination.

CONCLUSION

Awake, behaving infants move their legs in coordinated and often rhythmical ways. The form and pattern of those movements are a function of the maturational status of the neural and skeletomuscular apparatus and the particular physical and task context of the infant. Neither developmental status nor situation alone determines coordinative outcome. This context-sensitivity demands that the neuromotor system continually monitor the periphery and adjust to it. We presented evidence that this ability was present very early in ontogeny. We further suggested that the dialogue with the periphery selected new patterns of coordination from a larger universe of movement possibilities, so that some patterns become preferred, but not obligatory. By this "outside-in" process, new forms can emerge in development without the system specifically anticipating them.

ACKNOWLEDGEMENT

Supported by National Institutes of Health Grant RO1 22830 and a Research Scientist Development Award to E. Thelen from the National Institutes of Mental Health.

REFERENCES

Bernstein, N. (1967). The Co-ordination and Regulation of Movement. Pergamon Press, New York.

Edelman, G. M. (1987). Neural Darwinism: The Theory of Neuronal Group Selection. Basic Books, New York.

Forssberg, H., Grillner, S., Halbertsma, J., & Rossignol, S. (1980). The locomotion of the low spinal cat: II. Interlimb coordination. Acta Physiol. Scand., 108, 283-295.

Hasan, Z., & Stuart, D. G. (1988). Animal solutions to problems of movement control: The role of proprioceptors. Ann. Rev. Neuroscience., 11, 199-223.

Kugler, P. N., & Turvey, M. T. (1987). Information, Natural Law and the Self-Assembly of Rhythmic Movement. Erlbaum, Hillsdale, N.J.

Kulagin, A. S., & Shik, M. L. (1970). Interaction of symmetrical limbs during controlled locomotion. Biofizika, 15, 164-170.

Schoner, G., & Kelso, J. A. S. (1988). Dynamic pattern generation in behavioral and neural systems. Science, 239, 1513-1520.

Schneider, K., Zernicke, R. F., Ulrich, B. D., Jensen, J. L., & Thelen, E. (1988). Control of lower limb intersegmental dynamics during spontaneous kicking in 2-month-old human infants. Submitted for publication.

Thelen, E. (1979). Rhythmical stereotypies in normal human infants. Anim. Behav., 27, 699-715.

Thelen, E. (in press). Evolving and dissolving synergies in the development of leg coordination. In Perspectives on the Coordination of Movement. (ed. S. A. Wallace). Elsevier, Amsterdam.

Thelen, E., Kelso, J. A. S., & Fogel, A. (1987). Self-organizing systems and infant motor development. Dev. Rev., 7, 39-65.

Thelen, E., Ridley-Johnson, R., & Fisher, D. M. (1983). Shifting patterns of bilateral coordination and lateral dominance in the leg movements of young infants. Dev. Psychobiol., 16, 29-45.

Thelen, E., Skala, K., & Kelso, J. A. S. (1987). The dynamic nature of early coordination: Evidence from bilateral leg movements in young infants. Dev. Psychol., 23, 179-186.

Thelen, E. & Ulrich, B. D. (1988). Hidden Precursors to Skill: The Development of Treadmill Stepping during the First Year. In preparation.

Thelen, E. Ulrich, B.D., & Niles, D. (1987). Bilateral coordination in human infants: Stepping on a split-belt treadmill. J. Exp. Psychol.; Hum. Percep. Perform., 13, 405-410.

Whiting, H. T. A. (Ed.)(1984). Human Motor Actions: Bernstein Reassessed. North Holland: Amsterdam.

Zelazo, P.R. (1983). The development of walking: New findings and old assumptions. J. Mot. Behav., 15, 99-137.

11
Infant Stepping and Development of Plantigrade Gait

Hans Forssberg

BIPEDAL PLANTIGRADE GAIT

Upright bipedal locomotion is only found in human beings, although other animals may walk on two legs occasionally. All other primates are basically quadrupedal judged from the structure of their musculo skeletal system and their locomotor pattern. The anatomy of pelvis and femur (Lovejoy, 1988) as well as preserved foot prints in volcanic ashes (White, 1980) indicate that hominids living about 3 millions years ago were the first to use bipedal gait.

The adaptation of the musculo skeletal system to the upright position has resulted in an unique gait pattern (see Forssberg, 1985) with several plantigrade determinants reducing the energy expenditure of bipedal walk (Table 1)(Saunders et al., 1953). A

1 .... Heel Strike
2 .... Knee Flexion Wave During Stance Phase
3 .... Desynchronized EMG Pattern
4 .... Desynchronized Joint Movements
5 .... Pelvic Rotation and Translation

Table 1. Plantigrade determinants

significant feature is the control of the foot-ankle movement producing a prominent heel strike due to a maintained active dorsiflexion of the ankle during the end of the swing phase. The heel strike induces an extending torque around the ankle, which plantar flexes the foot against a lengthening contraction of pretibial muscles. A forward thrust is produced by a forceful contraction of the calf muscles during the end of the stance phase. The knee flexes passively during hip flexion in the beginning of the swing phase and is passively extended when the forward movement of the leg is decelerated by hip extensors. At heel strike the knee is subjected to a flexing torque resisted by lengthening contractions

119

of the knee extensors. This results in a well controlled flexion of the knee during midstance when the body is passing over the leg. The effective leg length is shortened during midstance and lengthened at heel strike and lift off. This is due primarily to knee-ankle kinematics which results in reduced vertical oscillation of the body and energy expenditure.

The actions of knee and ankle result in a specific kinematic pattern in which they move out of phase during most of the step cycle. The diverging movements are controlled by specific temporal and spatial muscle contractions. The onset, duration and envelope of the EMG vary considerably between flexor and extensor muscles also at the same joint. This should be compared to the locomotor pattern of quadrupeds and non-human primates, in which hip, knee and ankle joints are moved in phase while flexor muscles are active during the swing phase and extensor muscle during the stance phase (Forssberg et al., 1980a, Vangor and Wells, 1983).

The patterns of muscle activity, reaction forces, torques and movements around the joints are the product of the neural activity of the central nervous system and the properties of the musculo-skeletal system (Bernstein, 1967). In humans, the mechanical system is different from other mammals, including non-human primates, and might cause some of these differences. The marked difference of the muscle activation pattern of the limb (hind) muscles and the reversed movements of some joints suggest, however, a considerable reorganization of central circuits generating the basic locomotor synergy during the phylogeny of human plantigrade gait.

INFANT STEPPING

A newborn infant can perform locomotor-like movements if held erect with the feet contacting a horizontal surface. Similar alternating leg movements are induced even in the fetus moving in utero (Precthl this volume). Infant stepping can be elicited during the first neonatal period. It deteriorates in most infants after two months, but remains in some, especially if they are trained daily (Zelazzo, 1983). Locomotor movements are then hard to elicit until 7 - 9 months of age when voluntary locomotion begins to develop. During this period of supported locomotion children need external support or take support with their arms to maintain equilibrium. Most children begin to walk without support at approximately one year of age.

The locomotor pattern of a newborn differs markedly from the plantigrade pattern of adults described above (Forssberg, 1985). The leg is relatively flexed during the whole step cycle. It is rotated forwards during the swing phase and the foot is kicked high above ground. This is followed by a backward rotation of the leg, as the forefoot is placed on the ground. The hip, knee and ankle joints move in phase during the larger part of the step cycle; however, the characteristic adult coordination of the knee and ankle is absent.

Flexor and extensor muscles have a uniform activity with a main burst during the stance phase in all muscles and peaks of activity at touch down and lift off. The activity of the ankle extensors, concomitant to the other extensor muscles prior to touch down, plantar flex the foot and contribute to the placing of the forefoot. The flexor muscles have almost the same activation pattern as the extensors with main bursts during the stance phase and weaker tonic activity during the swing phase. Antagonistic muscles are co-activated during a large part of the step cycle.

It is obvious that the locomotor pattern of supported infants clearly differs from the adult plantigrade gait, although the basic alternating movements are similar. Part of the difference could be due to different mechanical constraints. The infant is supported under it's arms, leaned forward and does not bear all the body weight on the legs. However, the uniform EMG pattern and the synchronized joint movements suggest that a simpler neuronal organization (fewer degree of freedoms) could be used for infant stepping compared to the complex pattern of adults.

DEVELOPMENT OF PLANTIGRADE GAIT

Basically the infantile pattern reoccurs when children begin to walk with support during the later part of the first year. The leg is hyperflexed and the joints are rotated in phase, although the ankle starts to move more independent with respect to the other joints. The foot is placed on the forepart, followed by a dorsiflexion of the foot. All muscles are uniformly activated and there are brisk reflex peaks of activity directly after foot strike with extensors and flexors co-activated. One important difference between infant stepping and supported locomotion is that the latter is voluntarily initiated and controlled by the will of the child, while the former is reflexive in nature. The infantile pattern is present also during the first period of independent walk. The pattern may regress during the first weeks with more co-activation of antagonistic muscles and stronger synchronization of muscle activity and joint movements (Okamato and Goto, 1985). A seemingly effortless quality of stepping develops rapidly after the establishment of an independent gait. The step length and duration of single-limb support increase almost linearly up to three years of age (Sutherland et al., 1980). The gait pattern is gradually transformed into the plantigrade pattern. Several plantigrade determinants develop before the child is two years old. At this age the degree of synchronized joint movements is decreased and the ankle is moved in an opposite direction to the knee and hip joints. The leg is no longer rotated backwards during the end of swing and the ankle joint is maintained in flexion resulting in a placement with the posterior part of the foot (Burnett and Johnson, 1971; Sutherland et al., 1980). The flexion directly after foot strike, present in infants, is at the same time reversed to a brisk plantar flexion. The jerky and short flexion of the knee directly after foot placement is slowly prolonged to a smooth flexion continuing over midstance (Fig. 2). The uniform EMG pattern is changed

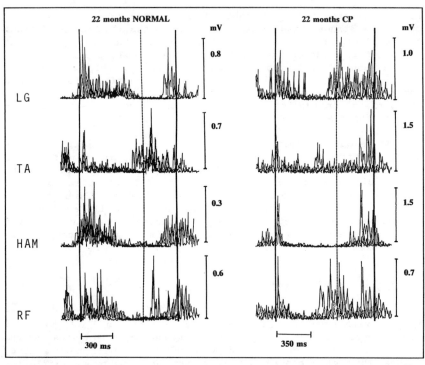

Fig. 1. Muscular activation pattern during independent walking on a treadmill in two 22 months old children, one of which has cerebral palsy. EMG was recorded by surface electrodes from the lateral gastrocnemius (LG), tibialis anterior (TA), hamstring (HAM) and rectus femoris (RF) muscles. The EMG recordings of several (n=5) step cycles are normalized and superimposed. Vertical lines indicate foot fall (continuous line) and lift off (hatched line). Note the tendency to form discrete bursts, biphasic in TA and RF, in the normal child. Bursts are formed also in the child with cerebral palsy but not in appropriate phases of the step cycle (modified from Leonard et al., 1988)

to discrete bursts at determined phases of the step cycle. The antagonistic co-activation is gradually decreased and the reflex spikes following foot placement disappear.

DEVELOPMENT OF LOCOMOTION AFTER PERINATAL BRAIN DAMAGE

During supported locomotion, children with cerebral palsy perform an infantile pattern similar to that of normal children. Depending on the severity of the cerebral damage the onset of independent gait varies but it is always delayed in relation to normal children. Clear differences between cerebral palsy and normal children begin to occur during the early period of independent locomotion. While the locomotor pattern of normal children develops in a determined way towards the plantigrade pattern, this is not seen in children with cerebral palsy (Leonard et al., 1988). Even after several years of independent locomotion no plantigrade features develop (Figs. 1, 2). There are changes in the pattern, but these changes are quite different and probably depend on the nature of the brain damage. Interestingly, they never develop a prominent heel strike and often maintain a digitigrade foot placement with a premature activation of the calf muscles during the swing phase (Fig. 1). Some children with cerebral palsy actually develope a pure digitigrade gait pattern walking on their toes during the whole stance phase. Muscle activity is often changed from the uniform pattern to one with more distinct bursts, but these are longer and not activated during the same phase of the step cycle as during normal gait (Fig. 1). The high degree of antagonistic co-activation is partly maintained as well as the short latency reflex bursts directly after touch down.

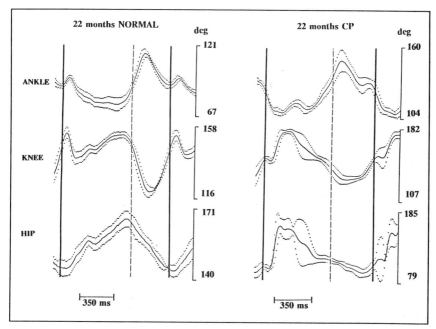

Fig. 2. Joint movements during independent locomotion in the sagittal plane from two children, one with cerebral palsy. Movements were recorded by a SELSPOT system for off-line computer analysis. The recordings of 5 step cycles are normalized and averaged with the mean and SD plotted. Vertical lines indicate foot fall (continuous line) and lift off (hatched line). Note the reciprocal ankle movements in both children and the ankle joint extension after foot fall and the knee flexion in the normal child (modified from Leonard et al., 1988)

DEVELOPMENT OF SEGMENTAL REFLEXES

Following a tap to the achilles tendon human infants have a short latency (20 ms) reflex response in the antagonist ankle flexor TA and in proximal synergistic muscles (e.g. HAM) in addition to the stimulated gastrocnemius and soleus muscles (Myklebust et al., 1986; Leonard et al., 1988). This wide distribution of reflex effects is present in children until four years of age, when the amplitude of the reflex in antagonistic and proximal muscles are reduced. There is a large variation of reflex distribution between children and recent experiments have shown antagonist activation also in some adults without neural impairment. The reflexes are evoked by dynamic muscle spindles and group Ia afferents from the calf muscle since taps with the reflex hammer adjacent to the tendon, activating a similar cutaneous stimulation and vibration of the leg, do not evoke any reflex responses. There obviously must be a neuronal correlate to the wide distribution of the reflex during the neonatal period and its subsequent reduction during normal development, i.e. direct or indirect projection of group Ia afferents to several antagonistic and synergistic motoneurone pools. Two different mechanisms may be involved in the abolition of the reflex effects: i) retraction of exuberant Ia afferent projections or ii) inhibition of the transmission in remaining afferent pathways by supraspinal or spinal centers.

All tested children with cerebral palsy (n=11) had a strong antagonist reflex activation of the anterior tibialis muscle after a tap to the achilles tendon, regardless of age and type of damage (Leonard et al., 1988). Some of the children also retained the reflex response in proximal synergists (hamstring). There is considerable evidence of exuberant neuronal projections during the neonatal period and its retraction during ontogeny. Neonatal sensorimotor cortex damage in the cat prevent the normally occurring exuberant projections from retracting (Leonard and Goldberger, 1987). There is some evidence that exuberant Ia projections are present at birth and that they fail to retract during development, secondary to damage to the central nervous system (Thor, 1982). The retraction of exuberant projections may reflect the competitive interactions known to exist between supraspinal and spinal projections (Goldberger, 1986). The maintenance of the wide distribution of short latency reflexes in children with cerebral palsy may thus be the result of sparing of exuberant group Ia projections which remain in the absence of competitive descending nerve fibers. Another explanation for the remaining infantile reflex pattern would be that the transmission in the reflex pathways normally are inhibited by descending supraspinal system which are damaged in children with cerebral palsy.

NEURAL CONTROL OF LOCOMOTOR DEVELOPMENT

Higher brain centers are not needed to generate the basic synergy of locomotion in several vertebrates such as lamprey (Grillner et al., 1986), chicken (Bekoff, this volume) and cat (Forssberg et al., 1980a). The spinal cord contains neuronal circuits that have the potential for generating alternating locomotor movements in the limbs in the absence of descending and peripheral influence (Grillner, 1981). These circuits, known as central pattern generators, are controlled and influenced by supraspinal centers and peripheral signals, which can modify the pattern. These mechanisms have been studied in walking spinal and mesencephalic cats. The speed of the treadmill belt modulates the intensity of the locomotor activity in a spinal cat by peripheral feed back mechanisms e.g. from hip and calf muscle (Grillner and Rossignol, 1978; Pearson and Duysens, 1976). The cycle duration, the intensity and duration of the muscle activity as well as the interlimb coordination, i.e. walk, trot and gallop, are modified. The peripheral influence is actually strong enough to drive the two hindlimbs of a spinal cat at different speed, when it is walking on a split treadmill with different speeds on the two belts (Forssberg et al., 1980b). When lifted in the air a spinal cat will perform air stepping (Sherrington, 1910), probably produced by the central pattern generator for locomotion, but with another relation between flexion and extension phases due to the changed mechanical constraints (Miller et al., 1975). Similarly, the locomotor pattern in mesencephalic cats with brainstem stimulation change when they are swimming in water, due to the changed mechanical condition (Miller et al., 1975).

The spinal locomotor mechanisms, i.e. the central pattern generator and the peripheral reflex interaction, are normally controlled by several descending supraspinal systems. They can conceptually be divided into i) locomotor driving systems and ii) adaptive systems. The driving systems originate from the brainstem and are controlled from basal ganglia and cerebral cortex (Garcia Rill 1986). They can initiate and control the speed of the basic locomotor activity. Corticospinal systems can modify the steps e.g. according to visual information (Armstrong, 1988; Drew, 1988). Rubrospinal, vestibulospinal and reticulospinal systems are the descending part in a spino-cerebellar-spinal loop, which also is used for adaptation of the locomotor synergy, e.g. for postural compensations (Arshavsky and Orlovsky, 1986).

Earlier I suggested that human locomotion is controlled in a similar hierarchical organization as in other vertebrates (Forssberg, 1982, 1985, 1986). The early fetal stepping movements (see Prechtl this volume) and the infant stepping probably express the autonomous activity of the spinal locomotor generator, programmed for a basic alternating rhythm with a synchronized and uniform EMG pattern. This is supported by the fact that anencephalic infants perform stepping movements and that fetal stepping has been observed in a fetus with a lethal cervical cord lesion (Prechtl pers. comm.). It is obvious that there is a dramatic modification of the locomotor pattern during the subsequent development but what kind of mechanisms are responsible for this change?

In the previous paper Thelen (this volume) argues that the same neural circuits are used both during infant stepping movements and during adult plantigrade gait. In her perspective the disappearance of the stepping movements after the first weeks of life is not due to changes of the neural control but rather reflect disparity in muscle strength. The change of the locomotor pattern should again not be due to a remodelling of the neural control circuits but reflect changes in muscular and inertial characteristics of the limb segments. The unique plantigrade pattern of adult human gait should simply be the result of the structure of the human body segments to which the output from the central nervous system should adapt during ontogeny in each human being.

It is beyond doubt that there is a powerful influence from peripheral afferents that can modify the locomotor output from the central pattern generator (see above). But could solely such peripheral mechanisms be responsible for the dramatic change of muscle activity and movements?

The chicken has a similar development with synchronized muscle activity and joint movements during hatching to a more specialized pattern during post hatched walking (Bekoff this volume). The change occurs within a few hours after completed hatching. Bekoff suggests that the same neuronal circuits are responsible for both hatching and walking. Interestingly the hatching leg motor output can be re-elicited from a post hatching chick by bending its neck (Bekoff and Kauer, 1984). When neck bending is released walking reappears. The pattern from neck afferents can thus switch between two different motor patterns, presumably generated from shared spinal circuits. Neck bending provides a peripheral stimulus but it is unrelated to the phasic afferent activity from the limbs. Hence, there are central mechanisms that can change a primitive locomotor pattern into a complex and specific one.

Since the infantile gait pattern is also used during supported locomotion and the first period of independent gait, I have earlier suggested (Forssberg, 1982, 1985, 1986) the same original circuits are used also during these stages of the development. The subsequent gradual transformation of the pattern should then reflect a change of the locomotor generating circuits including peripheral and supraspinal influence; a change from a synchronous uniform output to a specific temporal and spatial pattern. In humans there is a gradual transformation during several years. It is likely that central influences, acting with similar mechanisms as neck bending in the chicken, also contribute to the modification and specialization of the motor output. The lack of plantigrade transformation of the gait pattern in children with cerebral palsy supports a central origin of the transformation. Known damages of higher brain centers in some of these children, including lesions of the corticospinal tract, would imply that these brain structures are directly or indirectly involved in the transformation process. It has been shown that these damages in the same subjects also causes disturbances in segmental reflexes as well as reciprocal inhibition during voluntary movements (Leonard et al., 1988). These effects have obviously neuronal correlates, supraspinal as well as secondary spinal changes. It is therefore likely that structural changes within central nervous system also are causing the transformation to plantigrade gait and that damages to these structures impair the normal development.

ACKNOWLEDGMENTS: These studies have been suppoted by the Swedish Research Council (4X-5925), First Mayflower Annual Campaign for Childrens Health, Stiftelsen Allmänna BB:s Minnes fond and Norrback-Eugenia Stiftelsen. The fruitful comments of Virgil Stokes is gratefully acknowledged.

REFERENCES

Armstrong, D.M. (1988) The supraspinal control of mammalian locomotion, J Physiol, 405, 1-37.

Arshavsky Y.I. and Orlovsky G.N. (1986) Role of the cerebellum in the control of rhythmic movements. In S. Grillner, G.S. Stein, D. Stuart, H. Forssberg, R.M. Herman. Neurobiology of Vertebrate Locomotion. Wenner-Gren International Symposium Series, Stockholm, 677-689.

Bekoff, A. and Kauer, J.A. (1984) Neural control of hatching: fate of the pattern generator for the movements of hatching in the post-hatching chicks. J Neurisci, 4, 2659-2666.

Bernstein, N.A. (1967) The Coordination and Regulation of Movements. Pergamon Press, Oxford.

Burnett, C.N. and Johnson, E.W. (1971) Development of gait in childhood: Part II. Dev Med Child Neurol, 13, 207-215.

Drew, T. (1988) Motor cortical cell discharge during voluntary gait modification, Brain Res, 457, 181-187.

Forssberg H. (1982), Spinal locomotor functions and descending control. In B. Sjölund, A. Björklund Brain Stem Control of Spinal Mechanisms. Elsevier Biomedical Press, Amsterdam, 253-271.

Forssberg, H. (1985) Ontogeny of human locomotor control I. Infant stepping, supported locomotion and transition to independent locomotion., Exp Brain Res, 57, 480-493.

Forssberg, H. (1986) A developmental model of human locomotion. In S. Grillner, P. Stein, D. Stuart, H. Forssberg, R. Herman. Neurobiology of Vertebrate Locomotion. Macmillan Press, Hong Kong, 485-501.

Forssberg, H., Grillner, S., Halbertsma, J. (1980a) The locomotion of the spinal cat. 1. Coordination within a hindlimb, Acta Physiol Scand, 108, 269-281.

Forssberg, H., Grillner, S., Halbertsma, J., Rossignol, S. (1980b) The locomotion of the spinal cat. 2. Interlimb coordination. Acta Physiol Scand, 108, 283-295.

Garcia-Rill, E. (1986) The basal ganglia and the locomotor regions Brain Res Revs, 11, 47-63.

Goldberger M.E. (1986), Autonomous spinal motor function and the infant lesion effect. In M.E. Goldberger, A. Gorio and M. Murray M. Development and Plasticity of the Mammalian Spinal Cord. Springer Verlag, New York, 363-378.

Grillner, S. and Rossignol, S. (1978) On the initiation of the swing phase of locomotion in chronic spinal cats. Brain Res, 146, 269-277.

Grillner, S. (1981). Control of locomotion in bipeds, tetrapods, and fish. In V.B. Brooks Handbook of Physiology - The Nervous System II, Motor Control. American Physiological Society, Bethesda, 1179-1236.

Grillner, S., Brodin, L., Sigvardt, K., Dale, N. (1986) On the spinal network generating locomotion in lamprey: transmitters, membrane properties and circuitry. In S. Grillner, P. Stein, D. Stuart, H. Forssberg, R. Herman. Neurobiology of Vertebrate Locomotion. Macmillan Press, Hong Kong, 335-352.

Leonard, C.T. and Goldberger, M.E. (1987) Consequences of damage to the sensorimotor cortex in neonatal and adult cats. II. Maintenance of exuberant projections, Dev Brain Res, 32, 15- 30.

Leonard, C.T., Hirschfeld, H., Forssberg, H. (1988) Gait acquisition and reflex abnormalities in normal children and children with cerebral palsy. In B. Amblard Development, Adaptation and Modulation of Posture and Gait. Elsevier Press, Amsterdam, 33-45.

Lovejoy, C.O. (1988) Evolution of human walking, Sci American, Nov, 82-89.

Miller, S., Van Der Burg, J., Van Der Meche, F. (1975) Coordination of the hindlimbs and forelimbs in different forms of locomotion in normal and decerebrate cats. Brain Res 91, 217-237.

Myklebust, M.B., Gottlieb, L.G., Agarwal, C.G. (1986) Stretch reflexes of the normal infant, Dev Med Child Neurol, 28, 440-449.

Okamoto T. and Goto Y. (1985) Human infant pre-independent and independent walking. In S. Kondo. Primate Morphology, Locomotor Analyses and Human Bipedalism. Univ. Tokyo Press, Tokyo, 25-45.

Pearson K.G. and Duysens I. (1976) Function of segmental reflexes in the control of stepping in coakroaches and cats. In R.M. Herman, S. Grillner, P. Stein, D. Stuart. Neural Control of Locomotion. Plenum, New York, 519-538.

Saunders, M., Inman, V., Eberhart, H. (1953) The major determinants in normal and pathological gait. J Bone Jt Surg, 35A, 543-558.

Sherrington, C.S.(1910) Flexion-reflex of the limb, crossed extension reflex and reflex stepping and standing. J Physiol, 40, 28-121.

Sutherland, D.H., Olshen, R., Cooper, L., Woo, S.Y. (1980) The development of mature gait, J Bone Jt Surg, 62-A, 336-353.

Thor, S. (1982) Exuberant dorsal root projections at birth in cat. Neurosci Abs, 8, 305.

White, T.D. (1980) Evolutionary implications of pliocene hominid footprints. Science, 208, 175- 176.

Vangor, A.K. and Wells, J.P. (1983) Muscle recruitment and the evolution of bipedality: evidence from telemetered electromyography of spider, woolly and patas monkeys. Ann Sci Nat Z, 5, 125-135.

Zelazo, P.R. (1983) The development of walking: New findings and old assumptions, J Motor Behav, 15, 99-137.

12

The Organization of Arm and Hand Movements in the Neonate

Claes von Hofsten

INTRODUCTION

Observing an alert neonate in a supine or semireclining position
reveals a large variety of arm and hand movements. It is clear
that these movements are differently organized and differently
controlled than in the mature adult. However, in what respects
are they different? Is it that neonatal arm and hand movements are
purely involuntary reflexes elicited by tactile, proprioceptive,
or vestibular stimuli as the traditional view conveys? The view of
the present paper is that the involuntary character of neonatal
manual movements has been grossly overestimated in the past. At
least some movements produced by neonates are better described as
goal directed actions.

In adults, vision plays a most important role in controlling the
movements of the arm and hand. It is puzzling that the basis for
this sensorimotor system has been supposed to be non-existent in
the neonate (Piaget, 1953). I intend to show that vision is indeed
connected to the manual system in the neonate. The third and final
aim of the present paper is to try to describe in what ways the
immature neuromotor system will constrain and delimit the movement
repertoir of the neonate.

HAND MOVEMENTS

In terms of the neural organization of hand movements, the
immaturity of the pyramidal tract is one of the most striking
differences between adults and neonates (Yakovlev and Lecours,
1967). Behavioral data indicates that this system which is
responsible for the control of the pincer grasp and other
relatively independent finger movements mature during the second
half of the first year of life in humans. There are excellent
anatomical and behavioral studies performed on the rhesus monkey
by Kuypers and his group (Kuypers, 1962; Lawrence & Hopkins, 1976)

that demonstrate how crucial the corticomotoneuronal connections are for fractionated finger movement control. The rhesus monkey is a reasonable model because it has an opposing thumb and is able to perform relatively independent finger movements. The newborn rhesus monkey has almost no corticomotoneuronal connections. These form postnatally and reach an adult level around 8 months of age (Kuypers, 1962). Lawrence and Hopkins (1976) showed that bilateral pyramidalotomy performed on 1-4 week old rhesus monkeys had little immediate effects but prevented the development of fractionated finger control in these animals.

The relative absence of corticomotoneuronal connections in the neonate only implies absence of precise spatial control of fractionated finger movements as needed for manual actions. Grasping in neonates when it occurs is a gross movement of the whole hand as observed in the grasp reflex. However, already Halverson (1937) observed that the index finger often failed to participated in this response.

Closer inspection of spontaneous finger movements in newborns actually reveal a large variety of them. Hofsten and Rönnqvist (1988) videorecorded the finger movements of 10 newborns during two 5 minute periods, one where the mother was present in front of the infant and one where an object was presented in front of the infant. Altogether 2530 movements were scored from the videorecordings. Slightly less than half of these or 49% were opening or closing of the whole hand. The next most numerous kind of movement only involved the thumb and the index finger (22%). Almost all of these movements were thumb-indexfinger oppositions. Finally there were a number of less frequent types of movement like flexion of the two central digits of the hand, an increased flexion or increased extension from Digit 2 to Digit 5, and extension of just the index finger like in pointing.

Many of these movements will play important roles in later appearing manual skills. The thumb-indexfinger opposition is a good example. Around nine month of age the infants will start using the pincer grasp in picking up small artifacts. However, in the neonate these movements do not seem to have a manual function. The existence of fractionated finger movements appears to constitute a manual vocabulary organized at a low level which the corticomotoneuronal connections can exploit and combine into skillful movements.

The fact that fractionated finger movements do not combine into skillful manual movements in the neonate does not mean that they lack function altogether. The two conditions studied showed systematic differences in hand movement patterns. The most clear difference was frequency of movements. When the mother was present, the subjects performed more than twice as many movements as when presented with an object. Quality of movements was also

much different. There were,for instance, more opened hands and
thumb-indexfinger oppositions in the Object condition and more
continuous opening-closing or closing-opening hand movements in
the Mother condition. Thus, there is a possibility that the two
main functions of the hand, as a manual device and as a gesturing
device, are to a certain extent differentiated in the neonate
(Trevarthen, 1979) and that its social function is more advanced
than its manual function at that age.

SYNERGIES

Arm-hand synergy.

In the neonate, the movements of the arm are coupled to the
movements of the hand in a synergistic way. This is clearly seen
in the traction response which can be elicited by pulling the
infant's arm by the wrist. The response is flexion of all the
segments of the arm and the digits of the hand. According to
Twitchell (1965), all neonate grasping are of this kind. He
states that "finger flexion cannot be elicited reflexly as an
isolated response, but occurs as a part of a synergy of the upper
extremity with simultaneous flexion of the wrist, elbow and
shoulder"(p. 250). According to Twitchell (1965) the grasp
response cannot be elicited by pure tactile stimulation.
According to him, contact stimulus alone will only elicit an
avoidance response. Also Halverson (1937) points out how
ineffective tactile stimulation is in eliciting a grasp response
and how the hand rather had a tendency to withdraw from the
tactile stimulus. Pressure on the palm seems to be required that
will stretch the tendons in the hand and induce a traction
response.

In the Moro response, two kinds of synergistic movement patterns
occur depending on how the response is elicited (Prechtl, 1965).
Elicited in the classical way by a small head drop, the segments
of the arm and the digits of the hand extend together. However as
Prechtl (1965) observed, if the infant is held by the wrist or the
hand and a mild traction is exerted as the head drop stimulation
is given, a dramatic change takes place. The arm and the hand
will not extend together anymore but flex. This is illustrated in
Figure 1. Prechtl observed that the traction of the arm is
necessary. Stimulation of the palms alone is not effective.

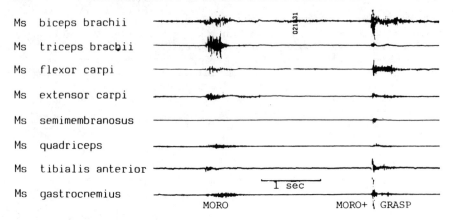

Figure 1. EMG from arm and leg muscles of an infant making "Moro" movements. At "Moro" on the left side of the recording, a head drop was carried out with the infant's arms free. At "Moro + Grasp", a head drop was applied when the infant grasped the examiner's fingers and mild traction was applied in upward direction. The recording shows the shift in activity from extensor muscles (left) to flexor muscles (right). Age 6 days. From Prechtl (1965).

The coupling between arm and hand movements are also clearly reflected in the spontaneous movements of the neonate. In studying visually directed behavior in neonates, Hofsten (1984) monitored the movements and posture of the hand in extended arm movements of 18 neonates aged 4-8 days. In these studies as in the other studies of neonatal arm and hand movements that I have performed, the infant was placed in a semireclining infant seat which allowed free movements of the arms while supporting the head and trunk. The inclination of the chair was 50 deg. The movements of arms and hands were monitored by two video cameras placed 90 deg to each other. The recording arrangement is shown in Figure 2. In the experiment, an object of about 4 cm in diameter (a tuft made of bright red, blue, and yellow yarn was either moved slowly in front of the infant or remained stationary at a nearest distance of 12 cm.

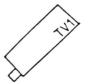

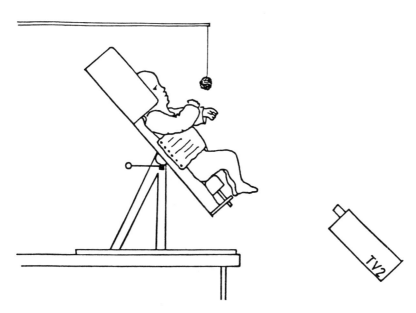

Figure 2. The experimental situation used to study neonatal arm movements by Hofsten (1982, 1984, 1985).

Every arm movement extending forward more than 7.5 cm from the body of the infant was scored from the videotape, except those originating from startles or Moro reflexes, or those associated with yawning, sneezing, or sudden forward head movements. Altogether 225 forward extended movements were monitored. Each movement was scored with respect to the looking behavior of the infant and the posture and movement of the hand. The following four categories of hand behavior was used: **fisted (F)**, all the fingers were fully flexed before and during the movement; **half-open (HO)**, the fingers were semiflexed before and during the movement; **open-before (OB)**, the fingers were extended before the movement started; **open during (OD)**, two or more digits extended during the forward extension of the arm.

The result is shown in Table 1. Table 1 shows that the hand was most often opened in the extended phase. The fingers were fully flexed in less than 10% of the movements. Some extension of the fingers during the forward extension of the arm was observed in more than a third of the cases whereas flexion of the fingers was never observed during arm extension.

Table 1: Percentages of different kinds of hand behavior during arm extension. Separate figures are presented for those movements where the subject fixated the object and for those where the object was not fixated.

Looking behavior	Hand behavior			
	OD	OB	HO	F
Fixation of object	38	31	23	8
Non-fixation	33	31	27	9

It can be seen from Table 1 that hand behavior during arm extension is rather unaffected by the looking behavior of the infant. Thus, hand behavior during reaching movements at this age does not appear to be visually regulated. It seems more appropriate to conceive of it as a part of an extension synergy. This synergy, however, is not rigidly organized. Rather, it expresses itself as a behavioral bias.

Synergy between the arms.

The movements of the two arms are synergisticly coupled too. They adduct and abduct together and are raised and lowered together. An example of this characteristic behavior is shown in Figure 3.

Synergy between head and arm.

The coupling between head and arm movements in early infancy is well known and traditionally observed through its expression in the asymmetric tonic neck reflex. However, this response is not easily elicited in the neonate. In the spontaneous behavior of the neonate, the asymmetric neck posture is more often expressed but not at all in a rigid way (Casaer, 1979). It can easily be broken up as the subject put his or her hand into the mouth.

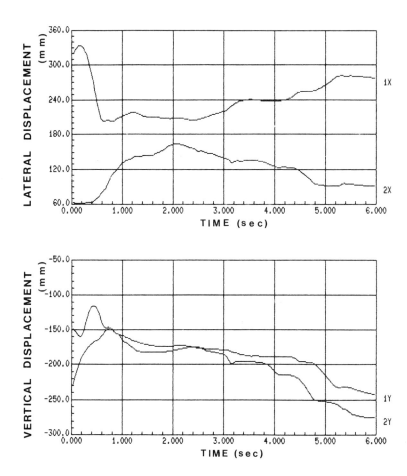

Figure 3. Tracings of a movement involving both upper limbs of a 5-day-old boy. The upper graph shows the displacements of the hands in the lateral dimension and the lower graph shows the displacements of the hands in the vertical dimension.

COORDINATED ACTION

Visual control.

In spite of what has been traditionally believed, vision exerts quite a clear influence on the arm movements of the infant. This influence was studied by myself in a series of experiments using the setup shown in Figure 2.

In one experiment the object was present and absent on alternative minutes. Altogether, the object was present during 4 minutes and absent during 4 minutes. When present, it moved slowly and irregularly in front of the infant. Fourteen neonates were tested. They were between 5 and 9 days old. Any movement exceeding 5 cm, whether adduction, abduction, upward, downward, or forward movement was scored from the video recordings. Those movements extending more than 7.5 cm forward were separately noted. It was found that the number of movements decreased when the object was present but not the number of forward extended movements. In fact, when looking behavior was taken into account, it was found that the proportion extended movements performed when the target was fixated was twice as high as when the object wasn't fixated. This result fits well with the definition of the orienting response as defined by Sokolov (1963). An important part of the orienting response consists of a decrease in general activity and an increase in focused activity.

The result reported above shows that looking behavior and arm hand activity of the neonate are closely related. However it does not tell us whether the forward extended movements performed while an infant watches the object in front of him or her are in any sense directed toward it. To be able to answer this question it was necessary to get a description of how the reaching hand moved in space over time. This was accomplished by transcribing the movements from video to a computer. Second, to calculate the aim of forward extensions, it was critically important to find and isolate units of movement. The unit chosen was based on an analysis of the acceleration profiles. Each unit consisted of one acceleration phase and one deceleration phase (Brooks, 1974). Finally, an estimation was made of how the forward movement was aimed relative to the object. The aiming was estimated from the unit that carried the hand closest to the trajectory of the object. This part of the movement should be directed at the object if there is visual directedness but not otherwise. The aiming was expressed as a space angle between the position of the object at the start of the movement unit, the position of the hand at the same time, and the position of the hand at the end of the unit.

Two studies were carried out (Hofsten, 1982, 1985). In the first study (Hofsten, 1982), 16 infants participated. A maximum of 40 forward extended movements were identified and analyzed for each infant. Altogether 232 movements fulfilled these requirements. Although the object was within reach most of the time, reaching rarely resulted in physical encounter with the object. It was touched 22 times, 12 times when it was fixated and 11 when it was not fixated. The analysis showed that when the object was fixated, the movements were, on the average, aimed 32.1 deg from the target while the figures for the movements performed while the infant did not fixate the object and for those where the infant had his or her eyes closed was 51.9 and 54.3 deg respectively. Thus the movements performed while fixating the object were aimed significantly closer to it.

As the object changed position only laterally and as the head moved with the object as it was fixated, the result could have been a function of these lateral adjustments only. In other words, we could be dealing with a head-arm synergy instead of visually directed movements. To be able to rule out this possibility, the vertical components of the movements were further examined. In the vertical plane, the aiming of the movements while fixating was 25.3 deg, on the average, while corresponding figures for the movements performed while looking elsewhere or closing the eyes were 37.2 deg and 40.2 deg respectively. Also in this case, the movements performed while fixating the target was aimed closer to it.

This result was replicated in a study with 11 neonates between 4 and 8 days of age (Hofsten, 1985). In this study the average aiming for the movements performed while fixating the target was found to be 34.1 deg while the corresponding figure for movements performed while not fixating the target was 60.0 deg. To determine the tendency to reach in the direction of the head, an imaginary object straight in front of the head was defined for each non-fixating movement and the aiming for this point calculated. This figure was found to be 55.0 deg, on the average, which was not significantly smaller than the aiming calculated on true object positions.

These results support the contention that the sensorimotor system of the upper limbs is coordinated with vision in the neonate. There is a clear effect of vision on direction of forward movements. The obtained differences in approach angles between different types of looking behavior were not the result of any tendency to reach out in the direction of the head. The results show that the visuomotor space within which neonate reaching movements are guided has a well-defined directional structure. This is the same kind of structuring as in visuo-oculomotor space. The neonate has an ability to direct both his or her eyes and hands toward a visually detected external event. The system seems to work not only from the eye to the hand but also from the hand to the eye. Several cases were observed in which the infant accidently touched the object and immediately afterward turned his or her eyes toward it.

The results do not show clearly to what degree reaching space is structured with reference to distance in depth as that aspect was

not manipulated in these studies. However, studies by Granrud
(1988) suggest that at least some aspects of perceptual space is
structured in depth. He showed that neonates take into
consideration the distance to the object when perceiving its
size.

Proprioceptive control.

There are arguments that newborn arm movements may be controlled
by proprioception only, i.e. the position of the arm as well as
the target being specified proprioceptively. The evidence comes
from the ability of the neonate to place the hand in the mouth.
This coordination has been known for a long time but received
little study until recently. The close relation between the hand
and the mouth is reflected in the peculiar "Babkin reflex"; when
the neonate s palm is pressed the mouth opens. Another evidence
for the close relationship between hand and mouth are the group of
cells found by Rizzolatti (1988) in the rostral part of agranular
frontal cortex (inferior area 6) of the Macaca Nemestrina that
respond to movements either of the hand or the mouth region.
Butterworth (1986) found that about 15 % of the spontaneous arm
movements of the neonate result in the hand being placed in the
mouth. Butterworth (1986) and Rochat et   al. (1987) found that
these movements did not just happen to end up in the mouth but
that they were directed there. Butterworth reported that the
mouth was significantly more likely to be open before and
throughout the arm movement when the hand ended up in the mouth
than when the hand did not end up in the mouth. Butterworth also
found that even though the hand did not always go directly to the
mouth but sometimes contacted other parts of the face first, it
still had a distinct goal directed character. He found no
evidence of rooting after contact, the head was held still and the
hand moved "immediately in the direction of the mouth" (p. 28).

The nature of neonatal reaching.

The adult manual system exploits both vision and proprioception
for its control. The research reviewed above suggest that
both these modes of control are, in principle, also functioning in
the neonate.

In most manual skills, vision and proprioception both contribute
to the efficiency of the action. When initiating a reach, for
instance, the predominant strategy is to define the position of
the object visually and the position and movement of the reaching
arm proprioceptively. This mode of control seems to be the one
used by neonates too. As the arm is not placed in a stereotyped
position before the initiation of the movement, both the position
of the target and the position of the arm needs to be defined for
the production of an aimed movement. The infant fixates the target
which means that the starting position of the arm needs to be
defined by some other means, i.e. proprioceptively. This suggests

that visual space and proprioceptive space are connected and compatible at this age.

Whereas the movement of the arm in mature reaching is defined in proprioceptive space during the early phase of the approach, it will be defined in visual space during its later phase. As the hand enters into the visual field toward the end of the approach, the position and movement of it will be defined visually relative to the target. This enables the subject to perform delicate and precise adjustments of the hand as the object is about to be captured. The described two phases of the approach really seems to be two different modes of control deeply engraved into the sensorimotor system. Jeannerod (1981) has shown that the deceleration of the reaching movement toward the end of the approach is marked by a discontinuity where tangential velocity tends to become constant or even increase. The possibility that the discontinuity was simply an effect of visual correction for undershooting was found to be less likely because reaccelerations also occurred in the absence of visual feedback from the reaching hand (Jeannerod & Biguer, 1982). At the same time as the reacceleration occurred, the hand was found to have its peak aperture (Jeannerod, 1981). In other words, preparation for grasping the object is an integrated aspect of the visually guided secondary part of the approach.

The neonate does not seem to master the secondary mode of reaching in which both the position of target and of the hand may be visually defined. In the studies by me on neonatal reaching the hand was not observed to come progressively closer to the target with successive accelerative phases of the movements after the hand had entered the visual field. In the extended phase of the arm the subjects were never observed to flex the hand to grasp the target, not even when the hand ended up with the object on its palm. This part of the reaching action matures between the third and fourth month of life (Hofsten, 1984).

SOURCES OF INCOORDINATION

The various sensorimotor coordinations described above are seldom distinct and clear. Although vision has a substantial effect on directing neonates forward extended movements relative to a seen target, the precision is poor. On the average, they were off the target by 32 deg. One obvious reason for incoordination in the neonate is that the different perception-action systems need to be calibrated and stabilized in their new environment which impose very different biomechanical constraints on the system than the womb. The question of calibration is especially crucial for visually linked perception-action systems which for obvious reasons have not been functioning before birth.

A specific coordination may require a certain amount of postural control which the neonate doesn't have and will therefore only be

possible to demonstrate if the neonate is supported in certain
ways. Again, neonate walking is a good example of that. To be
able to walk freely the infant need to master the balancing of
upright posture and integrate that with the production of walking
movements. Neonates will not do that but when supported under the
arms they will produce walking movements. Another example of the
same phenomenon has been given by Fentress (1984). When supporting
neonatal mice in an upright position, already from day one, rich
but poorly coordinated grooming-like movements was seen.   In line
with this, Grenier (1980,1981) has suggested that the inability of
the infant to control the neck muscles and stabilize the head is
hampering the neonate's ability to control the movements of the
arm. Grenier held the neonate's neck in position for a certain
time and found much more coordinated reaching than otherwise.

Needless to say, the most important reason for a sensorimotor
system not to function appropriately at birth is that the neuro-
structures involved are not mature enough. An appropriately
coordinated reach and grasp requires the arm to extend and the
hand to flex around the object. The neonate will not do that.
Instead, the arm and hand will extend and flex in a synergy
(Hofsten, 1982). It is not until the third month of life that
infants' reaching and grasping movements get differentiated
(Hofsten, 1984) and it is not until nine months of age that
infants start to be able to control relatively independent finger
movements.

ACKNOWLEDGEMENT

This paper was prepared while the author was a fellow at the
Center for Advanced Study in the Behavioral Sciences at Stanford.
The reported research was made possible by grants to the author
from the Swedish council for Research in the Humanities and Social
Sciences, and from National Science Foundation # BNS 87-00864.

REFERENCES

Brooks, V.B.(1974) Some examples of programmed limb movements.
Brain Research, 71, 299-308.

Butterworth, G.(1986) Some problems in explaining the origins of
movement control. In M.G. Wade and H.T.A. Whiting (Eds.) Motor
Development in Children: Problems of Coordination and Control.
Dordrecht:Martinus Nijhoff.

Casaer, P.(1979) Postural Behavior in Newborn Infants.
London:Spastics society and William Heinemann.

Fentress, J.C.(1984) The development of coordination. _Journal of Motor Behavior_, _16_, 99-134.

Granrud, C. (1988) Size constancy in newborns. ICIS, Washington, April 1988

Grenier,A.(1980) Revelation d'une expression motorice differente par fixation manuelle de la nuque. In A. Grenier and C. Amiel-Tison (Eds.) _Evaluation Neurologique du Nouveau-Ne et du Nourrison_. Paris: Masson

Grenier, A. (1981) "Motoricite liberee" par fixation manuelle de la nuque au cours des premieres semanes de la vie. _Archives Francaises de Pediatrie_, _38_, 557-561.

Halverson, H.M. (1937) Studies of the grasping responses of early infancy: III. _Journal of Genetic Psychology_, _51_, 425-449.

Hofsten, C. von (1982) Eye-hand coordination in the newborn. _Developmental Psychology_, _18_, 450-461.

Hofsten, C. von (1984) Developmental changes in the organization of prereaching movements. _Developmental Psychology_, _20_, 378-388.

Hofsten, C. von (1985) Visual guidance of arm movements in the prereaching infant: A longitudinal study. Unpublished manuscript.

Hofsten, C. von and Rönnqvist, L. (1988) Finger movements in the neonate. Manuscript in preparation.

Jeannerod, M. (1981) Intersegmental coordination during reaching at natural visual objects. In J. Long & A. Baddeley (Eds.) _Attention and Performance IX_, Hillsdale:Erlbaum. pp. 153-168.

Jeannerod, M. and Biguer, B. (1982) Visuomotor mechanisms in reaching within extrapersonal space. In D.J. Ingle, M.A. Goodale and R.J.W. Mansfield (Eds.) _Analysis of visual Behavior_. Cambridge:Mit press

Kuypers,H.G.J.M. (1962) Corticospinal connections: Postnatal development in the rhesus monkey. _Science_, _138_, 678-680.

Lawrence, D.G. and Hopkins, D.A. (1976) The development of motor control in the rhesus monkey: Evidence concerning the role of corticomotoneuronal connections. _Brain_, _99_, 235-254.

Piaget, J. (1953) _The origins of intelligence in the child_. New York: Routledge.

Prechtl, H.F.R. (1965) Problems of behavioral studies in the newborn infant. In _Advances in the Study of Behavior, Volume 1_. New York: Academic Press

Rizzolatti, (1988) Premotor control of arm and hand movements. In M. Goodale (Ed.) Vision and Action: The control of grasping. Norwood, NJ: Ablex.

Rochat, P. Blass, E.M. and Hoffmeyer, L.B. (1987) Oropharyngeal control of hand-mouth coordination in newborn infants. Manuscript.

Sokolov, Ye.N. (1963) Perception and the conditional reflex. London:Pergamon Press

Trevarthen, C. (1979) Instincts for human understanding and for cultural cooperation: their development in infancy. In M. von Cranach, K. Foppa, W. Lepenies and D. Ploog (Eds.) Human Ethology. Cambridge:Cambridge university press

Twitchell, T.E. (1965) The automatic grasping responses of infants. Neuropsychologia, 3, 247-258.

Yakoley,A. and Lecours, A.R. (1967) Myelogenetic cycles of regional maturation of the brain. In Minkowski, A. (Ed.) Regional development of the brain in early Life. Philadelphia:Davis,F.A., pp.3-70.

13

Looking: The Development of a Fundamental Skill

David N. Lee, Brigid M. Daniel and Deborah J. Kerr

Precise visual control of limb and whole body movements requires the ability to stabilize gaze on moving objects of interest and on salient aspects of the environment when the body is moving. In humans this is normally accomplished by coordinated movements of the eyes and head. To measure the development of eye–head coordination, subjects looked at a target moving in an arc in front of them or looked at a stationary target when their chair was oscillated gently from side to side. Longitudinal experiments with infants from 11 to 29 weeks of age indicated that, during this period, prospective control of movement of the head relative to the target develops to near adult level. Eye control, however, does not develop to adult level. Further studies measured eye–head coordination in cerebral–palsied children with congenital hemiplegia, in normal children and in adults. The eye and head control of the cerebral palsied children was found to correspond to an earlier developmental level. The results indicate that for infants with known or suspected brain damage, the early assessment of looking skill could provide basic information about movement dysfunction for use in treatment.

Gearing action to the environment and to objects and events is a prime need of any organism. In general, it requires coordinating limb, head and trunk movements into an appropriate action system (Reed, 1982).

The gearing together of body movements to form an action system and the gearing of the action system to the environment both require prospective control and depend on information. The former requires *propriospecific* information about the position, orientation and movement of the body parts relative to each other: the latter requires *expropriospecific* information about the position, orientation and movement of the body parts relative to the environment. Vision is by far the most powerful source of *expropriospecific* information. It also appears to play an important role in *proprioception.* While

143

the mechanoreceptors in the joints, muscles and skin are most important in proprioception, since they are a *constant* source of information, experiments indicate that they are subject to drift and need to be tuned by vision, which provides very accurate propriospecific information, when needed (Lee, 1978).

The foundation of vision is the optic flow field, the changing pattern of light incident at a moving point of observation (Lee, 1980). The task of the visual system is to optimise the pickup of information from the optic flow field. This is far from being a passive process. It requires precise control of the direction of gaze through coordinated eye, head and body movements, as well as control of accomodation of the lens and convergence of the eyes. Thus seeing is a complex perceptuo-motor skill in its own right, on which many other perceptuo-motor skills depend.

A basic prerequisite for perceptuo-motor development is, therefore, *gearing vision to the environment and to moving objects (including parts of the body)* in order to optimise the pickup of information for controlling actions .

Research on how gaze is stabilized on moving objects and on the environment during body movement has generally been limited by a failure to examine the role of active head movements. Instead, the head has usually been artificially constrained in order to study "reflexes" such as the vestibular-ocular reflex (see, e.g., Barnes, 1980; Eviatar et. al., 1979), though the relation of such assumed reflex action to normal stabilization of gaze is far from clear (Biguer and Prablanc, 1981; Owen and Lee, 1986). Those few studies with infants that have not restricted head movements have shown a variety of patterns of coordination in which the head plays an active role (Tronick and Clanton, 1971; Goodkin, 1980; Regal et. al., 1983).

In a recent study of the development of gaze stabilization in infants with freely mobile heads and eyes, we found that head movement, in fact, plays a *precisely controlled* role (Daniel & Lee, 1988). We here summarize those developmental results and compare them with new data on cerebral palsied children (Lee et al, 1988). The data were collected in an attempt to uncover basic perceptuo-motor dysfunctions in cerebral palsy, the assessment and treatment of which (e.g. Brown et. al., 1987; Palmer et. al., 1988) need to be founded on principles of development of movement, since cerebral palsy is a developmental disorder.

METHOD

The subject sat on a chair mounted on a horizontal turntable which could be rotated to and fro. The turntable and subject's head were centred within a framework which supported a vertical adjustable strut that could be moved in an arc around the chair. On the strut, at the subject's eye level and at a distance of 44 cm, was mounted a target onto which the subject was encouraged to stabilize gaze, either with the chair moving and the target stationary or the reverse. The motions of the target and chair (which were moved by hand) were monitored together with the subject's head and eye movements (eog) on a Selspot system (detail in Daniel & Lee, 1988). The data were sampled during a period of 3 ms, at a rate of 62.5 Hz and recorded on a computer. Each session was also videotaped.

Four groups of subjects were run in separate experiments:
1. Six normal healthy infants, three girls and three boys, tested between the ages of about 11 and 29 weeks.
2. Five normal children, 3yr 2mth to 4yr 6mth of age.
3. Five cerebral palsied children with congential hemiplegia (2 left, 3 right), 2yr 2mth to 7yr 8mth of age.
4. Six normal adults, 24yrs to 40yrs old.

The infants sat on their mother's lap on the chair and were presented with a small toy, about 6cm across, as target. The toy was stuck with Velcro onto the shaft of a small electric motor pointing toward the child. This meant that toys could be rapidly changed and briefly spun in order to maintain the infant's attention. For the young children, who sat alone on the chair, the target was a miniature (2cm x 1.5cm) video screen showing a favourite cartoon film. The adults simply had a 1cm diameter fixation spot to look at.

Infants were tested every three weeks between the ages of about 11 and 29 weeks giving a total of six sessions per baby. A session comprised five blocks of four 15 sec trials. In each block there were four conditions presented in random order: either the target or the chair was moved approximately sinusoidally, at about 0.2 Hz, +50° either side of the subject's medial plane, or the movement was irregular within the same ±50° range and with the same peak velocity of about 125 deg.s^{-1}.

The procedure for the adults was similar except that they were each tested in only one 20-trial session. They were simply asked to keep looking at the fixation spot. The procedure for the children was somewhat different. Only regular sinusoidal movements (0.2 Hz, ±50°) of the target and chair were used since the regular and irregular movements used with the infants and adults had yielded similar results. Depending on how attentive the child was, he or she was given between two and five 45 sec trials in each condition until a sufficient quantity of valid data had been collected.

PERFORMANCE MEASURES

Analyses were based on the following two basic measures computed from the Selspot records.

Target/Chair Angle: the direction of the target with respect to the chair; the angle is zero with the target straight in front of the chair and positive when it is to the right.

Head/Chair Angle: the direction of facing of the head with respect to the chair; the angle is zero when facing straight ahead and positive when facing right.

To obtain valid measures of performance, sections of the records were omitted where, as judged from the video records, the attention of the infant or child subjects was not on the target. The following performance measures were then computed on each data section.

Head/Target Movement Ratio: the ratio of the standard deviations of the head/chair angle and the target/chair angle time series. This measures how much the head moves compared with how much it would need to move to keep facing the target.

Head/Target Correlation: the cross-correlation between the head/chair angle and the target/chair angle time series. This measures how precisely the head movement is geared to the relative movement between the target and chair. (Note that the gearing ratio – estimated by the head/target movement ratio – need not be 1:1.)

Gearing the head to the target requires visual prospective control. More detailed measures of that control were derived by considering how the gearing might be accomplished. Assuming a visuo-motor delay between registering and putting into action the visual control information, then the information must predict the position and motion of the target relative to the chair at this delay time ahead and the head must be controlled on the basis of this information. There are thus two components to the prospective control, which were measured by:

Head/Target Peak Correlation: the maximum cross-correlation obtained by time shifting the head/chair angle and target/chair angle time series. This measures how precisely the head movement is geared to the relative movement between target and chair, independently of synchronising with it.

Head/Target Lag: the time-shift yielding the maximum head/target correlation. This measures the error in intrinsic information on visuo- motor delay. Positive lag means the delay has been underestimated.

Finally, accuracy of eye control was measured by

Gaze Velocity Error: the root mean square difference between the time series of the calibrated eog velocity and the eye angular velocity necessary to stabilize the image of the target on the retina (eog was calibrated on the basis of sections of the experimental record which . showed good eye tracking).

RESULTS

Fig. 1 shows typical records from the different subject groups and Fig. 2 shows the means and standard deviations of subjects' average scores on the performance measures. Individual scores were averaged across experimental conditions, since there was little difference between conditions and the pattern of results in each condition matched the average shown in Fig. 2. For the infants, only the values at 11wks and 29wks of age are plotted, since intermediate ages gave intermediate values (Daniel and Lee, 1988). The results may be summarised as follows:

Head Control

Between 11 and 29 weeks of age, the infants turned their heads increasingly more in stabilizing gaze (Fig. 2a) and, concurrently, improved to near adult level in prospectively gearing the head movement to the target or chair movement (Fig. 2 b,c and d). Most of the increase in degree and precision of head movement in fact took place before about 16 weeks (Daniel and Lee, 1988), which, interestingly, is the age when visually guided reaching and catching normally starts developing (von Hofsten, 1980; 1986). The video records, in fact, frequently showed the infants at 16 weeks and older actively orienting towards the target as if to possess it.

The cerebral palsied and the normal children showed comparatively poor head control (Fig. 2 b,c,d). It seems unlikely that the normal children's poor showing was due to inability, since there seems no reason why ability should decline after infancy. A more likely explanation is that their evident shyness in the experiment tended to constrain their movements; they, in fact, moved their heads less than any of the subjects (Fig. 2a). The cerebral palsied children, on the other hand, were not particularly shy and moved their heads significantly more than the normal children. It is possible, therefore, that their ability to control their heads was at about the level of the 11 week olds, as Figs. 1 and 2 would indicate.

Eye Control

The infants' eye control did not improve with age, and was significantly poorer than the adults' (Fig. 2e). The normal children's performance was similar to the infants'. As with head control, shyness may have caused the children's low performance by constraining their movements. Alternatively this could be interpreted as no developmental change from infancy up to 4 yrs or more.

The cerebral palsied children showed very poor eye control compared with all other subjects, even the 11 week old infants (Fig. 2e). This disorder could

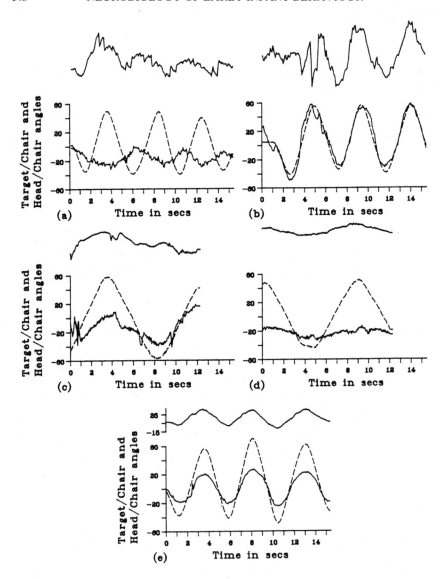

Fig. 1 Typical gaze stabilization records when chair was turning through ±50°
(a) 11 week old infant, (b) same infant, 29 wks old, (c) hemiparetic child aged
5yrs 9 mths, (d) child aged 3yrs 11mths, (e) adult, aged 23yrs. Upper record in
(a) – (d) is uncalibrated eog; in (e) it is calibrated eog. Broken line =
target/chair angle.

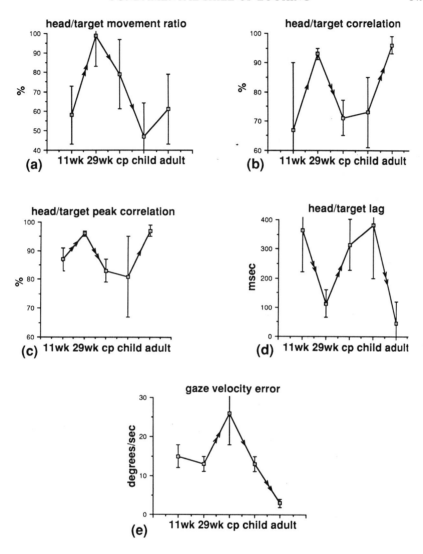

Fig. 2 Means and standard deviations of gaze stabilization performance measures for the different subject groups: 11wk and 29wk – six normal infants tested at these ages; cp – five cerebral palsied children with hemiparesis aged 2yr 2mth to 7yr 8mth; child – five normal children aged 3yr 2mth to 4yr 6mth; adult – six normal adults aged 24 to 40yrs. Single and double arrows on the graph lines indicate significant differences on t– test at p<0.05 and p<0.01 respectively.

have a common origin with their apparent disorder of head control. On the other hand, it could well be that their poor eye control (which presumably was similar in infancy) handicapped the development of head control in stabilizing gaze, since that requires good visual information.

CONCLUSION

Looking is not simply done with the eyes but "with the eyes in the head on the shoulders of a body that gets about" (Gibson, 1979). It is a fundamental skill that is necessary for obtaining control information for most other skills. Therefore, it makes sense that looking skill should develop early, as we have found, in preparation for other visually guided activities. Moreover, the prospective control and coordination required in turning the eyes, head and body to visually apprehend a moving object is formally similar to that required to articulate the limbs in catching, securing footing, and so on. Thus, in developing control of looking, the infant is not only learning how to acquire visual information, but is also developing general control processes that will be needed later in other skills. Early assessment of looking skill in young infants with known or suspected brain damage could, therefore, provide basic information about movement dysfunction for use in treatment.

Acknowledgements. We thank Audrey van der Meer, Jane Turnbull, David Young and the departmental technical staff for help with the apparatus and experiments; Keith Brown and Robert Minns for helpful discussions and providing the patients; and the parents, infants and children for their good-natured participation. The work was supported by grants to the first author from the Medical Research Council and the European Office of Aerospace Research and Development, and by a postgraduate studentship to the second author from the Science and Engineering Research Council.

REFERENCES

Barnes, G.R. (1980). Vestibular control of oculomotor and postural mechanisms. Clin. Phys. Physiol. Meas., 1, 3–40.

Biguer, B. & Prablanc, C. (1981). Modulation of the vestibulo-ocular reflex in eye-head coordination as a function of target distance in man. In Progress in Oculomotor Research. (eds. A.F. Fuchs & W. Becker). North Holland, Amsterdam.

Brown, J.K., van Rensburg, F., Lakie, M. & Wright, G.W. (1987). A neurological study of hand function of hemiplegic children. Dev. Med. Ch. Neurol., 29, 287–304.

Daniel, B. & Lee, D.N. (1988). Development of looking with head and eyes. Submitted for publication.

Eviatar, L., Miranda, S., Eviatar, A., Freeman, K. & Borkowski, M. (1979). Development of nystagmus in response to vestibular stimulation in infants. Ann. Neurol., 5, 508–514.

Gibson, J.J. (1979). The Ecological Approach to Visual Perception. Houghton Mifflin, Boston.

Goodkin, F. (1980). The development of mature patterns of head–eye coordination in the human infant. Early Hum. Dev., 4, 373– 386.

Hofsten, C. von (1980). Predictive reaching for moving objects by human infants. J. Exp. Ch. Psych., 30, 369–382.

Hofsten, C. von (1986). The emergence of manual skills. In Motor Development in Children: Aspects of Coordination and Control. (eds. M.G. Wade & H.T.A. Whiting). Martinus Nijhoff, Dordrecht.

Lee, D.N. (1978). The functions of vision. In Modes of Perceiving and Processing Information. (eds. H.L. Pick & E. Saltzman). Erlbaum, Hillsdale, NJ.

Lee, D.N. (1980). The optic flow–field: the foundation of vision. Phil. Trans. R. Soc. London B, 290, 169–179.

Lee, D.N. Daniel, B.M., Turnbull, J.D. & Cook, M.L. (1988). Basic perceptuo–motor dysfunctions in cerebral palsy. In Attention & Performance X111: Motor Representation & Control. (ed. M. Jeannerod). Erlbaum, Hillsdale, NJ.

Owen, B.M. & Lee, D.N. (1986). Establishing a frame of reference for action. In Motor Development in Children: Aspects of Coordination and Control. (eds. M.G.Wade & H.T.A. Whiting). Martinus Nijhoff, Dordrecht.

Palmer, F.B., Shapiro, B.K., Wachtel, R.C., Allen, M.C., Hiller, J.E., Harryman, S.E., Mosher, B.S., Meinhert, C.L. & Capute, A.J. (1988). The effects of physical therapy on cerebral palsy. The New Eng. J. of Med., 318(13), 803–808.

Paneth, N., Kiely, J.L.,Stein, Z. & Susser, M.(1981).Cerebral Palsy and newborn care. Dev. Med. Ch. Neurol., 23, 801–807.

Reed, E.S. (1982). An outline of a theory of action systems. J. Mot. Behav., 14(2), 98–134.

Regal, D.M., Ashmead, D.M. & Salapatek, P. (1983). The coordination of eye and head movements during early infancy: a selective review. Behav. Brain. Res., 10, 125–132.

Tronick, E. & Clanton, C. (1971). Infant looking patterns. Vis. Res., 11, 1479–1486.

IV. Sensory Systems

14

Development of Cortically Mediated Visual Processes in Human Infants

Richard Held

Early infancy is clearly a period of extremely active growth of all organ systems including the brain. The development of the visual system entails growth of the eyeball, the retina, the optic nerve, various nuclei of the brain stem, the midbrain, the thalamus, and the cerebral cortex. These organs constitute the optical and neuronal substrates for the development of vision in infants. For the purposes of this conference, strongly concerned as it is with the central nervous system, it seems appropriate to concentrate on a few selected aspects of the development of vision of infants in which the role of the cerebral cortex can be inferred. These aspects relate to several of the topics addressed by other speakers including the anatomical development of parts of the cerebral portion of the visual nervous system, principles of central neuronal development including plasticity, and the modulation of such development by neurohumoral factors.

Investigators of the visual system generally prefer to view information flow in the system as bottom-up although there is much evidence of flow in the opposite direction. According to the preferred view the flow consists of a series of stepwise transformations beginning with the light energy entering the eye transduced into neuronal signals at the retina and proceeding upstream by synaptic transmission in the various nuclei as far as it can be traced. The great advances in our knowledge of the visual system during the last few decades have shown us that certain forms of processing of this information occur only at particular levels in the stream of processing. Accordingly, selected functions can be attributed to processing in the cerebral cortex. With a few caveats, vision scientists generally agree that processing of information combined from the two eyes begins in earnest only in the cerebral cortex where anatomical connections imply, and physiological responses show, that information from the two eyes has converged. Such convergence is necessary for the processing of the combined inputs that characterizes mature binocular vision.

Similar arguments can be advanced concerning sensitivity to the
orientation of edges. Sharply tuned frequency selective cells
with clear orientation selectivity are not found below the level of
the cortex. Hyperacute spatial discriminations, such as vernier
acuity, are also thought to be processed at the cortical level
because of the very high positional resolution demanded (see
discussion in Zak and Berkley (1986) and below). Consequently,
these are some of the processes which are currently of interest
from the point of view of cortical processing. We shall consider
two of them: binocularity and hyperacuity.

Binocularity

Studies of the development of stereopsis in infants have shown
remarkable agreement across methods and experiments (see recent
review by Timney, 1988). Stereopsis has not been demonstrated in
the very young infant (less than 2 months of age). Coarse
stereopsis has an abrupt onset in most infants between two and five

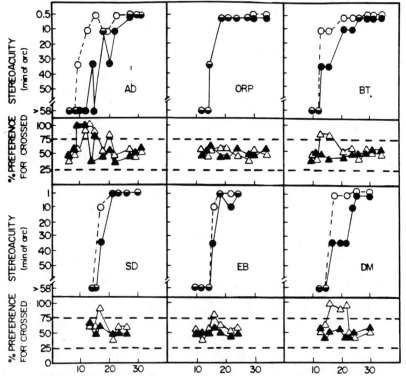

Figure 1: Development of uncrossed (●) and crossed (○) stereoacuity. Data obtained from direct crossed-uncrossed stimulus
pairings are also shown: 34 min crossed versus 34 min uncrossed
(▲); 10 min crossed versus 10 min uncrossed (△). From Birch, et
al, 1982.

months of age with a mean of three and a half months (see Figure 1).

It has been suggested that the delay from birth to the onset of stereopsis results from a lack of precise control of verging movements of the eyes. Good alignment of the two eyes is of course required for providing the precise and consistent dispari- ties among retinal images, as a function of the distances of objects, which are required for stereopsis. That surmise is negated by the finding that stereopsis has the same age of onset and threshold values even when stimuli are used that are relatively insensitive to the accuracy of convergence (Birch, Gwiazda, Held, 1983). Consequently, we may infer that the onset of stereopsis is the consequence of a neuronal development which facilitates the processing of disparities and their consequences for the control of eye movements (Held, 1988).

Following the onset of coarse stereopsis (30 or more minutes of disparity), stereoacuity rises rapidly so that within a few weeks after onset, sensitivity to disparity appears to reach at least one minute of arc (Held et al, 1980; Birch et al, 1982). These authors have also shown that discrimination of crossed disparities appears significantly earlier than that of uncrossed disparities (see Figure 1). In other words, targets nearer than the point of convergence of the two lines of sight at the fixation point are discriminated at an earlier age and their acuity thresholds remain lower than those of more remote targets during the period of development. In addition, it has been shown that male infants lag behind females in these developments by several weeks during these early months (Gwiazda et al, 1988).

The abrupt onset of stereopsis calls for some sort of explanation in terms of underlying neuronal development. So do the results showing rapid development of stereoacuity, the lag in discriminating uncrossed disparity, and the significantly later onset age of stereopsis in male compared to female infants. Based upon inferences from animal experiments, we have previously argued that the early lack of segregation of the ocular dominance columns in layer 4 of striate cortex could preclude stereopsis (Held, 1985). Segregation would be a necessary but not sufficient condition for stereopsis. In human infants it could also produce non-selective combination of the central representations of the images in the two eyes of human infants, an implication which was confirmed (Shimojo et al, 1986). These ideas were based upon the work of Levay and others who have studied the actual process of segregation by anatomical and physiological means. Rakic has studied the beginning of segregation of the ocular dominance columns in the pre-natal monkey (1976). Levay et al (1980) have described the process of post-natal segregation of the columns which is not complete until an age of at least six weeks. In the absence of segregation, the thalamocortical afferent fibers from

the two eyes overlap in layer 4 and often synapse on the same
cells in striate cortex of monkey (Levay, et al 1980). Thus
signals from the two eyes become mixed and further processing of
differences in the interests of extracting disparity information is
precluded. In the cat behavioral measures show that the onset of
stereopsis occurs between three and six weeks of age (Timney,
1981). Segregation of the columns is occurring during this period
(Levay et al, 1978) and disparity selective cells are appearing in
striate cortex of the cat (Pettigrew, 1974). According to
information available, segregation of the dominance columns occurs
in human infants between two and six months of age (Hickey &
Peduzzi, 1987). This timing is in concordance with the acquisition
of mature binocularity discussed above (Held et al, 1980; Birch et
al, 1982; Shimojo et al, 1986).

Recently, Levay and Voight (in press) have shown a clear
relation between ocular dominance and disparity in the visual
cortex of the cat. This result confirms the hypothetical
contention that the ocular dominance columns carry information
which is selective for the extraction of disparity. Recording from
single cells in striate cortex they showed that among cells with
receptive fields near the vertical meridian, those preferring far
disparities (uncrossed) tended to be dominated by the contralateral
eye while those preferring near disparties (crossed) were dominated
by the ipsilateral eye. This result makes sense if we consider the
optics of binocular vision and the projections of the retinas to
the cortex. For targets beyond the fixation point but near the
midline, images fall on nasal retinas and hence project centrally
to the contralateral cortices. Consequently, a responding cell in
one cortex receives direct input from the contralateral retina but
input from the ipsilateral retina only via indirect callosal
connections. Similarly, for targets closer than the fixation point
images fall on temporal retinas and project centrally to the
ipsilateral cortex. The direct connection is from the ipsilateral
retina which dominates responsive cells. In general, the direct
connections appear to dominate the response of most cells.

Most procedures, including our own, for measuring stereopsis
in infants test stimuli presented close to the midline.
Consequently, the results are subject to the considerations
advanced by Levay and Voight. Although there is no evidence that
segregation of information from ipsilateral cortex can occur before
that from contralateral cortex, if it were the case, we should
have a potential explanation for the earlier onset of crossed
stereopsis in human infants. This conclusion follows from the
discussion of the results of Levay and Voight. Preservation of the
address of an ipsilateral, but not contralateral, eye origin of
signals in layer 4 would imply the existence of regions containing
only afferents from the ipsilateral eye. This could conceivably
occur if thalamocortical afferents from the contralateral eye
segregated out to form strips while those from the ipsilateral eye

remained either uniformly distributed through layer 4 or at least less segregated then the contralateral afferents. The consequence would be strips in layer 4 in which the ipsilateral afferents were relatively isolated. This result could be the outcome of competition between thalamic afferents if the ipsilateral fibers were initially more successful than the contralateral fibers in maintaining their distribution throughout layer 4. In other words, the initial outcome of the competition would have to be asymmetric. In fact, Levay et al (1980) found just the reverse in the monkey. They report that segregation was evident in ipsilateral cortex earlier than contralateral cortex. However, they argued that this developmental difference was only an artifact resulting from greater spread of label in the projection system to the contralateral cortex yielding less clear and later delineation of the columns. Consequently, this idea remains a rather far-fetched attempt to explain the earlier onset of crossed disparity detection in infants.

Stereopsis is not the only binocular visual function which requires selective processing of inputs from the two eyes. At about the same age as the onset of stereopsis, infants show a selective response to rivaling as opposed to fusible binocular stimuli (Birch, Shimojo & Held 1983). The transition to discrimination of binocularly rivaling stimuli presumably requires central circuitry whereby information originating from each eye may inhibit that from the other eye. Just as in stereopsis, a necessary, but not sufficient condition for such a process is the existence of channels carrying information from the separate eyes. Prior to segregation of the ocular dominance columns the mutually inhibitory process cannot exist. In its absence what happens to the central projections of the two eyes ?   Our experiments suggest that the central representations are non-selectively combined (Shimojo, 1986). Moreover, these experiments have demonstrated a very precise age marker for the transition to mature binocularity. Using it we have again shown earlier development of binocularity in females by approximately four weeks (Bauer et al, 1986).

Hyperacuity

When the detectable distance in a visual task is significantly less than the minimal detectable separation of two points or lines (visual resolution), the performance is called hyperacute (Westheimer, 1979). Distances may be discriminated that are as small as a few seconds of visual angle and as much as an order of magnitude smaller than the minimum resolvable separation of edges. Detection of these very small distances is said to be based upon precise localization of features of the stimulus. While the information necessary for this sort of discrimination must be present at lower levels in the system, its processing is said to require cortex (see discussion in Zak and Berkley, 1986). However, the neuronal mechanism responsible for hyperacute performance remains controversial.

Recently, the development of two forms of hyperacuity, namely vernier acuity (Shimojo et al, 1984; Manny and Klein , 1984) and stereoacuity (Held et al, 1980; Birch et al, 1982) have been studied in human infants.   Shimojo and Held (1987) found that vernier acuity did not become hyperacute until an average age of approximately four months.   In fact it appears that before three months of age vernier acuity is generally less than grating acuity and hence is hypoacute.   Measures of stereoacuity showed a comparable age of onset of signficant hyperacuity.   When both vernier and stereo acuity measures are scaled with respect to grating acuity measures, both show the same rates of development of hyperacuity (see Figure 2).   This result suggests a common mechanism of cortical development for the achievement of very precise localization.   Recently, Stanley et al (in press) adapted the procedure of Shimojo et al (1984) to test a group of intra-uterine growth retarded infants averaging 40 weeks of age. They showed a significantly lower vernier acuity than a comparable group of normal infants, although grating acuities did not differ. Moreover, vernier acuity was significantly correlated with the

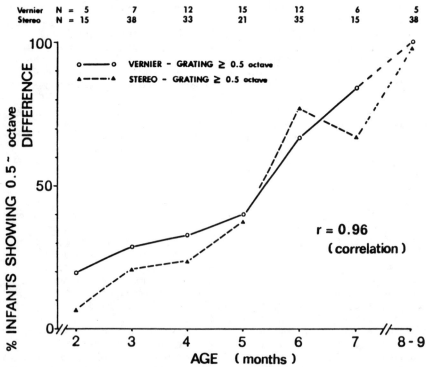

Figure 2: Vernier superiority and stereopsis superiority.   From Shimojo, et al, 1984.

inverse of head circumference. As the authors conclude, these results confirm a cortical locus for processing this form of hyperacuity.

Sex Difference and the Testosterone Hypothesis

We first discovered in measurements of vernier acuity a significant sex difference (Held et al, 1984). Females between four and six months of age were significantly superior to males. No such difference appears when data on the development of grating acuity during this period are analyzed. But as previously mentioned, both measures of the onset of binocularity show the sex difference.

Visual resolution (grating acuity and contrast sensitivity) is largely determined by properties of the retina (Banks et al, 1988; Wilson, 1988). Much of its increase during infancy can be ascribed to changes in the retina in sampling density of receptors and receptor sensitivity. We find no sex difference in resolution. On the other hand, so far in all measurements of visual function in which cortex is implicated, the sex difference has been found. The implication is, of course, that cortex is subject to some influence which varies with sex while retina is not. Sexual dimorphism is generally established during periods of intense synaptogenesis. Moreover, hormones frequently modulate the development of the dimorphism. Thus, the neurotrophic effects of testosterone are key to the masculinization of the brain pre-natally and in some cases post-natally. Recognizing these facts, we have suggested that it is the post-natal surge of testosterone in male infants in conjunction with the intense rate of synaptogenesis during the early weeks of life (Huttenlocher et al, 1982) that is responsible for their delayed onset of cortical-visual function (Held et al, 1984). The segregation of the ocular dominance columns, implicated in development of mature binocularity, is an example of the pruning of overproliferated synaptic connections so common in early neuronal development. We suggest, as one alternative among others, that testosterone may slow the rate of pruning of synapses in the process of segregation.

In an effort to confirm the alleged role of testosterone, using means at our disposal, we have performed the following experiment. Both testosterone levels in the blood and the ages of onset of binocularity vary considerably among male infants. Consequently, if testosterone has the hypothesized effect, the two measures should be correlated. Accordingly, we have simultaneously measured plasma testosterone levels and tested for binocularity at bi-weekly intervals through the early weeks in a population of male infants. The results to date are encouraging but not definitive. We have established significant correlations between testosterone levels and age of onset of binocularity during the very early weeks of life (5 through 8)(Held et al, 1988).

After these early weeks the correlation drops to insignificance, suggesting that the neurotrophic effects of testosterone are exerted many weeks before the achievement of mature binocular processing.

Conclusion

We have tried to bridge some gaps between our knowledge of the development of cortically-mediated vision in infants and the development, mostly inferred from animal studies, of parts of the visual nervous system. Many other aspects of vision such as edge orientation sensitivity and meridional variations in acuity, velocity, and phase sensitivities involve cortical mediation. In time they also will be correlated with underlying neurobiological developments. Vision science is ripe for this sort of unification and we may expect exciting developments.

Acknowledgment

The preparation of this manuscript and research reported from the author's laboratory have been supported by grants from the National Institutes of Health (No. 2RO1-EY-1191, No. SP30-EY02621, and BRSG 2SO7RR0747-18) and the Educational Foundation of America.

REFERENCES

Banks, M., Bennett, P. and Schefrin, B. (1988). Inefficient cones limit infants' spatial and chromatic vision. Invest. Ophthalmol. Visual Sci. Suppl., 29, 59.

Bauer, J., Shimojo, S., Gwiazda, J. and Held, R. (1986). Sex differences in the development of binocularity in human infants. Invest. Ophthalmol. Visual Sci. Suppl., 27, 265.

Birch, E.E., Gwiazda, J. and Held, R. (1982). Stereoacuity development for crossed and uncrossed disparities in human infants. Vision Res., 22, 507-513.

Birch, E.E., Gwiazda, J. and Held, R. (1983). The development of vergence does not account for the onset of steropsis. Perception, 12, 331-365.

Birch, E.E., Shimojo, S. and Held, R. (1983). The development of aversion to rivalrous stimuli in human infants. Invest. Ophthalmol. Visual Sci. Suppl., 24, 92.

Gwiazda, J., Bauer, J. and Held, R. (in press). Binocular function in human infants: Correlation of stereoptic and fusion-rivalry discriminations. Journal of Pediatric Ophthalmology and Strabismus.

Held, R. (1985). Binocular vision - Behavioral and neural development. In: Neonate Cognition: Beyond the Blooming Buzzing Confusion. (eds. J. Mehler and R. Fox). Lawrence Erlbaum Associates, Hillsdale, NJ.

Held, R. (1988). Normal visual development and its deviations. In: Strabismus and Amblyopia, 49, pp. 247-257, The MacMillan Press, Ltd., London.

Held, R., Bauer, J. and Gwiazda, J. (1988). Age of onset of binocularity correlates with level of plasma testosterone in male infants. Invest. Ophthalmol. Visual Sci. Suppl., 29, 60.

Held, R., Birch, E.E. and Gwiazda, J. (1980). Stereoacuity of human infants. Proc. Nat. Acad. Sci. USA, 77, 5572-5574.

Held, R., Shimojo, S. and Gwiazda, J. (1984). Gender differences in the early development of human visual resolution. Invest. Ophthamol. Visual Sci. Suppl., 25, 220.

Hickey, J.L. and Peduzzi, J.D. (1987). Structure and development of the visual system. In Handbook of Infant Perception. (eds. P. Salapatek and L. Cohen). Academic Press, New York.

Huttenlocher, P.R., de Courten, C., Garey, L.J. and van der Loos, H. (1982). Synaptogenesis in human visual cortex-Evidence for synapse elimination during normal development. Neurosci., 33, 247.

LeVay, S., Stryker, M.P. and Shatz, C.J. (1978). Ocular dominance columns and their development in layer IV of the cat's visual cortex: A quantitative study. J. comp. Neurol., 179, 223-244.

Levay, S. and Voight, T. (in press). Ocular dominance and disparity coding in cat visual cortex. Visual Neurosci.

LeVay, S., Wiesel, T.N. and Hubel, D.H. (1980). The development of ocular dominance columns in normal and visually deprived monkeys. J. Comp. Neurol., 191, 1-51.

Manny, R. and Klein, S. (1984). The development of vernier acuity in infants. Current Eye Research, 3, 453-62.

Pettigrew, J.D. (1974). The effect of visual experience on the development of stimulus specificity by kitten cortical neurones. J. Physiol., 237, 49-74.

Rakic, P. (1976). Prenatal genesis of connections subserving ocular dominance in the rhesus monkey. Nature, 261, 467-71.

Shimojo, S., Bauer, J.A., O'Connell, K.M. and Held, R. (1986). Pre-stereoptic binocular vision in infants. Vision Res, 26, 501-510.

Shimojo, S., Birch, E.E., Gwiazda, J. and Held, R. (1984). Development of vernier acuity in infants. Vision Res., 24, 721-728.

Shimojo, S. and Held, R. (1987). Vernier acuity is less than grating acuity in 2 and 3-month-olds. Vision Res., 27, 77-86.

Stanley, O.H., Fleming, P.J. and Morgan, M.H. (in press). Abnormal development of visual function following intra-uterine growth retardation. Early Human Development.

Timney, B.N. (1981). Development of binocular depth perception in kittens. Invest. Ophthal. Visual Sci., 21, 493-496.

Timney, B.N. (1988). The development of depth perception. In Advances in Neural and Behavioral Development. (ed. P. Shinkman). Ablex Publishing, New Jersey.

Westheimer, G. (1979). The spatial sense of the eye. Invest. Ophthal. Visual Sci., 18, 893-912.

Wilson, H.R. (1988). Development of spatiotemporal mechanisms in the human infant. Vision Res., 28, 611-628.

Zak, R. and Berkley, M.A. (1986). Evoked potentials elicited by brief vernier offsets: Estimating vernier thresholds and properties of the neural substrate. Vision Res., 26, 439-451.

15

Development of Visual Cortical Selectivity: Binocularity, Orientation and Direction of Motion

Oliver Braddick, Janette Atkinson and John Wattam-Bell

INTRODUCTION

Visual behaviour shows remarkable advances in the first six months of human life. Some of this development (e.g. of acuity) requires maturation of the peripheral visual pathway. However, the infant's ability to perform complex visual tasks must depend on the development of central processing. A wide range of evidence has suggested that the cortex may play a minor role in neonatal visual function, but come to achieve dominance over subcortical vision between about 2-4 months (Bronson, 1974; Atkinson, 1984; Braddick and Atkinson, 1988). Evidence on early cortical function is therefore critical for our understanding of visual development. Cells of the mature visual cortex have highly selective responses to various attributes of the stimulus. Anatomically, there is a great increase in the connectivity of visual cortex up to 6 months postnatal (Garey & De Courten, 1983) and presumably these new synapses serve to define the selectivity of cortical cells. Our goal has been to look at the development of cortical selectivity functionally. We use stimuli, each specially designed to elicit a response only from cortical neurons that have developed particular selective properties. These responses may be detected either by means of visual evoked potentials (VEP) or by behavioural discriminations.

BINOCULARITY

Probably the strongest body of evidence for the postnatal development of a specific visual cortical function comes from responses that depend on binocular interaction. For example, the VEP elicited by alternations of a dynamic random-dot pattern between binocular correlation and anticorrelation (Julesz, Kropfl & Petrig, 1980) must arise after signals from the two eyes come together on cortical neurons. Such correlogram responses are first seen on average around 3-4 months of age (Braddick et al,

1980; Petrig et al, 1981; Braddick et al, 1983; Wattam-Bell et al, 1987b). Sensitivity to binocular correlation does not necessarily imply stereopsis, but work from a number of laboratories agrees that by around four months postnatally most infants can be shown to discriminate disparities (Atkinson & Braddick, 1974; Fox et al, 1980; Held, Birch & Gwiazda, 1980; Birch, Gwiazda & Held, 1983; Birch, Shimojo & Held, 1985; see review by Braddick & Atkinson, 1983). However, there is quite a wide range between individuals (2-6 months) in the onset times for both functions. Current work in our laboratory (Smith et al, 1988) is comparing correlation and disparity detection by the same infants under the same conditions; so far it shows no systematic difference in age of onset, either on VEP or behavioural measures.

ORIENTATION SELECTIVITY

Besides binocularity, a property that is not found in primate visual neurones prior to the cortex is orientation selectivity. This selectivity can be identified in infants with the dynamic stimulus illustrated in Figure 1 (Braddick, Wattam-Bell & Atkinson, 1986). A significant VEP response, time locked to the orientation changes, indicates that the infant's cortex has produced a response specific to orientation change and not just to the local contrast changes which occur on every frame. This orientation-specific VEP is usually first detected at around 6 weeks postnatal age, even though significant pattern-appearance VEP responses can be recorded from infants in the first few days of life. Figure 2 shows an example of an orientation VEP response in a normal 7-week old. These results were obtained with orthogonal oblique orientations; however, we find no

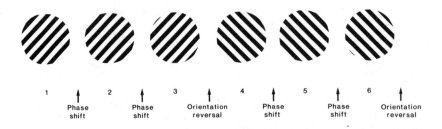

Figure 1. A sample from the display sequence designed to evoke orientation-specific responses. With each new frame (25 per second) the pattern undergoes a random displacement (phase shift). Between frames 3 and 4 (and every third frame) its orientation is changed.

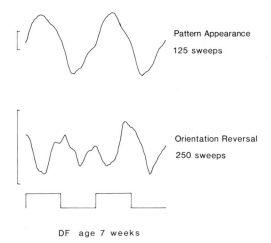

DF   age 7 weeks

Figure 2 Orientation and pattern-appearance VEP responses, from a normal 7 week old infant. The bottom trace indicates the timing of the stimulus alternations (total duration = 0.5 sec). Each record is the averaged response of the number of sweeps indicated. Vertical scale = 5 microvolts.

difference in age of onset for the response to horizontal/ vertical orientations (Wattam-Bell et al, 1987a). Anisotropies between horizontal-vertical and oblique responses do occur with this response, but they emerge later (3–5 months) and may be associated with the differential significance of vertical and horizontal contours for stereopsis.

Behavioural orientation discrimination

If, as the VEP results suggest, cortical orientation detectors are not functioning in newborns, we might expect newborns to have difficulty discriminating orientations. In the 'infant control habituation' method, the infant is shown one orientation repeatedly, and looking times decline until a criterion of visual habituation is reached. Following this, longer looking time to a novel than to the familiar orientation provides evidence that the infant can discriminate them. Using sequential presentation of familiar and novel patterns, with the distinctive feature of the new pattern being the presence of orientation changes, we found that newborns showed no discrimination whereas 5–6 week olds did (Atkinson et al, in press), in line with the VEP result. However, in a variant on the procedure, in which novel and familiar orientations are presented side by side following habituation, even newborns show an initially longer looking time to the novel orientation (Slater et al, in press; Atkinson et al, in press). The discrimination is truly related to orientation and not simply to the position of features within the display, since the phase of the grating can be changed on each presentation. However, this discrimination is possible despite the absence of the neural events reflected in the VEP signal. We discuss below possible bases for this dissociation.

DIRECTIONALITY

A third property of many visual cortical neurons is selective responsiveness to direction of motion. We might expect motion sensitivity to be present very early in development, since it is often thought of as a very basic and primitive visual function. We have studied the development of direction selectivity with a VEP method analogous to those for orientation and binocularity (Wattam-Bell, 1987). The method looks for a VEP component synchronized with periodic reversals in the up-down motion of a random-dot field. These direction reversals are embedded in a sequence of pattern changes, so that any signal at the correct frequency must be linked to direction of motion and not simply to flicker or pattern change. Surprisingly, this measure shows directional selectivity emerging after (10-12 weeks postnatal age) rather than before the orientation selective VEP response. (However, the age of onset is earlier for 5 deg/sec motion than for 20 deg/sec, so the age might be reduced further if still lower velocities could be tested.)

Directionality, then, is another visual cortical function which appears to emerge in the course of the immediately postnatal months. In the mature cortex, orientation- and direction-selectivity are closely associated, but our results suggest that orientation selectivity may come first in human development. Studies of how these dimensions are mapped in cat cortex (Swindale et al, 1987) show discontinuities between opposite directions in the direction map, within regions where the orientation map is continuous; this is consistent with the idea that, in the development of cortical columnar organization, the orientation map may be laid out prior to that for direction of motion. Hopefully, more detailed study of the developmental sequence will help us understand better how these selective properties of cortex become established and organized.

OVERVIEW

Our results have shown that some essential aspects of visual cortical function, namely binocularity, orientation-, and direction-selectivity, are at best extremely immature at birth and develop greatly over the first few months of human life.

What is the nature and degree of this immaturity? The simplest
and most radical suggestion, first made by Bronson (1974) and
developed by Atkinson (1984), is that the visual behaviour seen
before about six weeks is subcortically mediated.   This view has
to be reconciled with the finding of orientation-based
behavioural discriminations at birth. A key element of
Atkinson's (1984) proposal was the development of pathways by
which visual cortical activity could control subcortical
oculomotor and orienting function.   Immaturity in this respect
might explain why the demonstration of orientation selectivity is
so sensitive to the behavioural test procedures, but it is
difficult to see how neonates could discriminate as they do
without some kind of orientation-selective, presumably cortical
structures.

Developmental dissociations between distinct cortical pathways?

It is possible that discriminative behaviour can occur with
very few, or very sluggish, orientation-selective neurones,
insufficient to yield a measurable VEP. Alternatively, the two
methods may depend on different specific populations of neurones.
One possibility is that our VEP responses may depend primarily on
the spatial non-linearity of complex cells (Movshon et al, 1978).
A simple cell with linear summation within its receptive field,
even if oriented, could give as large a response to the
displacements in Figure 1 as to the orientation reversal, and so
show little or no specific response to the reversal. Neonates'
behavioural discrimination might then depend on these cells,
which could be relatively silent in the VEP.

Maurer and Lewis (1979) speculated, largely on the basis of
evidence from cat, that neonatal vision might reflect an absence
of Y-cell input to the cortex. We now know that the primate
system is not quite analogous, but does include an apparently
far-reaching separation of different kinds of visual information
between parvo- and magnocellular pathways (see e.g. Livingstone &
Hubel, 1988). The relatively late development of directional
responses, especially for higher velocities, raises the
possibility that the magnocellular pathway, which is believed to
be the primary route for motion information, may be slower in
development. If so, the non-linear response reflected in the
orientation VEP might also arise in this pathway, albeit at a
somewhat earlier age. The thick CO-staining stripes in area V2,
which receive input largely from the magnocellular system, are
also reported to be the predominant location of disparity-
selective cells. This raises the possibility that the
development of sensitivity to binocular correlation and disparity
around 3-4 months may also be a function of the development of
the magno pathway.

To evaluate any of these hypotheses, we shall need a fuller

understanding what different classes of cortical cell contribute to adult human vision, and how their functions develop in other primates.

ACKNOWLEDGMENTS

We thank Shirley Anker, Carol Evans, Bruce Hood, Jocelyn Smith, and Jo Tricklebank for their help with the work described here. We acknowledge the support of the Medical Research Council of Great Britain.

REFERENCES

Atkinson, J. (1984). Human visual development over the first 6 months of life: A review and a hypothesis. Human Neurobiol., 3, 61-74.

Atkinson, J. & Braddick, O.J. (1974). Stereoscopic discrimination in infants. Perception, 5, 29-38.

Atkinson, J., Hood, B., Wattam-Bell, J., Anker, S. & Tricklebank, J. (in press). Development of orientation discrimination in infancy. Perception.

Birch, E.E., Gwiazda, J., & Held, R. (1983). The development of vergence does not account for the development of stereopsis. Perception, 12, 331-336.

Birch, E.E., Shimojo, S., & Held, R. (1985). Preferential-looking assessment of fusion and stereopsis in infants aged 1-6 months. Invest. Ophthalmol. vis. Sci., 2, 366-370.

Braddick, O.J. & Atkinson, J. (1983). Some recent findings on the development of human binocularity: a review. Behav. Brain Res. 10, 71-80.

Braddick, O. J. & Atkinson, J. (1988). Sensory selectivity, attentional control, and cross-channel integration in early visual development. In 20th Minnesota Symposium on Child Psychology (ed. A. Yonas) Hillsdale, NJ: Lawrence Erlbaum.

Braddick O.J., Atkinson J., Julesz B., Kropfl W., Bodis-Wollner I., & Raab E. (1980). Cortical binocularity in infants. Nature, 288, 363-65.

Braddick, O.J., Wattam-Bell, J. & Atkinson, J. (1986). Orientation-specific cortical responses develop in early infancy. Nature, 320, 617-619.

Braddick O., Wattam-Bell J., Day J., & Atkinson, J. (1983). The onset of binocular function in human infants. Human Neurobiol. 2, 65–69.

Bronson, G.W. (1974). The postnatal growth of visual capacity. Child Devel. 45, 873–890.

Fox, R., Aslin, R.N., Shea, S.L. & Dumais, S.T. (1980). Stereopsis in human infants. Science, 207, 323–324.

Garey, L. & De Courten, C. (1983). Structural development of the lateral geniculate nucleus and visual cortex in monkey and man. Behav. Brain Res., 10, 3–15.

Held, R., Birch, E. E., & Gwiazda J. (1980). Stereoacuity of human infants. Proc. Nat. Acad. Sci. USA, 77, 5572–5574.

Julesz, B., Kropfl, W., & Petrig, B. (1980). Large evoked potentials of dynamic random-dot correlograms and stereograms permit quick determination of stereopsis. Proc. Nat. Acad. Sci. USA, 77, 2348–2351.

Livingstone, M. & Hubel, D.H. (1988). Segregation of form, color, movement, and depth: anatomy, physiology and perception. Science, 240, 740–749.

Maurer, D. & Lewis, T.L. (1979). A physiological explanation of infants' early visual development. Canad. J. Psychol., 33, 232–252.

Movshon, J.A., Thompson, I.G. & Tolhurst, D.J. (1978). Receptive field organization of complex cells in the cat's striate cortex. J. Physiol., 283, 79–99.

Petrig, B., Julesz, B., Kropfl, W., Baumgartner, G., & Anliker, M. (1981). Development of stereopsis and cortical binocularity in human infants: electrophysiological evidence. Science, 213, 1402–1405.

Slater, A., Morison, V., & Somers, M. (1988). Orientation discrimination and cortical function in the human newborn. Perception, in press.

Smith, J., Atkinson, J., Braddick, O.J., & Wattam-Bell, J. (1988). Development of sensitivity to binocular correlation and disparity in infancy. Perception (in press).

Swindale, N.V., Matsubara, J.A., & Cynader, M.S. (1987). Surface organization of orientation and direction selectivity in cat area 18. J. Neurosci., 7, 1414–1427.

Wattam-Bell, J. (1987). Motion-specific VEPs in adults and infants. Perception, 16, 231.

Wattam-Bell, J., Braddick, O.J., Marshall, G., Atkinson. J. (1987a). Development and anisotropy of the orientation-specific VEP. Invest. Ophthalmol. vis. Sci. (Suppl.), 28, 5.

Wattam-Bell, J., Braddick, O., Atkinson J., & Day J. (1987b). Measures of infant binocularity in a group at risk for strabismus. Clin. Vis. Sci., 1, 327-336.

16
Some Clinical Aspects on Abnormal Visual Development

Gunnar Lennerstrand

The presentations by drs Rakic[*], Held and Braddick have covered a very substantial part of basic research on visual development, from the fetal stage onwards. I will bring up some clinical aspects on the material presented, related to a few common or serious conditions that cause visual problems in children. We pediatric ophthalmologists are indeed fully aware of the very important progress that has been made in basic vision research over the last two to three decades and we know that we are treating a dynamic process and not a static condition when we deal with retinal disease, cataract, strabismus etc. in children. It is not enough to make the diagnosis and do the surgery, if that is the appropriate treatment, but the child has to be followed closely with regard to its visual development for a long time onwards. It is hoped that the discussion will raise new ideas on how to reduce the harmful effects on visual development of pathological conditions in children s eyes.

1. Congenital cataract.

Bilateral cataracts or other types of bilateral opacities of the ocular media may lead to form deprivation and profound impairment of visual development (Boothe, Dobson and Teller 1985, von Noorden 1985), if the opacities are not removed during the first year of life. However, the results with regard to visual acuity are excellent with early operations and corrections of aphakia with contact lenses and glasses.

In cases of monocular cataract, occlusion therapy is also needed, in order to avoid deleterious effects of abnormal binocular interaction at the striate cortex level. With these

---

[*] manuscript not submitted

measures the visual development can be corrected and the visual outcome is also quite favourable (Birch et al. 1986). On the other hand normal binocular vision is seldom seen in otherwise successfully treated cases with bilateral cataracts.

2. Visual problems related to prematurity.

Prematurely born children with a birth weight below 1000 g sustain high risks of a specific retinal disorder, called retinopathy of prematurity (ROP). It is due to abnormal growth of the immature retinal vessels, which in the most severe cases leads to blindness as a result of fibroblastic invasion of the vitreous body and subsequent total retinal detachment. In the majority of prematures, ROP is arrested and the retinal changes reversed, at least partially. However, there are often clear signs of chronic ROP in the fundus of the eye, for example temporal displacement of the macula.

The arrested ROP evidently causes disturbances in the development of the eye itself, since reduced vision and re-fractive errors are much more common in prematurely born children than in full term children (Kushner 1982). Strabismus is also common in this group, but this is probably the effects of prematurity on the CNS and it does not seem linked with retinal defects.

With regard to abnormal visual development, ROP would seem to represent factors that affect both the optical and the image sampling mechanisms of spatial vision (Jacobs and Blakemore 1988). Image degradation by refractive errors probably leads to changes in the more central neural connections, mainly in the striate cortex. However, retinal structure is deranged by ROP and such impairment of the image sampling mechanisms must also affect visual acuity development. Perhaps this represents an abnormal development of retinal function similar to that seen in the albino visual system, where it is claimed that matura-tion of the foveal cones is arrested at the level of the 10 month old child with regard to both structure and function (Wilson et al. 1988).

In the context of refractive errors and the effect on growth of the eye, it was pointed out by dr Braddick that development of myopia in an eye occluded from birth and re-ceiving no formed images, probably is a cortical event. There might exist different mechanisms for producing refractive errors and particularly myopia, some mechanisms being retinal and others cortical.

3. Optic nerve hypoplasia

Underdevelopment of the optic nerve has proved to be a major cause of visual loss in infancy. It is generally bilateral and frequently associated with anomalies of the central nervous system of various kinds (Hoyt 1986). Visual acuity is reduced to a level that usually corresponds to the amount of CNS involvement.

The etiology of optic nerve hypoplasia is largely unknown. Different teratogenic substances can cause the malformation, the most wellknown being ethanol. Alcoholism of the mother may induce the fetal alcohol syndrome in her unborn child, with optic hypoplasia as an important ophthalmological characteristic (Strömland 1985).

With regard to pathogenesis of optic nerve hypoplasia, the mechanism of retrograde degeneration has attained much interest. Dr Rakic reported that there is an "overproduction" and later elimination of retinal axons around birth in all animals including man. One question that arises is then whether optic hypoplasia is a result of an exaggerated elimination of fibers or if it is a defect in the generation of retinal ganglion cells and therefore occurs early in embryogenesis.

4. Strabismus

Reduced visual acuity in strabismus is usually an effect of abnormal binocular interaction (von Noorden 1985), occurring in the striate cortex or even higher visual areas. Disorders at the same level are responsible also for disruptions of stereopsis and other binocular functions.

In treating strabismic as well as other types of amblyopia there are reports of a "trade-off" between acuities reached in the non-amblyopic and the amblyopic eye. Held and coworkers (Held 1988) have shown that the non-amblyopic eye often has supernormal acuity before treatment, and that it is reduced at the same rate as the amblyopic eye gains in function. This have not been confirmed by others (see Boothe, Dobson and Teller 1985). Maybe a "trade-off" could be explained in terms of changes in the competetive interaction between fibers from the two eyes for their brain target zones, as described by dr Rakic, although his experiments were mostly done during the fetal period of the animal, and strabismic amblyopia would presumably be due to abnormal visual inputs postnatally.

This leads to a problem that is even more puzzling to pediatric ophthalmologists. Why do children with the type of early onset convergent strabismus (Harcourt 1988) start to squint in the first place? It has been shown in extensive studies by Helveston and coworkers (Helveston 1986) on newborn babies that this type of strabismus is hardly ever congenital but appears at 2-6 months of age. Newborn babies have often strabismus and even esotopia, but it usually disappears within the first 2 months of life and then appears in some infants who mostly were not esotropic to start with.

So early onset esotropia evidently manifests itself at an age when the visual cortex starts to mature and binocular functions develop, as reported by drs Held and Braddick. There is no sex difference in this type of strabismus which probably excludes hormonal factors such as those suggested by dr Held for development of vernier acuity and binocularity.

Could the early onset strabismus be caused by a defective development of the fusion mechanism that should hold the two eye together, as postulated already at the turn of the century by Worth? Could this depend on a disregulation in fetal life of the competetive elimination of synaptic connections in the striate cortex, as described by dr Rakic? This could lead to a loss of the substrate for binocular cells and therefore no binocular function could develop at the proper age. This would disconnect the two eyes and motor mechanisms could drive them out of alignment into a convergent position. There are many postulates in this chain of events and it would be interesting to hear if there is any anatomical evidence to support the idea.

5. Summary

A very brief description has been given of some pediatric ophthalmology entities in which our attitudes towards diagnosis and treatment have been influenced by recent research on development of visual functions, and topics for further discussion have been suggested.

REFERENCES

Birch, E.E., Stager, D.R. and Wright, W.W., (1986). Grating acuity development after early surgery for congenital unilateral cataract. Arch. Ophthalmol., 104, 1783-1787.

Boothe, R.G., Dobson, V. and Teller, D. (1985). Postnatal development of vision in human and non-human primate. Ann. Rev. Neurosci., 8, 495-545.

Harcourt, B. (1988). Aetiology, classification and clinical characteristics of esotropia in infancy. In Strabismus and Amblyopia. (eds. G. Lennerstrand, G.K. von Noorden and E.C. Campos). Macmillan Press, London, pp 23–35.

Held, R. (1988). Normal visual development and its deviations. In Strabismus and Amblyopia. (eds. G. Lennerstrand, G.K. von Noorden and E.C. Campos). Macmillan Press, London, pp 247–257.

Helveston, E.M. (1986). Esotropia in the first year of life. In Pediatric Ophthalmology and Strabismus. Transactions of the New Orleans Academy of Ophthalmology. Raven Press, New York, pp 419–429.

Hoyt, C.S. (1986). Optic nerve hypoplasia: a changing perspective. In Pediatric Ophthalmology and Strabismus. Transactions of the New Orleans Academy of Ophthalmology. Raven Press, New York, pp 257–264.

Jacobs, D.S. and Blakemore, C. (1988). Factors limiting the postnatal development of visual acuity in the monkey. Vision Res., 28, 947–958.

Kushner, B.J. (1982). Strabismus and amblyopia associated with regressed retinopathy of prematurity. Arch. Ophthalmol., 100, 256–261.

von Noorden, G.K. (1985). Amblyopia: a multidisciplinary approach (Proctor Lecture). Invest. Ophthalmol. Vis., Sci. 26, 52–64.

Strömland, K. (1985). Ocular abnormalities in the fetal alcohol syndrome. Acta Ophthalmol. (Copenh), 63, suppl. 171.

Wilson, H.R., Mets, M.B., Nagy, S.E. and Kressel, A.B. (1988). Albino spatial vision as an instance of arrested visual development. Vision Res., 28, 979–990.

V. Psychobiology

17

An Overview of Selected Research Topics in Developmental Psychobiology

Norman A. Krasnegor

INTRODUCTION

By way of introduction it bears reiterating that while the 1980's can be described as the "decade of the brain," it is also fair to observe that research during the past 10 years has witnessed a veritable explosion of information concerning behavioral development of the human infant. More specifically, psychologists have made exciting discoveries that reveal WHAT human babies know and WHEN they acquire the capacity to know many facets about themselves, significant others and the ENVIRONMENT that surrounds them. Another general observation is that developmental neurobiology and developmental psychology as scientific disciplines are almost totally isolated from one another. One discipline, developmental psychobiology, is an exception to this finding. Developmental psychobiology forms a meaningful scientific bridge between developmental biology and developmental psychology (Hall and Oppenheim, 1987). As currently conceived of by Gottlieb (1983): "A psychobiological approach signifies the study of behavior from a broadly biological perspective. A broad biological point of view includes not only some interest in the physiological, biochemical, and anatomical correlates of behavior but also embraces ecological and evolutionary considerations as well." Thus developmental psychobiology is clearly an interdisciplinary endeavor that in terms of Bloom's (1987) conceptualization spans the dimension which he terms "integrative neuroscience."

This chapter presents a selective overview of topics in developmental psychobiology research that illustrate new trends in this field. The first of these is an emphasis upon the perinatal period of development. This phase includes the time span that, in the human infant, extends from the 28th week of gestation to the end of the first postnatal month. The focus is upon the behavioral development of the fetus and the first few

weeks of neonatal ontogeny. The questions of interest are
typical behavioral ones: WHAT is observed to happen WHEN. That
is, a characterization of the ontogeny of behavior and a
comparison of the in-utero findings with what occurs during the
first hours and days after birth. Some of the work involves
systematic description of the emergence of patterns of endogenous
behavior. Other work focuses upon experimental manipulation of
the fetus and neonate to assess capacity for learning and neural
substrates that subsume such behavior. Other work seeks to
analyze the relationships between ENVIRONMENT and behavior to
assess how such interactions may affect development.

A second trend is the development of elegant new methodological
techniques that have allowed systematic quantitative observations
to be made and correlative brain/behavior questions to be posed.

A third important trend is that some leaders in the field of
developmental psychobiology have begun to apply what they have
learned from research on neonatal animals to the study of
neonatal human babies.

These trends are presented in the form of a series of research
exemplars on the following topics: (a) Organization of prenatal
behavioral development and in-utero learning; (b) Organization
of an early parent-infant interaction system; and (c) Neural
substrates of early behavioral plasticity.

PRENATAL BEHAVIOR AND IN UTERO LEARNING

Recent studies reveal that during the prenatal period, organisms
exhibit both characteristic endogenous behavioral patterns and
the capacity for learning (Smotherman and Robinson, 1987;
Smotherman and Robinson, in press; Krasnegor, in press).

Fetal Behavioral Development

In the present context behavior is defined as the systematic
observation of what an intact organism does based upon a
catalogue of the frequency and duration of particular acts over
a specified period of development (Krasnegor, in press).
Smotherman and Robinson (1987) have investigated the ontogeny of
spontaneous movement in the fetal rat. The research was made
possible due to the advances made in preparations that allow the
fetus to be directly observed by the experimenter (Narayanan,
Fox, and Hamburger, 1971; Smotherman, Richards, and Robinson,
1984; and Smotherman, Robinson, and Miller, 1986). This entails
anesthetizing the dam using either a chemomyelotomy or reversible
lidocaine anesthesia. These procedures eliminate afferent
stimulation of the abdominal area thereby obviating the need for
general anesthesia. Upon completion of the anesthesia, the
female is placed in a holding device, her uterus is externalized

via a mid-ventral incision, and her hind quarters and uterus are immersed in a bath of warmed saline (Smotherman and Robinson, 1987). Twenty minutes later, one fetus (with umbilicus and membranes intact) from the ovarian end of the uterus is delivered through an incision in the uterine horn into the bath. This preparation allows clear and detailed viewing of the fetus and its movements (Smotherman, Robinson, and Miller, 1986).

Smotherman and Robinson (1987) have dichotomized the observed fetal movements into two broad categories, simple and complex. Their units of analysis are specific body movements such as forelimb, head, mouth, hind limb and trunk. Simple movements are any of those described that occur alone. Complex movements are those that occur in combination. The investigators found that spontaneous movement of the fetus first appears on Day 16 of gestation (Smotherman and Robinson, 1986). This movement pattern asymptotes on Days 17-18 and stays at its peak throughout the remainder of pregnancy. Modal movement units on Day 16 involve the forelimbs and lateral or ventral trunk flexions. Head and hind limb movements are most frequently observed between Days 17-19. Mouth movements peak on the 19th day of gestation. Straightening and extension of the trunk (stretch) begins to be observed by Day 20 (Smotherman and Robinson, 1987). By the same day eye blinks, ear-wiggles and synchronous wiping and forelimb-mouth patterns emerge. The investigators also found temporal patterning of movements that clustered in "bouts" or "bursts" of activity (Smotherman and Robinson, 1987). In summary, movement patterns of the fetal rat have a definite sequence that follows an ontogenetic trajectory.

Fetal Learning

In addition to describing systematic movement patterns of the rat fetus, Smotherman and his colleagues have demonstrated that the fetus can learn in utero (Stickrod, Kimble, and Smotherman, 1982; Smotherman, 1982; Babine and Smotherman, 1984; Kolata, 1984; Smotherman and Robinson, 1987; and Krasnegor, in press). Three basic findings have emerged. First, rat fetuses have the capacity for associative conditioning. Second, conditioned responses that are formed during gestation can be retained for up to two weeks post-natally. Third, associations initiated in utero on Day 17 are consolidated by Day 19 of gestation.

The approach used to condition rat fetuses employs the Garcia paradigm (Garcia, et al, 1985). On Day 20 of gestation, apple juice is injected into the amniotic fluid surrounding an externalized fetus and lithium chloride (LiCl) into its peritoneum (Stickrod, Kimble and Smotherman, 1982; Babine and Smotherman, 1984). A single pairing of an aversive stimulus (LiCl) with a neutral taste or odor (apple juice) causes adult rats so treated to avoid that taste or odor on subsequent presentations. The externalized uterus of the dam is reinserted, the abdomen sutured, and the fetuses delivered at term (Day 22).

Prenatal conditioning influenced suckling behavior two weeks after birth. Experimental pups attached less often than control pups to the dam's nipple that was painted with apple juice. It was shown in a second study that conditioned pups evidenced delays in crossing a runway to gain access to their mother when the air was suffused with the odor of apple juice. In a variant of the paradigm conditioned pups were shown to stay in the low concentration end of a box that contained the odor of apple juice (Stickrod, Kimble, and Smotherman, 1982). These results indicate both that conditioning occurred prenatally and that the conditioned response was retained for up to 14 days after birth.

Smotherman and Robinson (1987) demonstrated that rat fetuses exposed on Day 17 of gestation to a single pairing of a neutral stimulus (mint) and an interperitoneal injection of LiCl are conditioned two days later. Their observations demonstrated that mint solution alone does not suppress fetal movement on either Day 17 or 19 of gestation. But after the pairing with the unconditioned stimulus (LiCl) on Day 17, mint alone suppresses movement by itself on Day 19 of gestation. This finding demonstrates that associative conditioning is consolidated within 48 hours. What is also apparent is that the experiment and the results described would not have been possible unless the work on the ontogeny of fetal movement were carried out.

In summary, marked progress has been made in gaining an understanding of development of endogenous behavioral patterns and the capacity for learning in the rat fetus.

ORGANIZATION OF EARLY PARENT-OFFSPRING INTERACTIONS

Mother-offspring interactions during the perinatal period are dynamic processes that for example help prepare the young organism for social and emotional adaptation to their postnatal environment (Hofer, 1987). Some preparation for other aspects of adaptation takes place during gestation and the period immediately following birth. One such critical interaction involves the biobehavioral regulation of circadian rhythms.

Setting the Circadian Clock

The alternating day-night cycle entrains an organism's circadian rhythms to the 24 hour period. This clock helps an organism to adapt to the demands of its biological niche. Recent research by Reppert and his colleagues (1987) has begun to elucidate how a pregnant rat sets the clock of its fetuses during gestation.

The suprachiasmic nuclei (SCN) of the anterior hypothalamus are the brain structures which have been identified in mammals as the site of the biological clock that generates rhythms believed to be essential for triggering hormonal secretions and behaviors (Moore, 1983; Takahashi and Zatz, 1982). Reppert et al (1987) indicate that contemporary findings have identified that the necessary stimulus (light) reaches the SCN via a monosynaptic retinohypothalamic pathway. A number of investigators (see Reppert et al, 1987) have shown that in rodents (rats, mice, and hamsters) and in monkeys, a functional circadian clock exists during the perinatal period prior to the point at which the retinohypothalamic pathway makes operational connections to the SCN. The research findings reviewed below indicate that the mother serves the role as a photic transducer between the ambient light and the brains of her developing fetuses. The synchronization of the maternal clock with that of her soon to be born offspring ensures that the pups can quickly adapt to postnatal environmental conditions without having to wait for the appropriate neural pathways to be enabled (Reppert et al, 1987).

Prenatal Influences

While it is true that during gestation the fetus does not show circadian patterns (Davis, 1981) its SCN is nonetheless functional. Evidence for this assertion was first provided by Deguchi (1975; 1982).

He carried out two different types of experiments. He found that pups born and raised under constant conditions had a phase pineal gland N-acetyltransferase (NAT) rhythm that was in sync with their dam. When he cross fostered pups to dams whose circadian patterns were opposite to the biological mother, the pups' NAT rhythms shift toward the pattern of their foster dam. Thus the data suggest that the clock is oscillating at or prior to birth and the dam influences the phase (Reppert et al, 1987).

Reppert and Schwartz (1983) showed that an entrainable clock oscillates in the SCN of fetal rats. This is regulated by the light impinging on the mother and it is her circadian clock which entrains that of her fetus. Experimental evidence which employed autoradiographs of maternal and fetal SCNs showed that their metabolic profiles were in synchrony and that they both corresponded to the maternal day-night cycle. Reppert and Schwartz (1983) manipulated the lighting cycle of another group of dams so that the phase was shifted by 12 hours. Autoradiographs of dams and fetuses showed that the metabolic activity of mother and fetus were synchronous and in phase with the shift in dark-light cycle. In a final manipulation, the experimenters employed blinded dams. The results of their study showed that the fetal rhythm was synchronous with the circadian pattern of the mother rather than the ambient lighting.

Postnatal Influences

The dam continues to exert influence upon the circadian rhythm
of her offspring after birth. This is greatest during the first
postnatal week (Reppert et al, 1984; Takahashi and Deguchi,
1983). Reppert et al (1984) studied the circadian phase rhythms
of NAT of the pineal gland in pups and dams. Half of the pups
in the litter and the dam were blinded just after birth. The
remainder of the litter was intact. All animals were exposed to
a reversed light-dark cycle. The results indicated that after
the manipulation the pineal gland rhythms of the blinded pups
were in sync with the blinded dam; however, the circadian
rhythms of the intact pups were synchronized to the existing
light-dark cycle. These data indicate that social interaction
between litter mates does not regulate circadian patterns.
Subsequent experiments that employed cross fostering techniques
and systematic shifting of the light-dark cycle demonstrate that
the pups so treated showed circadian patterns akin to the dams
who were their care givers. The data also reveal that the
effects of maternal influence began to decrease after the fifth
postnatal day.

In summary, maternal influences are clearly evident throughout
the perinatal period regarding the setting of circadian rhythms.
It is still not known by what mechanism(s) the mother exerts her
influence. Reppert et al (1987) speculate hormonal signals may
be operative prenatally and behavioral ones postnatally.

NEURAL SUBSTRATES OF BEHAVIORAL PLASTICITY

Perinatal learning is a subject of intense interest among
developmental psychobiologists. As demonstrated by Smotherman
and Robinson (see above), the fetal rat has the capacity for
associative conditioning. Other researchers have begun to
investigate learning in the newborn rat pup and to analyze this
capacity at both the behavioral and neural substrate levels.

Neonatal Behavioral Analysis

Hall (1987) and his colleagues have been investigating the
neural basis of motivation, learning, and reward in the neonatal
rat pup. The focus of their investigation is an analysis of
early activation and conditioning associated with ingestion
behaviors of infants during their first 20 days of life. Hall
(1979a; 1979b) has shown that rat pups will actively ingest milk
and other foods from the first day of life. Such intake is
associated with an intense activation of behavior (licking,
mouthing, crawling, probing, and tumbling) (Hall, 1987). This
behavioral repertoire suggest that the milk was acting as a
reward. Based upon this observation, Johansen and Hall (1979)
and Johansen and Hall (1982) demonstrated the capacity of the

one day old pups for both operant and classical conditioning in which milk ingestion acted as the primary reinforcer.

Neural Substrates of Learning in Neonates

Hall and his co-workers have taken a novel approach to elucidating the neural substrates that underpin activation and conditioning observed in neonatal rat pups. They have begun a general mapping of neural systems that are altered during ingestion and appetitive learning. The investigators employ autoradiographic techniques that depend upon the uptake of 2 deoxyglucose (2 DG). Localized brain activity can be identified in terms of brain glucose metabolism as indicated by the relative amounts of 2 DG incorporated into tissue. Hall (1987) mapped areas of the brain during behavioral activation associated with the ingestion of milk. He found that in deprived pups (compared to controls) who received milk infusions that the activity is greatest in the brainstem and thalamus. These areas relate to the activity of ingestion. Most interesting however was the uptake in the basal forebrain (hypothalamus, amygdala, and medical forebrain bundle). These latter areas overlap with loci of rewarding brain stimulation (Hall, 1987).

In addition to measuring brain activity associated with appetitive learning, Hall (1987) also mapped 2 DG uptake in relationship to classical conditioning. He studied the effects of the conditioned stimulus (CS) alone compared to the pairing of the CS and US (unconditioned stimulus).

He also investigated the effects of previous conditioning and what happens during conditioning (compared to what was learned). A detailed listing of brain loci active during each of his experimental conditions can be found in Hall (1987). While most of the results reported by Hall are preliminary in nature, the technique he has pioneered with autoradiographic mapping of the neonatal rat's central nervous system provides an exciting new approach for gaining a deep understanding of the neural systems that may underpin early learning and motivation.

The three topics discussed above are representative of current psychobiological approaches for elucidating early behavioral development (for additional overviews see Hall and Oppenheim, 1987). Almost without exception this research entails the use of animal models. In the past five years, an interesting new trend has emerged (Krasnegor, 1987). Some of the leading developmental psychobiologists have begun to apply what they learned from research on neonatal animals to the study of human neonates. Blass et al (1984; see also Blass this volume) has undertaken studies to elucidate the capacity of human babies for learning only hours after birth. He has been using classical conditioning paradigms to ascertain the role of learning for the infant. His work is clearly derived from his earlier research on neonatal rat pups. This approach if successful could lead to a generalized understanding of behavioral mechanisms employed by newborns to identify their care givers and more readily adapt to their postnatal environment.

REFERENCES

1. Babine, A.M. and Smotherman, W.P. (1984). Uterine position and conditioned taste aversion. Behavioral Neuroscience, 96, 461–466.

2. Blass, E.; Granschrow, J.R. and Steiner, J.E. (1984). Classical conditioning in newborns 2–48 hours of age. Infant Behavior Development, 7, 223–235.

3. Bloom, F. (1987). The Physiologist, 39(4), 89.

4. Davis, F.C. (1981). Ontogeny of circadian rhythms in J. Aschoff (Ed.) Handbook of Behavioral Neurobiology, V4, Biological Rhythms, 257–274.

5. Deguchi, T. (1975). Ontogenesis of a biological clock for serotonin: acetyl coenzyme A N-acetyltransferase in the pineal gland of the rat. Proceedings of the National Academy of Sciences, 72, 2914–2920.

6. Deguchi, T. (1982). Sympathetic regulation of circadian rhythm of serotonin N acetyltransferase activity in pineal gland of infant rat. Journal of Neurochemistry, 38, 797–802.

7. Garcia, J.; Lasiter, P.A.; Bermudez-Rattoni, F. and Deems, D.A. (1985). A general theory of aversion learning. In N.S. Braverman and P. Bronstein (Eds.) Experimental Assessments and Clinical Applications of Conditioned Food Aversion. Annals of the New York Academy of Sciences, 443, 8–21.

8. Gottlieb, G. (1983). The psychobiological approach to development issues. In P.H. Mussen (Ed.) Infancy and Developmental Psychobiology. Handbook of Child Psychology, V2, 1–26. New York: Wiley.

9. Hall, W.G. (1979a). Feeding and behavioral activation in rats. Science, 205, 206–209.

10. Hall, W.G. (1979b). The ontogeny of feeding in rats: I. Ingestive and behavioral responses to oral infusions. Journal of Comparative and Physiological Psychology, 93, 977–1000.

11. Hall, W.G. (1987). Early motivation, reward and learning, and their neural bases: Developmental revelations and simplifications. In N.A. Krasnegor, E.M. Blass, M.A. Hofer, and W.P. Smotherman (Eds.) Perinatal Development: A Psychobiological Perspective, 169-193. Orlando, Florida: Academic Press.

12. Hall, W.G. and Oppenheim, R.W. (1987). Developmental Psychobiology: Prenatal, Perinatal, and Early Postnatal Aspects of Behavioral Development. Annual Review of Psychology, 38, 91-128.

13. Hofer, M.A. (1987). Shaping forces within early social relationships. In N.A. Krasnegor, E.M. Blass, M.A. Hofer, and W.P. Smotherman (Eds.) Perinatal Development: A Psychobiological Perspective, 251-274. Orlando, Florida: Academic Press.

14. Johansen, I.B. and Hall, W.G. (1979). Appetitive learning in 1-day-old rat pups. Science, 205, 419-421.

15. Johansen, I.B. and Hall, W.G. (1982). Appetitive conditioning in neonatal rats: Conditioned orientation to a novel odor. Developmental Psychology, 15, 379-397.

16. Kolata, G. (1984). Studying Learning in the Womb. Science, 225, 302-303.

17. Krasnegor, N.A. (1987a). Introduction. In N.A. Krasnegor, E.M. Blass, M.A. Hofer, and W.P. Smotherman (Eds.) Perinatal Development: A Psychobiological Perspective, 1-8. Orlando, Florida: Academic Press.

18. Krasnegor, N.A. (1987b). Developmental psychobiological research: A health scientist administrator's perspective. Developmental Psychobiology, 20, 641-644.

19. Krasnegor, N.A. (in press). Measurement of learning, sensory, and linguistic capacity early in life: A selective overview of recent research. In A. Galaburda (Ed.) From Neurones to Reading. Boston: MIT Press.

20. Krasnegor, N.A. (in press). On fetal development: A behavioral perspective. In W.P. Smotherman and S.R. Robinson (Eds.) Behavior of the Fetus. New Jersey: Telford Press.

21. Moore, R.Y. (1983). Organization and function of a central nervous system circadian oscillator: The suprachiasmatic hypothalamic nuclei. Federation Proceedings, 42, 2783-2789.

22. Narayanan, C.H.; Fox, M.W. and Hamburger, V. (1971). Prenatal development of spontaneous evoked activity in the rat. Behaviour, 40, 100-134.

23. Reppert, S.M. and Schwartz, W.J. (1983). Maternal coordination of the fetal biological clock in-utero. Science, 220, 969-971.

24. Reppert, S.M.; Coleman, R.J.; Health, H.W. and Swedlow, J.R. (1984). Pineal N-acetyltransferase activity in 10-day-old rats: A paradigm for studying the circadian system. Endocrinology, 115, 918-925.

25. Reppert, S.M.; Duncan, M.J. and Weaver, D.R. (1987). Maternal influences on the developing circadian system. In N.A. Krasnegor, E.M. Blass, M.A. Hofer, and W.P. Smotherman (Eds.) Perinatal Development: A Psychobiological Perspective, 343-356. Orlando, Florida: Academic Press.

26. Smotherman, W.P. (1982a). Odor aversion in the rat fetus. Physiology and Behavior, 29, 769-771.

27. Smotherman, W.P. (1982b). In-utero chemosensory experience alters taste preferences and corticosterone responsiveness. Behavioral and Neural Biology, 36, 61-68.

28. Smotherman, W.P.; Richards, L.S. and Robinson, S.R. (1984). Techniques for observing fetal behavior in-utero: A comparison of chemomyelotomy and spinal transection. Developmental Psychobiology, 17, 661-674.

29. Smotherman, W.P. and Robinson, S.R. (1986). Environmental determinants of behaviour in the rat fetus. Animal Behaviour, 34, 1859-1873.

30. Smotherman, W.P., Robinson, S.R. and Miller, B.J. (1986). A reversible preparation for observing the behavior of rat fetuses in-utero: Spinal anesthesia with lidocaine. Physiology and Behavior, 37, 57-60.

31. Smotherman, W.P. and Robinson, S.R. (1987). Psychobiology of fetal experience in the rat. In N.A. Krasnegor, E.M. Blass, M.A. Hofer, and W.P. Smotherman (Eds.) Perinatal Development: A Psychobiological Perspective, 39-60. Orlando, Florida: Academic Press.

32. Smotherman, W.P. and Robinson, S.R. (Eds.) (in press). Behavior of the Fetus. New Jersey: Telford Press.

33. Stickrod, G.; Kimble, D.P. and Smotherman, W.P. (1982). In-utero taste/odor aversion conditioning in the rat. Physiology and Behavior, 28, 5-7.

34. Takahashi, K. and Deguchi, T. (1983). Entrainment of circadian rhythms of blinded rats by nursing mothers. Physiology and Behavior, 31, 373-378.

35. Takahashi, J.S. and Zatz, M. (1982). Regulation of circadian rhythmicity. Science, 217, 1104-1111.

18

Development of Early Social Interactions and the Affective Regulation of Brain Growth

Colwyn Trevarthen

INTRODUCTION: THE BEGINNING OF HUMAN EMOTIONAL ENGAGEMENT

In the past 20 years, descriptive studies of free mother-infant interactions, made by analyzing film and television recordings with sound, have significantly clarified basic inherent features of communication underlying language (Bateson, 1975; Bullowa, 1979; Stern, 1971, 1974a,b, 1985 ; Trevarthen, 1974, 1977, 1979, 1986a; Trevarthen and Marwick, 1986). Specific adaptions of mind and behaviour in both infant and mother create an engagement of motives and emotions. This communication becomes the essential regulator of the child's learning and cognitive growth.

The words a mother speaks to her baby often spell out aspects of her motivation and awareness of the communication (Murray and Trevarthen, 1986; Rheingold and Adams, 1980; Snow, 1977); but the mutual engagement is regulated non-referentially, outside words, at the level of expressions of animation, affection and interest. It is conveyed by means of vocalizations, facial expressions, eye-to-eye contacts, hand gestures, touching and postural changes (Fernald, 1985; Fernald and Simon, 1984; Papousek et al, 1985, 1986; Stern, 1974a, 1986; Stern et al, 1982, 1983, 1985; Trevarthen, 1977, 1979, 1985, 1986a; Trevarthen et al, 1981).

Infant capacities for engagement with stimuli of a kind that are produced only by another human being, are distinctly precocious in comparison with the baby's perception and cognition of inanimate and emotionless physical objects and events. Regulated transfer of affection between mother and infant is set up within 2 months of birth, when the nerve circuits of the cerebral and cerebellar neocortices are immature in anatomy and function. A human baby is born with a brain mechanism for recognizing feelings in another person, and for joining in an exchange of expressions to regulate a mutual patterning of emotional states. In effect, this mechanism of the baby is

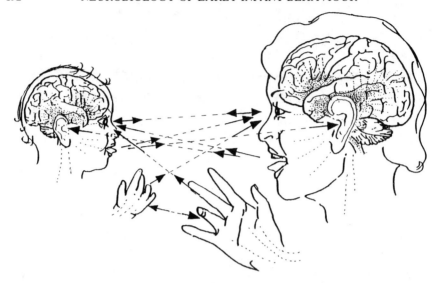

Figure 1:   Protoconversation between a mother and her 2- to 3-
month old infant is sustained simultaneously by many expressive
and receptive channels. The communication couples motivational/
emotional states in their brains.

adapted for linking with the brain states of a partner in
communication (Figure 1).   Presumably, interactive brain states
created in communication with the mother will have   powerful
effects on what the infant experiences and learns. The infant
very quickly learns to recognize and prefer the mother, or the
person who takes a mother's affectionate role as caretaker. An
attachment is formed between them that facilitates the infant's
development, mentally and physically (Bowlby, 1969; Winnicott,
1965).

    Here I am concerned with exploring how this early
communication, and the emotions it generates, might regulate the
child's psychological growth.   The traditional view of psychology
that general cognitive processes, adapted for conceiving objects
of any kind, become adapted to social life entirely through the
infant learning how to control the material or physiological
benefits from life with other people, as if persons were to be
used in the same ways as physical things, or as resource materials
such as food,would appear to be misleading.

'BODY LANGUAGE' OF EARLY COMMUNICATION

    The orientations and changes in motor activity of newborns
within minutes of birth, and of infants up to three months
premature while they are in intensive care, show that the baby is
responsive to being held in a mother's arms against her body, and

to being gently patted or stroked and spoken to softly in a
repetitive manner.   This basis for recognition of closeness to a
caretaker is innate.   Affectionate holding, moving, touching and
speaking has specific parameters or patterning that evoke a
positive response in the infant.   Insensitive handling, with more
abrupt movements that are not geared to the infant's state and
periodic activity, produces freezing of movement or negative,
avoidant reactions.   Newborns may show preferential visual
orientation to a mother's voice, seeking to see her face, but the
baby's eyes and retina are underdeveloped, particularly in the
fovea, and fixation is imprecise.   The eyes are not open for
long, and they close in bright light.   Orientation of head and
eyes, stilling of body movement, opening, closing and orienting of
the hands, and changes in respiration and heart beat can be used
as indicators of positive (or negative) attentional change.
Experiments with such reactions have shown that newborns can learn
to prefer their own mother's voice immediately after birth, and
they soon show preference for her personal odour in a breast pad.
These learned discriminations strenghten and refine the baby's
innate criteria for seeking proximity and communication with a
caretaker.

    In early communication, at 2 to 3 months, both mother and
infant make a variety of complex coordinated expressions that vary
predictably in form (physiognomy), timing (kinematics) and
strength (energetics) (Trevarthen, 1986a).

    Having orientated towards one another, mother and child go
through a process of reciprocal mirroring, each moving to reflect
the form, to synchronize with the timing and to balance the
intensity of the other's expression.   Then their matching of
feelings leads them to make brief complementary messages and to
build a dialogic 'proto-conversation' (Bateson, 1975), a
cooperative exchange made up of complementary utterances with
gestures.   Table IA summarizes the forms of mirroring by which
correspondence of feelings and an affectionate basis for
conversation are set up.   Table IB lists initiatives of
expression that appear to carry potential for informative messages
that are deictic (showing time or place) or referential (defining
an object or action).

    Table IA: Dimensions of Expression and Kinds of Mirroring

1. Of form   (physiognomics)   =   imitation

2. Of timing   (kinetics)   =   synchronization, or
                                          turn-taking

3. Of intensity (energetics)   =   equilibration, or
                                          balancing

Table IB: Rudiments of Deixis and Reference in Protoconversation

Infant Expression	Putative Future Functions
1. Cooing	Voicing for speech
2. Prespeech	Articulations of Words
3. Looking away after making contact	Transferring interest to the focus or topic of a comment
4. Gesturing	Pointing to, greeting, describing, inviting, challenging etc.

Note: All these positive infant utterances show
asymmetry, with a bias to the infant's right side that
indicates dominant activation in the left half of the
brain (MacKain et at, 1983; Studdert-Kennedy, 1983;
Trevarthen, 1988).   Defensive or self-regulatory infant
behaviours, including gaze avoidance, a 'hunching' of
the body, self-touching, hand regard, serve to reduce
contact with another person or to signal distress - e.g.
when the infant is tired, confronted by a stranger, or
when the mother stops responding.   Self-touching in
distress may be biased to the left hand, which would
appear to indicate greater involvement of the right half
of the brain (Trevarthen, 1986b, 1988).

INTERMODAL MATCHING OF EXPRESSIONS OF FEELING OR PURPOSE:
IMITATION

Imitations of expressive movements have been elicited from
infants within an hour of birth (Kugiumutzakis, 1985). Some
mirroring of facial expressions and vocalizations, with turn-
taking, has been recorded between a premature baby girl at 29
weeks gestational age and her very receptive father (unpublished
observations from a video by Saskia Van Rees;   Van Rees and de
Leeuw, 1987).   In imitation tests, a variant of 'baby-talk' is
used.   An adult repeats exaggerated model expressions after the
baby is alerted and aroused by rhythmic stimulation, then a pause
is made to wait for a response.   The infant reacts, therefore, in
a communication 'gap'.   Not all subjects imitate - some remain
observant, or become avoidant (Field, 1982, 1985).

Available evidence suggests that infants are more imitative at
two separate periods in the first 6 months.   In the first month,
facial expressions, mouth and tongue movements, vocalizations and
hand movements can be imitated (Field et al, 1982; Kugiumutzakis,
1985; Maratos, 1982; Meltzoff and Moore, 1977, 1983).   Only very
simple hand and voice patterns are reproduced.   It would appear
that, with models in the form of isolated expressions, the neonate

has a greater capacity to mirror the physiognomy of seen face
movements, a skill that can benefit from visual experience and
learning only after birth.   In any case, infants imitate
movements of expression that are close of those in their
spontaneous expressive repertoire.   These imitations are less
easily evoked at around 2 months after a fullterm birth, when the
infant's smiling is linked with an eager visual orientation to the
mother's eyes, and she can easily keep the baby in a
protoconversation.

Two-and-a-half to four-month-old infants are more likely to
imitate vocal patterns and finger movements than younger or older
subjects (Kuhl and Meltzoff, 1982; Kugiumutzakis, 1985; Maratos,
1982).   In months 4 to 6, infants participate with increasing
skill in musical action games and reciprocal vocalizing, and they
develop quick emotional reactions in teasing play which excites
their laughter (Sroufe and Waters, 1976; Stern, 1974; Trevarthen,
1983, 1986a; Trevarthen and Hubley, 1978).   Mothers respond by
increasing the range and vigour of baby talk, making larger
expressive movements of all kinds and using a far greater range of
voice qualities to express their feelings (Marwick et al, 1984).
Imitations occur, therefore, when the intersubjectivity mechanism
that regulates engagements is undergoing reorganization
preparatory to a new level of reciprocal or cooperative
engagement.   The first period of imitation occurs in the neonatal
phase, just before protoconversations.   The second period of vocal
and gestural imitation occurs just before the baby plays in games
and joins in 'baby songs'.   Imitation is common, again, between 7
and 9 months, the infant, at this age, beginning to imitate
conventional gestures, attitudes, and word-like sounds (Figure 2).

Intermodal functions regulating mother-infant engagements have
been demonstrated in imitation tests and in experiments that test
infant's abilities to match communicative expressions across
sensory modalities (Stern et al, 1985).   Infants under 6 months
make discriminations between normal and abnormal face
configurations (Carpenter et al, 1970; Fantz, 1963), imitate
different face expressions (Maratos, 1973, Meltzoff and Moore
1977, 1983; Field et al 1982) discriminate between faces of
different individuals (Carpenter, 1973; Field 1985), between
different vocalisations and vocal patterns (Mehler, 1985, Kuhl,
1987), between voices of different people (De Casper and Fifer,
1980; Mehler et al 1978), and between coincident and non-
coincident patterns of visible motion and sound variation (Spelke,
1985).   They can match visible mouth movements to appropriate
speech sounds (Kuhl and Meltzoff, 1982; MacKain et al, 1983).

Baldwin (1894) enunciated a theory of the development of
voluntary action and social coordination by means of 'circular
reactions' and 'self imitation'.   He thought such movements were
made to recreate previous experiences.   Piaget (1954) based his
theory of sensory-motor development and the formation of body and

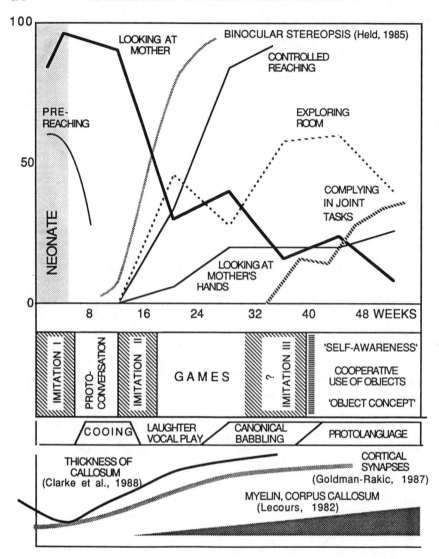

Figure 2: Developments in infancy; the first year (Trevarthen and
Marwick, 1986). Changes in communication, and some brain changes.

object schemata on Baldwin. Imitations of persons by neonates
show that the baby is born with some criteria for 'recognition'
that other people's expressions of feeling can be a consequence of
and equivalent to a matching expression (and feeling) of the baby.
They may be described as innate circular reactions in an
'interpersonal space', analogous to those involved in neonatal
pre-reaching which adjust an arm-and-hand movement to the position
of an object in the space round an infant's body. Imitations are
manifestations of 'altero-cognition', or awareness of other
persons (Trevarthen 1986a).

The intermodal, or supra-modal, standards for detecting
diagnostic invariants of the expressive behaviours and emotions of
people, which distinguish persons from every kind of physical
object, will be in parts of the brain that integrate inputs from
the different senses and outputs to the different motor organs.
Presumably these coordinators of intersubjectivity are defined
first, as emotions are, among interneurones of the brain's
reticular core, and they will have their functions elaborated in
limbic structures and basal ganglia (see Trevarthen 1985 for
references).

COORDINATION OF EXPRESSIONS ON A BEAT: PATTERNS OF 'MOTHERESE'

Timing or kinematic patterning is fundamental to
intersubjective coordination, as a central set of coupled
oscillators is for intracoordination of different sense organs and
body parts (Trevarthen, 1984a, 1986a). Using kinesic theory and
microanalysis of film, (Condon and Sander (1974) showed that the
limb movements of a newborn baby could become synchronous (i.e.
entrained) with stressed features in adult speech, even when the
infant was not being addressed by the speaker and was not
controlling the utterances. The suggestion was that the
synchrony between them (inter-synchrony) was caused by the infant
being passively paced. However, entrainment between oscillators
implies, for an engineer, not that the timing of phases is added
to the receiver, but that oscillators with matching periodicity
in emitter and receiver of energy are brought into phase. This
appears to be what happens when movements of an infant synchronize
with those of another person. Indeed, newborns and adults have,
independently, the same inherent autonomous periodicities in
movement. For example, intervals between oculomotor saccades of
intermediate size (5-30 degrees) are closely similar in newborns
and adults, and the timing of neonatal prereaching is close to
that of adult voluntary reaching (Trevarthen, 1974, 1984b).

Microanalyses of facial and gestural movements and sounds made
by quiet alert newborns who are responding to 'inviting'
expressions of a mother show that the two of them readily join in
movement on one beat. Proto-conversations with 2 to 3 month olds
have consistent timing (Beebe et al, 1985; Trevarthen, 1986a).
Both experienced caretakers and affectionate mothers with little

experience, make characteristic regular patterns of stroking, patting, jiggling and calling; to calm, comfort or arouse and attract infants.   Moreover, the regular forms and the timing of their expressions are similar in different cultures.   Closely similar expressive behaviours to these needed to communicate with young infants are used by skilled interactants with profoundly mentally handicapped adolescents to control their motivations and attention and to support them in play (Burford, 1988).   This kind of communication and empathy forms the basis of 'movement', or 'interactive', therapy.

Mothers vocalisations for young infants have a characteristic patterning called 'intuitive motherese', which is closely similar in Mandarin Chinese (a tonal language) and American English (non-tonal) (Grieser and Kuhl, 1988; Papousek, 1987).   Motherese, is also practised to obtain communication with a young infant by fathers, male pediatricians, nurses and children.   It is characterised by short, evenly spaced utterances with gently 'breathy' voicing and undulating fundamental frequency in a moderately high pitch range   (Fernald, 1984; Fernald and Simon, 1984; Marwick et al, 1984; Stern et al, 1982).   Motherese is preferred by young infants to less musical speech (Fernald,1985).

In baby talk, mothers exaggerate the self-synchrony and physiognomic matching of the movements of their different body parts, making similar shapes of expression by head rotations, eyebrow raising, mouth opening, voice glides and hand movement, their parts moving in synchrony.   The expressions of infants are coordinated, too.   In protoconversations such patterns within both mother and infant, become mutually entained between them, so that, for short intervals of time, very close inter-coordination (cooperative patterning) of expression is obtained.   This inter-coordination depends on a common beat and is assisted by mutual imitation and by matching or complementing of emotions.   Many of the mother's utterances and gestures in Motherese are imitations of the infant, often in a different modality, and the infant also moves into correspondence with the mother by imitating her. But, turn-taking and address-and-reply patterns are not driven by imitation. Indeed, protoconversation is formed by exchange of expressions that are complementary in form and feeling.

PROTOCONVERSATIONAL UTTERANCES FORESHADOW REFERENTIAL SPEECH AND GESTURES

In protoconversation, a mother will say her infant is 'talking' and 'telling a story',and she will reply with various degrees of agreement, surprise, praise, etc. to supposed utterances of her baby.   She seems to recognize signs of a motivation to speak.   In fact, the movements of the baby preceeding such utterances of the mother take the form of cooing vocalizations with a resonant 'core' resembling that of a speech syllable (Oller, 1981), or silent lip and tongue movements

resembling efforts at speech (pre-speech) (Trevarthen 1979, 1985),
and these utterances are accompanied by hand gestures (Trevarthen,
1986b).   Infant utterances (Table IB) are commonly made with a
brief orientation away from the mother, the baby breaking eye
contact for the duration of the utterance (approximately 3
seconds).   The mother's responses usually have a large excursion
of pitch and intonation, in either a questioning (rising) or
sympathetic (falling) form; then, after a pause she speaks more
invitingly again with falling-rising pitch contour to attract the
baby's attention back (Papousek et al, 1985, 1986; Stern et al,
1985; Trevarthen and Marwick, 1986).

     Typically, pronounced mutual orientation between mother and
baby, with sustained eye contact and smiling, is succeeded by the
expressive utterance of the baby, which appears to induce a
motive in the baby for referential expression.   Often the infant
orients from the mother to fixgaze on some 'topic' in their shared
environment.   After 6 months such re-orientation to refer
interest to something becomes quicker and more precise and
explicit, and the baby begins to combine distinctive vocal
requests or statements with pointing or reaching (see below).   I
believe that the cycles of orienting which, between conversing
adults, articulate interest in a topic with their interest in each
other, can be observed in protoconversation with an infant at 2
months.

UNIVERSAL PATTERNS OF BABY MUSIC

     Mothers sing to infants more than 3 months of age in many, if
not all, cultures and different languages have baby songs that are
similar in expressive structure (Trevarthen, 1986a, 1987).
Features of kinematics, (tempo and variation of the beat), rhythm
and melody, poetic form, rhyming and dramatic evolution appear to
transcend, and generate, cultural traditions.   Where
protoconversations with 2-month-olds are organised on a slower
adagio beat (1 1/3 beats/second), nearly all the songs with older
babies that we have analysed fall in the faster metronomic band of
andante near moderato (nearly 2 beats/second).   Many songs
integrate a vocal text with actions imposed on the baby's body.
It appears that the enjoyment infants get from joining in the
songs after 3 months derives from the increased body sense they
are gaining.   Such songs are rarely sung to younger babies.   By
5 or 6 months, baby songs and action games are common.   A
depressed mother will tend to sing in a way which does not engage
and please her infant; one case sang too slowly and regularly (an
even largo, (1/second) and with low mean pitch and little
variation of pitch or voice quality (Trevarthen, 1986a).   Babies
themselves are increasingly musical in their vocal expressions
(Papousek and Papousek, 1981).

UNIVERSALS OF EMOTION IN ENGAGEMENT

It is now well-established that, as Darwin proposed (Darwin, 1872), human emotions are expressed by a universal, and universally recognised, set of facial or motor action patterns (Ekman, 1973; Ekman et al, 1972). Vocal expressions also have universal patterns of quality, intensity and frequency variation related to different emotions. The same is true for body movements and hand gestures, though we have few systematic descriptions of these expressions. Infants shows their internal motivation state by vocal and facial patterns that partially match the ones adults use. The cries of newborns give information about central neural state in intricate variety (Lester, 1983). Facial expressions of joy, sadness, fear and annoyance are recognised from photographs of infants, and Facial Action Coding has been applied to describe emotional expressions like those of adults in newborns (Oster and Ekman, 1977).

In experiments with a double TV intercommunication technique and replay, it has been shown that a mother cannot converse with a recorded image of her 2-month old making utterances that was taped a few minutes previously. The engagement has to be live, with mutual awareness and mutual adjustment (Murray and Trevarthen, 1986). Infants, for their part, become distressed in pertubation tests in which the mother ceases to respond, or responds non-contingently (Cohn and Tronick, 1983; Murray and Trevarthen, 1985; Murray, 1988; Trevarthen 1985; Tronick et al 1978). The double video replay technique has shown that a 2-month old becomes similarly distressed when shown pre-recorded communicative behaviour of the mother, presumably because her image, though complete in physiognomic, kinematic and energetic patterning, is not synchronized, contingent or complementary with what the baby is doing (Murray and Trevarthen, 1985; Trevarthen, 1985). Observations with mothers suffering from severe depression show that their affective state is incompatible with successful face-to-face play and protoconversation with an infant, and indications are that this can cause at least temporary interference with the child's cognitive growth (Cohn and Tronick, 1983; Field, 1985; Fraiberg, 1980, Murray, 1988).

The double video communication technique has shown that, in face-to-face communication, the infant's emotions are in delicate equilibrium with the mother's expressions. Microanalysis of expressive forms in happy engagements and comparison with those when the infant's contact with the mother is broken or disrupted, or with the infant facing a stranger, has proved that a two-month-old has organized emotions adapted to regulation of contacts and relations with other persons.

Emotional attachment of the infant to a preferred caretaker, usually the mother, has been much studied with infants over 6 months of age. The foundation for such an attachment is established at birth.   Indeed, a mother's voice patterns may be distinguished and preferred in comparison with the voices of other women immediately after birth, which indicates that her voice characteristics had been learned in utero (De Casper   and Fifer, 1980).   Reactions of fear and caution with strangers are also evident in early months (Trevarthen, 1985, 1986b). The recent finding that infants as young as 3 months prefer people that adults find handsome or beautiful suggests that judgement of people's approachability or attractiveness depends, in part, on innate standards, presumably related to standard evaluations of emotional expression (Langlois et al, 1987).

Observations on hand movements of infants in circumstances that induce joy or distress indicate that the cerebral mechanisms for emotion may be laterally asymmetric at birth (Trevarthen, 1986b, 1988).   Infants 4 to 6 weeks of age make self-touching movements in distress with their left hands more, while their expressions in protoconventions more often combined with larger right hand movements.   Dichotic listening and evoked potential experiments also indicate that young infants are asymmetric in the auditory and visual perception of emotional expressions, and the data seems to indicate a precocity of the right half of the brain for emotional response.

FACTUAL COMMUNICATION ABOUT A SHARED AND 'INTERESTING' WORLD: LEARNING HOW TO 'MEAN'

After 9 months, infants acquire symbolic communication.   This requires a ready articulation between the child's cognition for objects and their purposeful use, on the one hand, and his or her communication with people on the other (Trevarthen and Hubley, 1978).   Symbols are motivated by a coorientation to people and to objective (factual) referents of potential joint interest (Trevarthen and Logotheti, 1987).   When infants of 7 to 9 months are about to embark upon the use of utterances with gestures to make 'acts of meaning' in communication with other people, they are both imitative and highly emotional, joining in excitable play and laughter with trusted companions and showing heightened fear and mistrust of strangers (Hubley and Trevarthen, 1979; Trevarthen and Hubley, 1978; Trevarthen, 1986b).   They address their rudimentary demands, refusals, enquiries, etc. with emotion, and they learn what other people refer to in speech or signing with particular attention to things that have emotional values attached to them, the child clearly looking and listening toward others, i.e. making 'emotional referencing', when confronted with any new experience (Bretherton et al, 1981; Dore, 1983, Halliday, 1975; Klinnert et al, 1983).   Stern et al (1982; 1985) have demonstrated how mothers give strong affective attunement to actions and interests of their infants and use language to name things or regulate actions with an exaggerated emotional gloss. Infants have been shown to use appropriate intonations in their photolinguistic utterances at about 1 year.

Emotions certainly play a part in the rapid development of toddlers' speech and understanding of language.   I would propose that the principles of affective and motivational engagement that have been elucidated by study of infants under 6 months of age are essential to the learning of language, and to the transmission of cultural knowledge.   Early speech, hand signing in deaf families and 'natural' reading before 3 years are all facilitated in play where the child can learn while sharing emotional evaluations, foci of interest and purposes of actions with trusted companions, who already know the language and who use it sympathetically and expressively with attention to the child's interest (Trevarthen, 1986b).

Towards the end of the first year infants are said to have acquired the concept of objects that have 'permanence', and this cognitive achievement is described as a precondition for many other behaviours that appear at about this age; such as, firm attachment to a caretaker, self-awareness, a 'theory of mind' for other people, and protolanguage.   These cognitive developments have been related to the formation of connections in the prefrontal cortex (Goldman-Rakic, 1987).   However, when the developments in manipulation, perception of people and object cognition are viewed in a perspective that recognizes the importance of communication in infant learning from birth, a different conclusion may be reached.   It seems likely that cognitive and problem-solving activities may develop at this age in coordination with changing motives for communication about experiences.   The interpersonal and affective dimension of the development may even be primary.   After the baby becomes cooperative and able to perform a joint task with the mother, the mother's language changes in a way that depends on her social class (Trevarthen and Marwick, 1986).   However, the fundamental change, common to all mothers of different cultures or sub-cultures, is that she uses more directives and instructions because the baby now complies willingly.   Her teaching changes because the baby's motives for communicating with her change.

GROWTH OF THE INFANT BRAIN

Primary communication behaviour is elaborated in the first 3 months before the dendro-synaptic organisation of the neocortex is achieved, and before the long association pathways within and between the hemispheres have differentiated (Trevarthen, 1986c). The main direct connection between the neocortices of the two hemispheres, the corpus callosum, goes through massive selective elimination of axons at this time and begins to gain myelin afterwards (Clarke et al, 1988).   Neocortical visual systems mature about the middle of the first year and auditory mechanisms of the neocortex develop more slowly, while speech is being learned (Lecours, 1982).   An infant starts to gain higher systems for control of posture and regulation of prehension between 3 and 6 months.   Effective walking begins after this.   Communications

by exchange of expressions of motivation and emotion and by mutual
engagement with other people is highly complex before these
developments in self-regulated mobility.

Recent studies of the development of the visual cortex of
kittens suggest that even the primary morphogenesis of the
neuronal system of visual perception, to build a mechanism capable
of binocular depth detection and vernier acuity (Held, 1985), is
regulated from the brain stem (Singer et al, 1982). It has been
known for 40 years that cortical activities are conditioned by
inputs from the reticular core of the midbrain that regulate
arousal and attention. Now we see that the development of
perceptual discrimination can be 'gated' by components of this
input from neurones in the reticular formation. The intricately
differentiated anatomy and chemistry of brainstem regulator
systems is established in late embryo and early fetal stages,
before the cortex begins to form. Limbic cortical tissues and
the basal ganglia mature prenatally, before neocortex (Chugani et
al, 1987). Monkeys learn to discriminate objects they see with
the aid of input from the limbic/emotional brain (Mishkin, 1982).
They require limbic input from the amygdala if they are to
associate visual and tactile experience of objects (Murray and
Mishkin, 1985). The parts of the temporal lobe cortex that are
essential to visual discrimination and learning and mature after
birth and their maturation is regulated by sex hormones as well as
by reticular and limbic inputs (Bachevalier and Mishkin, 1984;
Hagger et al, 1986). This is also true for visual functions of
human infants, male infants developing slower than females,
because they have more testosterone (Held, Bauer and Gwiazda,
1988).

Social communication depends upon limbic and meso-frontal
parts of the brain. The limbic and associated hypothalamic and
midbrain reticular components of the emotional system develop
prenatally but undergo modification for years, in adaptation to
the changing purposes of reproduction and parenting. Basal
ganglia systems important in control of instinctual motor patterns
and selective perception also develop their main organization
before the neocortex. Damage to limbic tissues and basal ganglia
cause disorders of communication and social coordination, and if
lesions occur in early life, effects may be seen only many months
later but their influence over other parts may manifest itself
long afterwards, indicating that postnatal maturation contributes
to the development of inherent social controls (Merjanian et al,
1986). Damage to reticular and hypothalamic centers of the
brainstem, and administration of pharmacological agents affecting
transmission of neurohormones from brainstem neurones, interfere
with motivation and emotion at their source. These structures
are organized in development prenatally. It has recently been
shown that neuro-hormones regulating brain growth in full term or
premature newborns respond to body contact and gentle tactile
stimulation, which therefore is a factor in support of brain

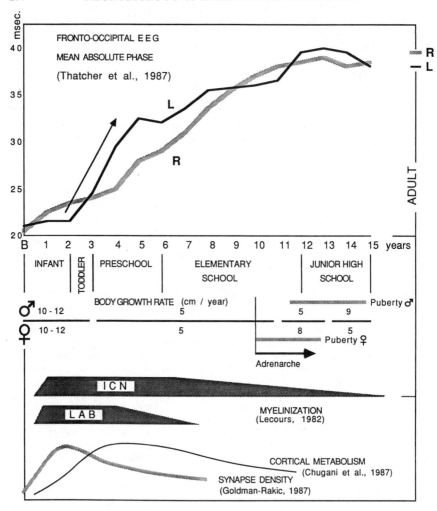

Figure 3: Postnatal developments in the brain. Left (L) and right (R) hemispheres show different profiles in rate of increase of connections, which are reflected in the EEG. There is a highly significant increase in the left hemisphere (arrow) between 2 and 4 years, when the vocabulary of the mother tongue is growing fastest. L A B – Long Association Bundles; I C N – Intracortical Neuropil.

maturation and function at this first stage of infancy (Schanberg
and Field, 1987).

Before birth, the human neo-cortex manifests left-right
differences in anatomy that are related to hemispheric
specializations for culturally important higher cognitive
functions, including language (Trevarthen, 1988).   Neocortical
territories are asymmetric in midfoetal stages, and postnatal
developments occur at different times on left and right sides.
In infants the right hemisphere appears more developed, but there
is a marked growth spurt in the left hemisphere between 3 and 5
years, when language is being learned most rapidly (Thatcher et
al, 1987) (Figure 3).   The origins of these asymmetries are
unknown, but they may be in subcortical systems, which are
different in size, organization or chemistry on the two sides, and
which may also lead to the increasingly evident hemispheric
differences in emotional processes (Fox and Davidson, 1984;
Gainotti, 1987; Tucker and Frederick, 1987).

DEVELOPMENTAL DISORDERS OF PSYCHO-SOCIAL GROWTH

Indirect evidence on the systems for emotion and
communication, which enter into the regulation of the maturation
of the neocortex after birth, comes from the children with
genetic disorders of brain development that simultaneously affect
communication and cognitive growth.

Autistic children lose the capacity for co-ordinating their
motivations with other people in the second or third year (Kanner,
1943).   They are unable to enter into cooperative activity,
failing to reciprocate with appropriate expressions.   They do
not play normally with their parents or siblings, may never speak
and tend to fall into self-absorbed stereotyped behaviour that
limits their opportunities for learning.   At all stages, autistic
children have difficulty in engaging with peers and teachers, and,
as they reciprocate poorly with emotions, they do not form close
relationships.   However, they do respond to a carefully adjusted
level of affectionate communication, often enjoy movement games
and music, and may respond to rough and tumble play.
Nevertheless, they rarely become competent members of society.
They do not grasp situations with normal curiosity and tend to
obsessional behaviour, and their cognitive and linguistic
development are abnormal, though to highly variable degrees.

As far as present evidence goes, autism is associated with
functional disturbance in limbic areas, hypothalamus, midline
thalamus, basal ganglia and parts of the cerebellum (Bauman and
Kemper, 1985; Courchesne et al, 1987; Damasio and Maurer, 1978).
Experiments with monkeys indicate that amygdala lesions sustained
soon after birth produce autistic symptoms 6 months later
(Merjanian et al, 1986).   In adult monkeys, mesofrontal lesions
cause deficiencies of emotional response and social isolation

comparable to autism (Myers, 1969).

Girls with Rett's syndrome appear nearly normal for the first 6 months then become somewhat autistic and lose motor coordination towards 12 months, as they begin to use protolanguage. After about 1½-2 years they drop back into a stable condition with a mental age of about 6 months, unlike autism because they orient readily to people and join in protoconversational and nursery song kinds of play (Hagberg et al, 1983; Kerr, 1987; Nomura et al, 1984). They seek eye contact and smile, and react appropriately to the prosody of speech. However, they remain profoundly mentally handicapped, do not speak or understand, cannot manipulate and rarely manage voluntary reaching and grasping of objects. Some are able to walk, but there are motor disorders. Their brains are smaller than normal after 2 years but appear normal to gross histological examination except for low pigmentation in the substantia nigra and locus ceruleus.

In Rett's syndrome, it appears that the genetic regulation of functions of the cortex beyond 6 to 9 months is defective, sparing the system that permits positive contact and communication at a level below language, while crippling cognition. Autism, with much more variable severity of cognitive and linguistic arrest, is a disorder that affects the motivation for communication more deeply, creating a deregulation of the control of attention to other people and of responses to their emotion. The mechanism of learning is retained, but deformed in a way that severely restricts and mastery of cultural conventions.

Defects in the X chromosomes (fragile-X sites) have been identified as one factor in both autism and Rett syndrome, and a similar fragile-X chromosome fault has been reported for Gerstmann's syndrome, in which the functions of the left hemisphere appear to be primarily affected, leading to finger agnosia, acalculia, failure to appreciate the relation of the body to that of another person and disturbance of abstract reasoning (Brown et al, 1986; Comings, 1986; Fisch et al, 1986; Grigsby et al, 1987; Hagerman et al, 1986). It would seem possible that a group of genes in the X chromosome is particularly important in the regulation of neocortical development by mechanisms of affective communication and intersubjectivity, which are highly active in early childhood.

REFERENCES

Bachevalier, J. and Mishkin, M. (1984). An early and a late
developing system for learning and retention in infant monkeys.
Behav. Neurosci. 98, 770-778.

Baldwin, J.M. (1894). Mental Development in the Child and the
Race. Macmillan, New York.

Bateson, M.C. (1975). Mother-infant exchanges: the epigenesis of
conversational-interaction. In Developmental Psycholinguistics
and Communication Disorders, Annals of the New York Academy of
Sciences, Vol. 263, (eds. D. Aaronson and R.W. Rieber).   New
York Academy of Sciences, New York.

Bauman, M.L. and Kemper, T.L. (1985).   Histoanatomic observations
of the brain in early infantile autism. Neurology, 35, 866-874.

Beebe, B. Jaffe, J., Feldstein, S., Mays, K. and Alison, D.
(1985). Inter- personel timing: The application of an adult
dialogue model to mother- infant vocal and kinesic interactions.
In Social Perception in Infants, (eds T.M. Field and N. Fox).
Norwood, NJ, Ablex.

Bowlby, J. (1969). Attachment and Loss, Volume 1; Attachment.
Hogarth Press, London.

Bretherton, I., McNew, S. and Beeghly-Smith, M. (1981).   Early
person knowledge as expressed in gestural and verbal
communication: When do infants acquire a "theory of mind"?
In Infant Social Cognition: Theoretical and Empirical
Considerations (eds. M.E. Lamb and L.R. Sherrod).   Lawrence
Erlbaum, Hillsdale N.J.

Brown, W.T.. Jenkins, E.C., Cohen, I.L., Fisch, G.S., Wolf-Schen,
E.G.,Gross A., Waterhouse, L., Fein, D., Mason-Brothers, A.,
Ritvo, E., Ruttenberg, B.A., Bentley, W. and Castells, S.
(1986). Fragile-X and autism: A multicenter survey. Am. J.
Med. Genet. 23, 341-352.

Bullowa, M. (ed) 1979. Before Speech; The Beginnings of Human
Communication. Cambridge University Press, London.

Burford, B. (1988). Action cycles: Rhythmic actions for
engagement with children and young adults with Profound Mental
Handicap. Europ. J. Spec. Needs Educ., in press.

Carpenter, G.C. (1973). Differential response to mother and
stranger within the first month of life. Bull. Brit. Psychol.
Soc., 26, 138

Carpenter, G.C., Tecce, J.J., Stechler, G. and Freidmann, S. (1970). Differential visual behaviour to human and humanoid faces in early infancy. Merrill-Palmer Quart., 16, 91-108.

Chugani, H.T., Phelps, M.E. and Mazzotta, J.C. (1987). Positron emission tomography study of human brain functional development, Ann. Neurol., 22, 587-497.

Clarke, S., Kraftsik, R., Van der Loos, H. and Innocenti, G.M. (1988). Forms and measures of adult and developing human corpus callosum. Is there sexual dimorphism? J. Comp. Neurol., in press.

Cohn, J.F. and Tronick, E.Z. (1983). Three-month-old infants' reaction to simulated maternal depression. Child Devel., 54, 185-193.

Comings, D.E. (1986). The genetic Rett Syndrome: The consequences of a disorder where every case is a new mutation. Am. J. Med. Genet., 24, 383-388.

Condon, W.S. and Sander, L.W. (1974). Neonate movement is synchronised with adult speech; interactional participation and language acquisition. Science, 183, 99-101.

Courchesne, E., Yeung-Courchesne, R., Hesselink, J.R. and Jernigan, T.L., (1987). Abnormal neuroanatomy in non-retarded person with autism. Archiv. Neurol, 44, 335-341.

Darwin, C. (1872). The Expression of Emotions in Man and Animals. Methuen, London.

Damasio, A.R. and Maurer, T.G. (1978). A neurological model for childhood autism. Arch. of Neurol., 35, 777-786.

DeCasper, A. and Fifer, W. (1980). Of human bonding: Newborns prefer mother's voices. Science, 208, 1174.

Dore, J. (1983) Feeling, form and intention in the baby's transition to language. In The Transition from Pre-linguistic Communication (ed. R. Golinkoff). Lawrence Erlbaum, Hillsdale N.J.

Ekman, P. (1973). Cross-cultural studies of facial expression. In Darwin and Facial Expression, (ed. P. Ekman). New York and London; Academic Press.

Ekman, P., Friesen W.V. and Ellsworth, P. (1972). Emotion in the Human Face. Pergamon Press, New York.

Fantz, R.L. (1963).   Pattern vision in newborn infants.
Science, 140, 296- 297.

Fernald, A. (1984).   The perceptual and affective salience of
mother's speech to infants.   In The Origins and Growth of
Communication (eds. L. Feagans, C. Garvey, R. Golinkoff and
others).   Ablex, Norwood, N.J.

Fernald, A. (1985).   Four-month-old infants prefer to listen to
motherese.   Infant Behav., 8, 181-195.

Fernald, A. and Simon, T. (1984).   Expanded intonation contours in
mothers'speech to newborns.   Devel. Psychol., 20, 104-113.

Field, T.M. (1982).   Individual differences in the expressivity
of neonate and young infants.   Development of Non-verbal
Behaviour in Children, (ed. R.W. Feldman).   Springer Verlag, New
York.

Field, T.M. (1985).   Neonatal perception of people: Maturational
and individual differences.   In Social Perception in Infants,
(ed. T.M. Field and N. Fox).   Ablex, Norwood, N.J.

Field, T.M., Woodson, R., Greenberg, R. and Cohen, D. (1982).
Discrimination and imitation of facial expressions by neonates.
Science, 218, 179-181.

Fisch, G.S., Cohen, I.L., Wolf, E.G., Brown, W.T. and Jenkins,
E.C. (1986) Autism and fragile-X syndrome.   Am. J. Psychiat.,
143, 71-73.

Fox, N.A. and Davidson, R.J. (1984) (Eds.)   The Psychology of
Affective Development.   Lawrence Erlbaum, Hillsdale, N.J.

Fraiberg, R. (1980).   Clinical Studies in Infant Mental Health:
The First Year of Life.   Tavistock, London.

Gainotti, G. (1987).   Disorders of emotional behaviour and of
autonomic arousal resulting from unilateral brain damage.   In
Duality and Unity of the Brain (ed. D. Ottoson) (Wenner-Gren
International Symposium Series, No. 47).   Macmillan, London.

Goldman-Rakic, P.S. (1987).   Development of cortical circuitry and
cognitive function.   Child Development, 58, 601-622.

Grieser, D.L. and Kuhl, P.K. (1988).   Maternal speech to infants
in a tonal language: Support for universal prosodic features in
motherese.   Devel. Psychol, 24, 14-20.

Grigsby, J.P., Kemper, M.B. and Hagerman, R.J. (1987).
Developmental Gerstmann syndrome without aphasia in fragile-X
syndrome. Neuropsychologia, 25, 881-891.

Hagberg, B., Aicardi, J., Dias, K. and Ramos, O. (1983). A
progressive syndrom of autism, dementia, ataxia and loss of
purposeful hand use in girls.   Rett syndrome: report of 35
cases.   Annals Neurol., 14, 471-479.

Hagerman, R.J., Jackson, A.W.III, Braden, M., Rimland, B. and
Levitas, A. (1986).   An analysis of autism in fifty males with
fragile-X syndrome.   Amer. J. Med. Genet., 23, 353-358.

Hagger, C., Bachevalier, J., and Bercu, B.B. (1986).   The effects
of perinatal testosterone on the development of habit formation
in infant monkeys.   Soc. Neurosci. Abst., 12, 23.

Halliday, M.A.K. (1975).   Learning How to Mean, Arnold, London.

Held, R. (1985).   Binocular vision - behavioural neuronal
development.   In Neonate Cognition: Beyond the Blooming, Buzzing
Confusion (eds. J. Mehler and R. Fox).   Erlbaum, Hillsdale, NJ.

Held, R., Bauer, J. and Gwiazda, J. (1988).   Age of onset of
binocularity correlates with level of plasma testosterone in
male infants.   Invest. Opthal. and Vis. Sci. (Suppl.), 29, 60.

Hubley, P. and Trevarthen, C. (1979).   Sharing a task in infancy.
In Social Interaction During Infancy, New Directions for Child
Development, Vol. 4 (ed. I. Uzgiris). Jossey-Bass, San
Fransisco.

Kanner, L. (1943).   Autistic disturbances of affective contact.
Nervous Child, 2, 217-250.

Kerr, A.M. (1987).   Report on the Rett Syndrome Workshop:
Glasgow, Scotland, 24-25 May 1986.   Ment. Defic. Res., 31, 93-
113.

Klinnert, M.D., Campos, J., Sorce, J., Emde, R. and Svejda, M.
(1983).   Emotions as behaviour regulators: Social referencing in
infancy.   In Emotion: Theory, Research and Experience, Vol. 2.
Emotions in Early Development (eds. R. Plutchik and H.
Kellerman).   Academic Press, New York.

Kugiumutzakis, J.E. (1985).   The Origins, Development, and
Function of the Early Infant Imitation.   Uppsala University,
Ph.D. Thesis.   Acta Universitatis Uppsaliensis, 35.

Kuhl, P.K. (1987). Perception of speech and sound in early infancy. In Handbook of Infant Perception, Vol. 2, From Perception to Cognition. (eds. P. Salapatek and L. Cohn). Academic Press, New York.

Kuhl, P.K. and Meltzoff, A.N., (1982). The bimodal perception of speech in infancy. Science, 218, 1138-1141

Langlois, J.H., Roggman, L.A., Casey, R.J., Ritter, J.M., Rieser-Danner, L.A. and Jenkins, V.Y. (1987). Infant preferences for attractive faces: Rudiments of a stereotype?   Devel. Psychol. 23, 363-369.

Lecours, A.R. (1982). Correlates of developmental behaviour in brain maturation. In Regression in Mental Development: Basic Phenomena and Theories. (ed. T.G. Bever). Erlbaum, Hillsdale, NJ.

Lester, B.M., 1983. A biosocial model of infant crying. Advances in Infancy Research, Vol. 3. (eds L.P. Lipsitt and R. Roves-Collier). Ablex, Norwood, N.J.

MacKain, K., Studdert-Kennedy, M., Speiker, S. and Stern, D.N. (1983). Infant intermodal speech perception is a left-hemisphere function. Science, 219, 1347-1349.

Maratos, O. (1973). The Origin and Development of Imitation in the First Six Months of Life.   Ph.D. thesis, University of Geneva.

Maratos, O. (1982). Trends in the development of imitation in early infancy. Regression in Mental Development, (ed. T.G. Bever) Erlbaum, Hillside, N.J.

Marwick, H., Mackenzie,J., Laver J. and Trevarthen, C. (1984). Voice quality as an expressive system in mother-to-infant communication: A case study. Work in Progress, No. 17. University of Edinburgh, Department of Linguistics.

Mehler, J. (1985). Language related dispositions in early infancy. In Neonate Cognition, (eds. J. Mehler and R. Fox). Erlbaum, Hillsdale, NJ.

Mehler, J., Bertoncini, J. and Barriere, M. (1978). Infant recognition of mothers voice. Perception, 7, 491-497.

Meltzoff, A.N. and Moore, M.H. (1977). Imitation of facial and manual gestures by human neonates. Science, 198, 75-78.

Meltzoff, A.N. and Moore, M.H. (1983). Newborn infants imitate adult facial gestures. Child Devel., 54, 702-709.

Merjanian, P.M., Bachevalier, J., Crawford, H. and Mishkin, M. (1986). Socio-emotional disturbances in the development rhesus monkey following neonatal limbic lesions. Soc. Neuro. Sci. Abstr., 12, 23.

Mishkin, M. (1982). A memory system in the monkey. Phil. Trans. Soc. Lond., Series B, 298, 85-95.

Murray, E.A. and Mishkin, M. (1985). Amygdalectomy impairs cross-modal association in monkeys. Science, 228, 406-606.

Murray, L. 1988. Effects of post-natal depression on infant development: Direct studies of early mother-infant interactions. In Motherhood and Mental Illness, Vol. 2 (eds I. Brockington and R. Kumar). John Wright, Bristol.

Murray, L. and Trevarthen, C. (1985). Emotional regulation of interactions between two-month-olds and their mothers. In Social Perception in Infants, (eds. T. Field and N. Fox). Ablex, Norwood, NJ.

Murray, L. and Trevarthen, C. (1986). The infant's role in mother-infant communication. In Journal of Child Language, 13, 15-29.

Myers, R.E. (1969). Neurology of social communication in primates Proceedings of the Second International Congress of Primatology, Atlanta, Georgia, Vol. III. Karger, Basel, New York.

Nomura, Y., Segawa, M. and Hasegawa, M. (1984). Retts Syndrome - clinical studies and pathophysiological consideration. Brain and Devel., 6, 475-486.

Oller, D.K. (1981). Infant vocalizations: Exploration and reflexivity. In Language Behaviour in Infancy and Early Childhood (ed R.E. Stork) Elsevier, North Holland, Amsterdam.

Oster, H. and Ekman, P. (1977). Facial behaviour in child development. In Minnesota Symposia in Child Development (Vol. 11).

Papousek, M. (1987). Models and messages in the melodies of maternal speech in tonal and non-tonal languages. Abstracts, Society for Research in Child Development, 6, 407.

Papousek, M. and Papousek, H. (1981). Musical elements in infants' vocalization: Their significance for communication, cognition and creativity. In Advances in Infancy Research (Vol. 1). Ablex, Norwood, N.J.

Papousek, M., Papousek, H. and Bornstein, M.H. (1985). The naturalistic vocal environment of young infants: On the significance of homogeneity and variability in parental speech. In Social Perception in Infants, (eds T.M. Field and N. Fox). Ablex, Norwood, N.J.

Papousek, M., Papousek, H. and Koester, L.S. (1986). Sharing emotionality and sharing knowledge: A microanalytic approach to parent-infant communication. In Measuring Emotions in Infants and Children Vol. 2, (eds C.E. Izard and P.B. Read). Cambridge University Press, New York.

Piaget, J. (1954). Origins of Intelligence, Basic Books, New York.

Schanberg, S.M. and Field, T.M. (1987). Sensory deprivation stress and supplemental stimulation in the rat pup and preterm human neonate. Child Devol., 58, 1431-1447

Singer, W., Tretter, F. and Yinon. W. (1982). Central gating of developmental plasticity in kitten visual cortex. J. Physiol., 324, 221-237.

Snow, C.E. (1977). The development of conversation between mothers and babies. J. Child Lang., 4, 1-22.

Spelke, E.S. (1985). Perception of unity, persistence and identity: Thoughts on infants' conception of objects. Neonate Cognition: Beyond the Blooming Buzzing Confusion (eds J. Mehler and R. Fox), Erlbaum, Hillsdale, N.J.

Sroufe, L.A. and Waters, E. (1976). The autogenesis of smiling and laughter: A perspective on the organization of development in infancy. Psychol. Rev., 83, 173-189

Stern, D.N. (1971). A micro-analysis of mother-infant interaction: Behavioural regulation of social contact between a mother and her 3½ month old twins. J. Am. Acad. Ch. Psychiat., 10, 501-517.

Stern, D.N. (1974a). Mother and infant at play: The dyadic interaction involving facial, vocal and gaze behaviors. In The Effect of the Infant on Its Caregiver. (eds. M. Lewis and L. Rosenblum). John Wiley, New York.

Stern, D.N. (1974b). The goal and structure of infant play. Amer. Acad. Ch. Psychiat., 13, 402-421.

Stern, D.N. (1985). The Interpersonal World of the Infant. Basic Books, New York.

Stern, D.N. (1986). Affect attunement. In Frontiers of Infant Psychiatry, Vol. 2. (eds. J.D. Call. E. Galenson and R.L. Tyson). Basic Books, New York.

Stern, D.N., Spieker, S. and MacKain, K. (1982). Intonation Contours as signals in maternal speech to prelinguistic infants. Devel. Psych., 18, 191-195.

Stern, D.N., Speiker, S. Barnett, R.K. and MacKain, K. (1983). The prosody of maternal speech: Infant age and context related changes. J. Ch. Lang., 10, 1-15

Stern, D.M., Hofer, L., Hart, W. and Dore, J. (1985). Affect attunement: The sharing of feeling states between mother and infant by means of inter-model fluency. In Social Perception in Infants. (eds. T.M. Field and N. Fox). Ablex, Norwood, NJ.

Studdert-Kennedy, M. (1983). On learning to speak. Human Neurobiology, 2: 191-195.

Thatcher, R.W., Walker, R.A. and Giudice, S. (1987) Human cerebral hemispheres develop at different rates and ages. Science, 236, 1110-1113.

Trevarthen, C. (1974). The psychobiology of speech development. In Language and Brain Development Aspects, Neurosciences Research Programme Bulletin, 12, 570-585, (ed E.H. Lenneberg) Neurosciences Research Program, Boston.

Trevarthen, C. (1977). Descriptive analysis of infant communication behaviour. In Studies of Mother-Infant Interaction: The Loch Lomond Symposium, (ed. H.R. Schaffer). Academic Press, London.

Trevarthen, C. (1979). Communication and cooperation in early infancy. A description of primary intersubjectivity. In Before Speech: The Beginnings of Human Communication. (ed. M. Bullowa) Cambridge University Press, London.

Trevarthen, C. (1983). Interpersonal abilities of infants as generators for transmission of language and culture. In The Behavior of Human Infants. (eds. A. Oliverio and M. Zapella), Plenum, London and New York.

Trevarthen, C. (1984a). Biodynamic structures, cognitive correlates of motive sets and development of motives in infants. In Cognition and Motor Processes (eds W. Prinz and A.F. Saunders). Berlin, Heidelberg-New York: Springer Verlag.

Trevarthen, C. (1984b). How control of movements develops. In Human Motor Actions: Bernstein Reassessed. (ed. H.T.A. Whiting). Elsevier (North Holland), Amsterdam.

Trevarthen, C. (1985)   Facial expressions of emotion in mother-infant interaction.   Human Neurobiol. 4, 21-32.

Trevarthen, C. (1986a).   Development of intersubjective motor control in infants.   In Motor Developments in Children: Aspects of Co-ordination and Control.   (eds. M.G. Wade and H.T.A. Whiting).   Martinus Nijhof, Dordrecht.

Trevarthen, C. (1986b).   Form, significance and psychological potention of hand gestures of infants.   In The Biological Foundation of Gestures: Motor and Semiotic Aspects, (eds J.L. Nespoulous, P. Perron and A. Roch) M.I.T. Press, Cambridge, Mass.

Trevarthen, C. (1986c).   Neuroembryology and the development of perceputal mechanisms.   In Human Growth, (2nd Ed.) (eds F. Falkner and J.M. Tanner).   Plenum, New York.

Trevarthen, C. (1987).   Sharing makes sense: Intersubjectivity and the making of an infants meaning.   In Language Topics: Essays in Honor of Michael Halliday.   (eds. R. Steele and T. Threadgold).   John Benjamins, Amsterdam and Philadelphia.

Trevarthen, C. (1988).   Growth and education of the hemispheres. In Brain Circuits and Functions of the Mind: Essays in Honour of Roger W. Sperry.   (ed. C. Trevarthen).   Cambridge University Press, New York.

Trevarthen, C. and Hubley, P. (1978).   Secondary intersubjectivity: Confidence, confiding and acts of meaning in the first year.   In Action, Gesture and Symbol.   (ed. A. Lock) Academic Press, London.

Trevarthen, C. and Logotheti, K. (1987).   First symbols and the nature of human knowledge.   In Symbolism and Knowledge (eds. J. Montangero, A. Tryphon and S. Dionnet).   Jean Piaget Archives Foundation, Geneva.

Trevarthen, C. and Marwick, H. (1986).   Signs of motivation for speech in infants, and the nature of a mother's support for development of language.   In Precursors of Early Speech (eds B. Lindblom and R. Zetterstrom).   Macmillan, London/Stockholm Press, New York.

Trevarthen, C. Murray and Hubley, P. (1981).   Psychology of infants.   In Scientific Foundations of Clinical Paediatrics . (eds. J. Davis and J. Dobbing).   W. Heinemann Medical Books Ltd, London.

Tronick, E.Z., Als, H., Adamson, L., Wise, S. and Brazelton, T.B. (1978). The infant's response to entrapment between contradictory messages in face-to-face interaction. J. Amer. Acad. Ch. Psychiat., <u>17</u>, 1-13.

Tucker, D.M. and Frederick, S.L. (1987). Emotion and brain laterilization. In <u>Handbook of Psychophysiology: Emotion and Social Behavior</u>. (eds. H. Wagner and T. Manstead) John Wiley, New York.

Van Rees, S. and de Leeuw, R. (1987). <u>Born Too Early: The Kangaroo Method with Premature Babies</u>. Video by Stichting Lichaamstaal, Scheyvenhofweg 12, 6092 NK, Leveroy, The Netherlands.

Winnicott, D.W. (1965). <u>The Maturational Process and the Facilitating Environment</u>, Hogarth, London.

19

Ontogeny of Social Interactions in Newborn Infants

Hanuš Papoušek and Mechthild Papoušek

ADAPTIVE SIGNIFICANCE OF SOCIAL INTERACTIONS

Human newborns cannot survive without adequate social help. Temporarily, they may be left alone if there is no need for interventions. Even then, however, someone appears again under predictable conditions or may be called back by the newborn's cry: some kind of social interaction is still present. Any type of newborn behavior may elicit parental attention and intervention, and may thus become a part of social interactions.

In a broad sense, therefore, social interactions do not represent any special category of behaviors; rather, the term of social interactions indicates the observer's approach to infant behaviors. It says that the observer is not willing to analyse infant behaviors outside natural contexts, that he is aware of a dialogic interchange between infants and caregivers in which any observable behavior simultaneously functions as both a response and a stimulus, and thus, unlike in S-R designs, requires rather complex analyses. In addition, those analyses also necessitate a revision of the available knowledge on caregivers' behaviors.

In a narrow sense, early social interactions have been studied from the point of view of mother-infant bonding. Those studies have been influenced by ethological concepts of imprinting and emotional attachment, and to a certain degree biased by animal models: the mother has been seen as an exclusive representative of social environment. Preverbal communication has been under-researched, although human social interactions are hardly think-able without it. Comparative concepts, however, also pay atten-tion to the adaptive significance and evolutionary past of observed behaviors.

In humans, adaptation has been crucially influenced by the emergence of symbolic communication and speech. Verbal communica-tion allowed man to accumulate and integrate a vast amount of

information across generations and cultural borders without the
necessity to learn every piece of information from an immediate
experience. Consequently, man has been able to develop culture
and technology, and with their help to overcome various physiological constraints. Man is not the best runner, jumper, or swimmer
among animals, nor can man fly like birds. Human infants are
truly altricial in motor development. Due to technology, however,
man is able to distance all animals in locomotion, and it is the
communicative competence which accounts for the difference. As to
the communicative development, human infants are doubtlessly
precocious. Consequently, the role of social interactions in the
development of communication calls for a special attention.

HUMAN COMMUNICATION

Although nobody expects the newborn to speak, the significance of speech and discrepant interpretations of its origin call
for a close and comparative look at the very beginning of infant-
parent dialogues. In general, namely, a high degree of biological
relevance in adaptive capacities is usually expressed in their
universal distribution within the given species, in early appearance during ontogeny -- albeit in the form of elementary precursors -- as well as in co-evolution of supportive counterparts
in environment. These aspects of speech acquisition still lack
satisfactory interpretations.

The newborn's nutritive sucking can exemplify this argument.
The complex nervous regulation of sucking is fully functional
immediately after birth, allows the newborn to suck, breathe, and
swallow without suffocation in long periods of smooth performance
which an adult is unable to imitate. The functions of maternal
breast, the nipple in particular, have evolved as a harmonious
counterpart to the newborn's need, including maternal behaviors
which compensate for the newborn's constraints in locomotion.
Moreover, the secretion of prolactin in response to sucking on
maternal nipple fulfills important adaptive functions inasmuch as
it inhibits the maturation of further ovarian follicles and
effectively prevents further pregnancy in the mother as long as
she nurses frequently enough and in intervals shorter than 30
minutes (Konner & Worthman, 1980). In preurban human societies,
this form of contraception has regulated the rate of reproduction
within optimal physiological limits. Comparative and interdisciplinary approaches to this problem helped to elucidate the
co-evolution of biological determinants of breastfeeding and their
significance for human evolution in general.

If we now want to consider the role of social interactions in
the development of communication we first have to consider the
corresponding competencies which might have evolved both on the
side of the newborn and on the side of social environment. The
polar difference between the newborn, unable to speak and un-

experienced in social interrelations, and the caregiver, with his verbal competence and social experience, attributes to early social interactions the character of didactic interactions, if we assume that the newborn is intrinsically motivated for acquisition of knowledge, and the caregiver for sharing knowledge (Papoušek & Papoušek, 1987).

For various reasons, early social interactions have seldom been investigated from this point of view. One reason may be that comparative research could not provide stimulating examples from non-human animals. Another reason may be the lack of conscious evidence on past or present programs for teaching infants how to speak. Not a long time ago, Lenneberg (1971) complained that no convenient hierarchy in the structure of language and no learning order was known to offer a tool for teaching.

Crossculturally adopted infants prove that infants acquire speech through both innate prerequisites, and early learning; when they start speaking they use the language of adoptive rather than biological parents. If we view speech acquisition as a self-regulating process of development rather than a teleologically selected genetic preadaptedness, then it is difficult to interpret the experience with crossculturally adopted infants unless some form of a didactic lead is taken into account. If there is no clear evidence on conscious and rational programs for such support, we have to scrutinize nonconscious, intuitive behaviors.

In adults, the realm of nonconscious behaviors has attracted an increasing attention for several general reasons. Studies on motor skills have shown that a nonconscious integration of skills in innumerable repetitions during training is more effective than a rational guidance for achievement of a champion performance in sports or a virtuoso performance in music. Nonconsciously integrated skills seem to be much more resistant against amnesia than rationally integrated skills. Cognitive psychologists increasingly acknowledge that nonconscious integrations of experience play a crucial role in complex cognitive operations (Kihlström, 1987). The question of consciousness has also been reattacked in informatics and cybernetics since there, conscious-ness represents a keystone in attempts to construct artificial intelligence.

The authors' studies have concerned both aspects of the didactic potential in early social interactions: the newborn's integrative competence, and the caregiver's didactic competence.

THE NEWBORN'S INTEGRATIVE COMPETENCE

Earlier studies of the first author (Papoušek, 1977) elucida-ted several aspects of neonatal learning which are relevant to the present topic. Learning experiments involved head-turning which

is relatively well coordinated in newborns, and required integration of experience in several modalities: acoustic, gustatory, and
proprioceptive. Modifications of those designs also allowed to
study the earliest forms of intentionality in newborns. Following
the Konorski's model, learning designs included both elements of
contingency, and the necessity of adjusting instrumental acts to
environmental signals. Experimenting was motivated by interest in
the process of and interindividual differences in learning rather
than in the mere first signs of learning abilities.

Developmental differences in the rate of learning evidenced
that learning is slow in newborns but becomes substantially faster
during the first trimester, not only due to maturation but also
due to training. For instance, newborns were able to solve a
difficult task -- discriminative learning -- much faster if they
first learned how to solve easier tasks -- simple conditioning,
extinction, and reconditioning (Papoušek, 1977). Although the
study did not primarily focussed at didactic principles, it did
demonstrate for the first time that a proper arrangement could
have a didactic effect.

Changes in facial expressions and vocalization of learning
infants indicated that infants experienced unsuccessful learning
as unpleasant and successful learning as pleasant. Moreover,
having detected a contingent event, infants activated exploratory
efforts to a degree which was close to the limit of physiological
reserves. Only an intrinsic mechanism, which we called a "biological fuse", helped very young infants to avoid exhaustion of
reserves. Hypothetically, we concluded that infants were strongly
motivated to explore environment and accumulate information on it.

The fact that newborns can improve learning abilities through
practising helps understand the significance of infant learning
which is seemingly questioned by infantile amnesia. It is true
that most if not all information on infants' environment and
events gets lost due to amnesia. However, infants not only learn
the forms, dimensions or colors of things around them but they
also learn how to improve motor skills, learning and cognitive
operations, and communicative subroutines. In other words,
infants accumulate not only declarative, data-based information
but also procedure-based information. During the first postpartum
months learning concerns procedural information almost exclusively. Resistance against amnesia is higher in procedural learning
than in data-based learning as it is evident in both experimental
research and clinical studies (Cohen & Squire, 1980). Thus we can
speculate that infants mainly profit from procedural learning.
Learning how to learn and think may well be the most relevant
aspect of infant learning at all: the acquisition of speech is
hardly thinkable in the absence of fast perceptual and integrative
capacities. Profit in this area of learning is obviously not
affected by infantile amnesia.

THE PARENT'S DIDACTIC COMPETENCE

Our search for naturalistic situations in which infants might practise integrative operations revealed few in relation to physical enviroment but a plenty in dyadic interchanges between infants and parents or other caregivers (Papoušek & Papoušek, 1984). It soon became obvious that, with a remarkable univers- ality across sex, age, and cultures, not only parents but also children and strangers regularly and specifically modify behaviors and vocal utterances when interacting with newborns or infants. Modifications correspond to finely adjusted didactic interven- tions; however, caregivers carry them out unknowingly, are unable to report on them consciously, and find them difficult to control if they become aware of them.

We have detected and described several sets of such noncon- scious, intuitive behaviors and analysed their relations to various interactional contexts (Papoušek & Papoušek, 1987). We did so in microanalytic evaluations of audiovisual records of either naturalistic interactions or interactions in laboratory settings that were modified in order to verify working hypotheses. Studies involved mothers, fathers, or unfamiliar females of German origin, and mother-infant dyads in American Caucasian and Mandarin Chinese populations (M. Papoušek & Papoušek, 1987).

We have found that caregivers in general tend to display simple and repetitive behavioral patterns toward infants and to make those patterns contingent on infant behaviors. Thus care- givers make it easier to infants to conceptualize, to predict, or to manipulate caregiving activities. Caregivers offer similar chances not only abundantly but also with respect to the infant's behavioral state and attention. They test the infant's muscle tone in the area of fingers, chin and mouth when behavioral cues in infants signal potential changes in state, and they intervene to either keep infants in quiet waking state or to facilitate transitions to quiet sleep (Papoušek & Papoušek, 1984). In this way caregivers seem to contribute to the developmental decrease in transitional states of either fussiness and poorly coordinated, fidgety motor activities, or passivity with decreased responsive- ness. Those transitional states are known to be unfavorable for infant learning.

From the very beginning, caregivers tend to imitate infants' facial expressions and quiet vocal sounds. At the same time, caregivers display similar behavioral models, encourage infants to imitate those models, and consistently reward them for attempts to do so (M. Papoušek & Papoušek, in press). According to current knowledge, vocal imitation of novel sound patterns does not appear prior to 9 months of age. Nonetheless, reciprocal vocal matching and vocal play regularly participate in earlier parent-infant dialogues, and there, matching concerns only those sounds and sound features which are subjected to infantile practising during that time (Papoušek & Papoušek, in press). Thus, caregivers provide infants with a modelling/echoing frame which allows infants to link production and auditory-visual perception of newly acquired sounds. Interestingly, 4-to-5-month-old infants are capable of amodal audio-visual and audio-visual-motor integration of speech sounds, according to Kuhl & Meltzoff (1984). This ability has been considered a crucial prerequisite for both imitation of speech sounds, and speech acquisition (Studdert--Kennedy, 1986).

Considering the involvement of facial behaviors in the production of speech sounds and in the expression of affective states, it is not surprising that caregivers strongly tend to draw the infant's visual attention to the caregiver's face and to achieve eye-to-eye contact. This tendency is, however, very unusual among animals, including nonhuman primates, where a direct eye-to-eye contact signals threat and aggression. According to the present evidence, the tendency to achieve eye-to-eye contact for prosocial purposes, such as the intuitive didactic interventions, exemplifies species-specific components in human interactional behaviors (Papoušek, Papoušek, Suomi & Rahn, in press).

In general, the given examples of intuitive sets of behaviors adequately compensate for the initial constraints in infant integrative capacities and grant a didactic character to the caregiver's tendency to mediate the newborn's first confrontation with the novel environment. While doing so, the caregiver carefully follows the progress in infant capacities and supports practising and improving those which are most adaptive under the given cultural and ecological circumstances. It is astonishing to see how perfect the non-conscious didactic programs may be in comparison with the state of arts in the classical didactics which have been based upon rational, conscious knowledge. In no other example is this aspect as evident as in the parental support, related to the acquisition of speech.

THE BEGINNING OF VOCAL COMMUNICATION

Newborns cannot speak, of course, and their integrative competence -- although much higher than expected a few decades ago -- is still too far from the level enabling verbal symbolization. Nevertheless, caregivers treat newborns as potential thinkers and conversational partners. Both parents and strangers strongly tend to talk to newborns while using a very interesting modification of speech, called "babytalk" or "motherese". This modification distinctly deviates from adult linguistic principles and at the same time exemplifies the intuitive didactic tendencies in caregivers par excellence.

It is useful first to design a didactic script for the support of early speech prerequisites on the base of our present

-- and very young -- knowledge. The newborn's vocal tract is not yet developed enough to allow a fine differentiation of vocal sounds. It approximately corresponds to the developmental level of vocal tracts in Neanderthalians or chimpanzees (Lieberman, 1984). With the exception of cry, the newborn is merely able to produce a vowel-like "fundamental voicing" (Papoušek & Papoušek, 1981) -- a "quasi resonant nucleus", according to Oller (1986), -- which is only superimposed upon the momentary type of respiration, since the newborn is not yet able to prolongate expiration for the purpose of noncry vocalizations. Thus, it would be advisable to teach the infant how to prolongate the vowel-like sounds, improve their resonance, and finally produce distinct human vowels.

Before distinct consonants appear and enable segmenting the vowels into canonic syllables around seven months of age, too little is seemingly available for mediating symbolic information through vocalization. The only thinkable way would be to utilize the paralinguistic features of vowel-like sounds, such as the modulation of pitch, and on this base, to create the first elementary "vocabulary" of messages on the most relevant aspects of social interactions. Such didactic device would at least allow teaching the infant that vocal sounds may mediate information and that it is useful to learn them. Considering the preconditions of successful learning in newborns and very young infants (Papoušek & Papoušek, 1984), the caregiver would have to use a small number of distinct vocal patterns and patiently repeat them many times during the short periods of quiet waking state in infants.

If, with this hypothetical design in mind, we look at the qualities of vocal interchanges between infants and caregivers, we find an astonishing congruency between what the caregivers intuitively do, and what, at present, an infancy researcher could recommend them to do for didactic purposes.

In the babytalk, caregivers use simple, repetitive vocal utterances, slow down the tempo of speech, strikingly prolongate vowels and display them in an unusually melodic way. The melody of utterances -- the prosodic contours -- substantially differ from the complex, less conspicuous and multilevel prosody of speech between two adults. The prosody of babytalk disengages from its dependence on syntactic rules and starts functioning as a carrier of the first prototypical messages relating to the most relevant contextual aspects of social interactions between infants and caregivers (Papoušek, Papoušek & Bornstein, 1985).

For instance, distinct acoustic configurations indicate the presence and individuality of the caregiver, the caregiver's readiness to help and satisfy infant needs, the caregiver's need of more information from the infant, the caregiver's offer to engage in playful activities or to demonstrate vocal models worth imitating, etc. Melodic patterns may also tell the infant in general whether its behaviors are appropriate or inappropriate in

the given context (Papoušek, Papoušek & Koester, 1986). Caregivers use a relatively small number of prototypical contours but
repeat them many times in contingent relations to infant behaviors. The contours thus become the salient units of babytalk
which infants may detect and process very early. The verification
of this assumption is currently under the authors' investigation.

On the whole, the presented materials point to an aspect of
early social interactions which has long escaped attention,
although it concerns an important issue of human phylogeny and
ontogeny. According to our present evidence, we suggest that human
speech has evolved not only due to the selection of complex
integrative capacities and a suitable vocal tract but also under
the influence of a species-specific form of environmental support
resulting from the co-evolution of intuitive didactic capacities
in caregivers. We cannot yet say whether this support is an
unconditional prerequisite; a surplus in prerequisites is not
unusual in nature in relation to crucial means of adaptation. We
can say, however, that the support for speech acquisition starts
immediately after the infant's birth and represents a major part
of the first social interactions.

REFERENCES

Cohen, N.J. and Squire, L. (1982). Preserved Learning and
Retention of Pattern-analyzing Skill in Amnesia: Dissociation of
Knowing How and Knowing That. Science, 210, 207-210.

Kihlström, J.F. (1987). The Cognitive Unconscious. Science, 237,
1445-1452.

Konner, M.J. and Worthman, C. (1980). Nursing Frequency, Gonadal
Function, and Birth Spacing Among !Kung Hunter-gatherers.
Science, 207, 788-791.

Lenneberg, E.H. (1971). Of Language Knowledge, Apes, and Brains.
In Early Childhood. The Development of Self-regulatory Mecha-
nisms. (eds. D.N. Walcher and D.L. Peters). Academic Press, New
York.

Lieberman, P. (1984). The Biology and Evolution of Language.
Harvard University Press, Cambridge, MA.

Oller, D.K. (1986). Metaphonology and Infant Vocalizations. In
Precursors of Early Speech. (eds. B. Lindblom and R. Zetterström).
Wenner-Gren Center International Symposium Series, 44, 21-35.
Macmillan Press, Basingstoke, UK.

Papoušek, H. (1977). Entwicklung der Lernfähigkeit im Säuglings-
alter /Development of Learning Ability During Infancy/. In
Intelligenz, Lernen und Lernstörungen /Intelligence, Learning, and

Learning Disorders/. (ed. G. Nissen). Springer-Verlag, Heidel-
berg.

Papoušek, H. and Papoušek, M. (1984). Learning and Cognition in
The Everyday Life of Human Infants. Advances in The Study of
Behavior, 14, 127-163.

Papoušek, H., Papoušek M. and Koester L. S. (1986). Sharing
Emotionality and Sharing Knowledge: A Microanalytic Approach to
Parent-Infant Communication. In Measuring Emotions in Infants and
Children, Vol. 2. (eds. C.E. Izard and P. Read). Cambridge
University Press, Cambridge, UK.

Papoušek, H. and Papoušek, M. (1987). Intuitive Parenting: A
Dialectic Counterpart to The Infant's Integrative Competence. In
Handbook of Infant Development, 2nd edit. (ed. J. Osofsky). Wiley:
New York.

Papoušek, H., Papoušek, M., Suomi, S.J. and Rahn, C.W. (in press).
Preverbal Communication and Attachment: Comparative Views. In
Intersections With Attachment. (eds. J.L. Gewirtz and W.M.
Kurtines). Erlbaum, Hillsdale, NJ.

Papoušek, M. and Papoušek, H. (1981). Musical Elements in The
Infant's Vocalization: Their Significance for Communication,
Cognition and Creativity. In Advances in Infancy Research, Vol.1.
(eds. L.P. Lipsitt and C.K. Rovee-Collier). Ablex, Norwood, NJ.

Papoušek, M., Papoušek, H. and Bornstein, M. H. (1985). The
Naturalistic Vocal Environment of Young Infants: On The
Significance of Homogeneity and Variability in Parental Speech.
In Social Perception in Infants. (eds. T. Field and N. Fox).
Ablex, Norwood, NJ.

Papoušek, M. and Papoušek, H. (1987). Models and Messages in
Maternal Speech to Prelinguistic Infants in Tonal and Nontonal
Languages. Presentation at the Biennial Meetings of the Society
for Research in Child Development, Baltimore, MD.

Papoušek, M. and Papoušek, H. (in press). Forms and Functions of
Vocal Matching in Precanonical Mother-Infant Interactions. First
Language, Special Issue on Precursors to Speech.

Studdert-Kennedy, M. (1986). Development of The Speech Perceptuo-
motor System. In Precursors of Early Speech. (eds. B. Lindblom
and R. Zetterström). Wenner-Gren Center International Symposium
Series, 44, 205-217. Macmillan Press, Basingstoke, UK.

20
Early Cognitive Functioning

Elizabeth S. Spelke

Over the last 30 years, research has revealed that young human infants have considerable capacities to perceive the surrounding layout and to act in a coordinated manner. Until recently, however, research produced little evidence that young infants have any of the higher cognitive capacities of mature humans: capacities to represent the world and to reason about its behavior. In this respect, research on human infancy has remained consonant with the centuries-old view that capacities to think and know are constructed on a foundation of sensation and action. Development, on this view, progresses from the outside inward. First humans come to perceive the world and to act upon it. The experience of perceiving and acting then provides the basis by which humans come to think and reason.

Recent research has begun to call this view into question. This research provides evidence that young infants can represent hidden objects and make inferences about their behavior before they are able to reach for or locomote around objects, and even before they are skilled at perceiving objects and following their motions. This research suggests that central cognitive capacities develop from their own foundations, not from a foundation of perception or action. What is more, infants' first cognitive capacities appear to resemble the capacities of mature humans, as much as their earliest perceptual and motor capacities do.

Methods for studying cognition in infancy

How can we learn whether infants represent and reason about things they cannot see? Since the 1930s, Piaget and his followers have attempted to study the development of these abilities by focusing on infants' search for hidden objects (Piaget, 1954). Unfortunately, object-directed search emerges quite late in infancy and develops slowly thereafter. The development of search appears to depend largely on changes in the child's sensory-motor coordination (Piaget, 1952), strategic behavior (Wellman, et al, 1987), and ability to act on information in memory (Goldman-Rakic, 1987). Since these changes may be independent of the child's basic representational and reasoning capacities, object-directed search does not appear to offer the best means to study those capacities.

The method of the present experiments has been used to study perception throughout the infancy period. It focuses on infants' systematic tendency to look longer at objects or events that are novel. If infants are presented repeatedly with one visual display, their looking time to the display tends to decline. If infants are then shown a new display, their looking time increases. This preference for novelty has been used to investigate a variety of perceptual abilities, from pattern discrimination to size constancy to perceptual categorization (see Bornstein, 1985; Spelke, 1985). New and surprising research by Baillargeon (in press) indicates that the preference for novelty can also be used to investigate a more central cognitive ability: the ability to represent an object in its absence. Young infants have been found to show heightened looking not only to events whose novelty can be seen but to events whose novelty must be inferred, because the novel aspects of the event take place out of their view.

Representations of hidden objects

In Baillargeon's first experiment, 5 1/2-month-old infants were familiarized with an event in which a flat screen rotated 180° between two flat positions on a surface (Figure 1). When their looking time to successive presentations of the event declined to half its original level, a block was introduced behind the screen, and two test events were presented in

Figure 1

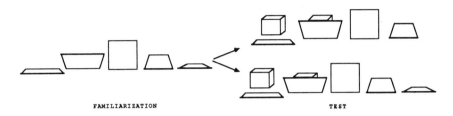

FAMILIARIZATION   TEST

alternation. In both events, the screen rotated upward
so as to hide the block, and it continued rotating toward
it. In one event, the screen stopped rotating when it
reached the hidden block's location. This event involved
a new visible motion (a rotation of about 120°) but was
the expected event for adults. In the other event, the
screen rotated the full 180°, revealing no object in its
path. This event involved a familiar visible motion but
was surprising to adults, since the block that had stood
behind the screen appeared to go out of existence.

If infants fail to represent the continuous existence
of a hidden object, the subjects were expected to look
longer at the first test event, because it involved a
novel motion. If infants represent hidden objects, in
contrast, the subjects were expected to look longer at
the second test event. The latter finding was obtained:
Infants looked longer at the impossible screen rotation.

Baillargeon's experiment provides evidence that 5
1/2-month-old infants can represent the existence of a
hidden object, and that this representation can be
studied by means of a preferential looking method. In
subsequent research using this method, Baillargeon has
investigated whether younger infants represent hidden
objects; her experiments provide evidence for this
ability in infants as young as 3 1/2 months (see
Baillargeon, in press). Baillargeon has also
investigated whether infants represent properties of a
hidden object such as its height, its location, and its
rigidity or elasticity: Seven-month-old infants were
found to represent all these properties, and younger
infants were found to represent at least one property:
object height. Long before infants can search for a
hidden object, they appear to represent the object's
continued existence.

Inferences about occluded object motion

In the above experiments, infants were presented with
an occluded object that was stationary and unchanging.
What happens, however, when a moving object is occluded:
Can infants infer how the object continues to move and
where it comes to rest? The next experiments
investigated these abilities.

When adults view an object that moves from view, we
often can infer how the object continues to move. These
inferences are guided by knowledge of physical
constraints on object motion. For example, adults infer
that a hidden object will move on a connected path, it
will change its motion if it encounters another object or
surface, it will not change its motion abruptly in the
absence of any object or surface, and it will move
downward if not adequately supported. These inferences
depend on knowledge that object motion is subject to a
continuity constraint (objects only move on connected
paths), a solidity constraint (objects only move through
space not occupied by other objects), an inertia
constraint (objects do not change their motion
spontaneously and abruptly), and a gravity constraint
(object motion is subject to a downward attraction).

Our first experiment investigated whether 4-month-old
infants make inferences about object motion in accord
with the continuity and solidity constraints (Spelke,
Macomber, & Breinlinger, 1989). At the start of the
study, infants were shown an open stage with a bright
floor. On each of a series of familiarization trials, a
screen was lowered over the bottom half of the stage, a
ball was dropped behind it, and the screen was raised to
reveal the ball on the floor (see Figure 2, top).
Looking time was recorded only after the ball was
revealed in its final position. When these looking times
declined to half their initial level, the test sequence
was given. A second surface was introduced above the
floor of the stage, the screen was lowered and the ball
was dropped as before, and the screen was raised to
reveal the ball either in a new position on the upper
surface or in its familiar position on the lower surface.
The second position was inconsistent with the solidity
and continuity constraints: the ball could only reach
this position if it passed through the surface or jumped
from one side of the surface to the other.

Figure 2   Figure 3

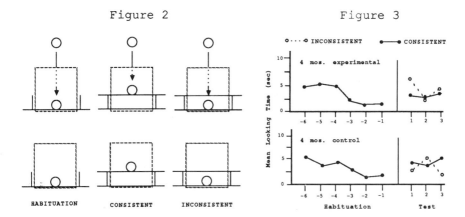

HABITUATION   CONSISTENT   INCONSISTENT

    Looking times during the test sequence were recorded
after the screen was raised. These looking times were
compared to the looking times of infants in a control
experiment who viewed events with the same final
positions in which the ball was simply placed in that
position (Figure 2, bottom). If infants infer that
occluded objects will move in accord with the solidity
and continuity constraints, then the infants in the main
experiment were expected to look longer at the
superficially familiar but inconsistent test position,
relative to the infants in the control experiment. These
were the results obtained (Figure 3). The experiment
provides evidence that 4-month-old infants infer that a
moving object will not pass through or jump over a
surface in its path: It will move in accord with the
continuity and solidity constraints.

    The next experiment investigated whether 2 1/2-month-
old infants would make the same inference (Spelke et al,
1989). The experiment used new events involving slower
object motion, so that the younger infants could follow
the motion (Figure 4). At the start of the study, the
infants were presented with an open stage bounded on the
right by a wall, a screen was lowered over the right side
of the stage, and a ball was introduced on the left. The
ball was tapped so that it rolled slowly behind the
screen, the screen was raised to reveal the ball at rest
beside the wall, and looking time was recorded. For the
test, a block was introduced in the center of the stage.
The screen was lowered as before, covering the block, the
ball was set in motion, and the screen was raised to
reveal the ball either in a new position beside the block
(consistent) or in its familiar position beside the wall

(inconsistent). Test trial looking times were compared
to those of infants in a control experiment, who viewed
the same final positions after events that were all
consistent with the continuity and solidity constraints.
The findings were the same as in the preceding study:
Infants in the main experiment looked longer at the
superficially familiar but inconsistent test position,
relative to infants in the control experiment (Figure 5).

These experiments provided evidence that 2 1/2- and
4-month-old infants represent the continued existence of
a hidden, moving object and make inferences about the
object's continued motion. The infants infer that the
object will move on a connected path through unoccupied
space: It will neither pass through nor jump over a
surface in its path. Young infants appear to be
sensitive to two important constraints on the motions of
physical bodies.

The above studies suggest that young infants can
represent objects and infer object motions much as adults
do. Further experiments, however, suggest substantial
differences between the inferences of young infants and
adults. For example, 4-month-old infants evidently do
not infer that a falling object will continue falling
until it reaches a surface in its path. If a falling
object has landed repeatedly on a surface and then the
surface is removed, the infants appear to expect the
falling object to land in the same position, now in
midair, rather than on a lower supporting surface
(Spelke, et al, 1989). Moreover, 5-month-old infants
evidently do not infer that a rolling object will

Figure 4   Figure 5

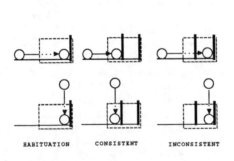

HABITUATION   CONSISTENT   INCONSISTENT

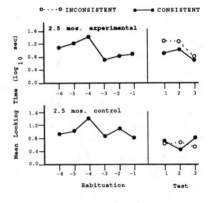

accelerate if it moves down an inclined plane. If an object has been propelled up an inclined plane repeatedly and has decelerated naturally as it moved, the infants appear to expect the object to decelerate once again if it is placed at the top of an inclined plane and allowed to roll downward (Kim & Spelke, 1989). Finally, 4- to 6-month-old infants evidently do not infer that an object moving rapidly on a flat surface will continue its motion in the absence of obstacles (Turner, Spelke, & Brunson, 1989), that it will move in a straight line (Katz, 1989), or that it will move at a constant or gradually changing speed (Spelke, Kestenbaum, & Wein, 1988). All these findings suggest that young infants fail to appreciate that object motion is subject to gravity or inertia. Knowledge of the inertia and gravity constraints appears to develop later than knowledge of the continuity and substance constraints.

Conclusions and suggestions

The experiments discussed here provide evidence that some central cognitive capacities arise early in infancy. Infants under 4 months of age can represent the existence of a hidden object that is stationary, and they can infer the motion and resting position of a hidden object that moves. These representations and inferences are subject to developmental change: as humans grow, we appear to represent more of the properties of hidden objects (e.g., Baillargeon, in press) and to make more inferences about hidden object motions (e.g., Spelke, et al, 1989). Nevertheless, young infants already possess some of the capacities and knowledge that are a hallmark of mature cognitive functioning.

How do cognitive capacities develop in infancy? Some of the most popular and influential answers to this question can be rejected, because of the ages of the subjects in the present studies. Four-month-old infants do not yet reach for objects or locomote around them, manipulate objects systematically, or communicate about objects with words or conventional gestures. Abilities to represent objects and infer object motion evidently can develop in the absence of these activities. Infants under 3 months, moreover, have poor visual acuity (Banks & Salapatek, 1983) and limited abilities to follow visible motion (Aslin, 1988). Abilities to represent and reason about objects evidently can develop in the absence of extensive or detailed visual experience. It remains possible that infants learn to represent hidden objects and infer their motions. In that case, however, learning would seem to occur on the basis of strikingly limited encounters with physical objects and events. Representational capacities appear to develop under considerable intrinsic constraints.

The present experiments suggest, therefore, that cognitive capacities, like perceptual and motor capacities, arise early in infancy from their own foundations. This suggestion does not imply that developing conceptions of the world are unaffected by perception or action. It is likely that conceptions of objects grow and change as infants observe how objects behave in particular circumstances and as they act on objects in particular ways. The present findings suggest, however, that interrelations among perception, action, and cognition will be found in all directions: Development will not proceed strictly from the periphery inward. For example, early conceptions of object motion may foster the development of event perception, by guiding infants' attempts to keep track of moving objects. Early conceptions of object motion may also foster the development of object-directed reaching, which must be adapted to constraints on object motion (see Hofsten, 1983). If action, perception, and cognition develop together, then each function can enhance the development of the others through a rich set of interactions. Initial cognitive capacities will be as fundamental to these interactions as are initial capacities of other kinds.

The present findings could serve as an invitation, to students of neurobiology, to investigate the biological structures and processes by which humans represent the world and its unseen behavior. If representational capacities emerged only at the pinnacle of human functioning and depended on structures and processes of great rarity and complexity, then it would be reasonable for neurobiologists to defer study of these structures until the more basic and universal structures of perception and action were better understood. The present studies suggest, however, that humans begin to represent the world and infer its behavior at or near the beginning of life. This evidence complements recent evidence for representational and inferential capacities in other animals, including primates (e.g., Premack, 1976), lower mammals (e.g., Cheng & Gallistel, 1986), and even invertebrates (see Gallistel, in press). Thus, some mechanisms of thought may be no more rare or complex than the mechanisms of perception or action. Research in neurobiology has led to great advances in our understanding of the latter mechanisms, their structure and development. One may hope that more neurobiologists will seek similar insights into the physical mechanisms of thought.

REFERENCES

Aslin, R. N. (1988). Anatomical constraints on oculomotor development: Implications for infant perception. In Perceptual development in infancy: The Minnesota Symposia in Child Psychology, Vol 20. (ed. A. Yonas). Hillsdale, NJ: Erlbaum.

Baillargeon, R. (in press). The object concept revisited: New directions. In Advances in child development and behavior, Volume 23. (ed. H. W. Reese). New York: Academic Press.

Baillargeon, R., Spelke, E.S., & Wasserman, S. (1985). Object permanence in five-month-old infants. Cognition, 20, 191-208.

Banks, M. S., and Salapatek, P. (1983) Infant visual perception. In Infancy and biological development, (eds. M. M. Haith and J. Campos), Volume 2 of Handbook of child psychology, (ed. P. Mussen). John Wiley and Sons, New York, pp. 435-472.

Bornstein, M. H. (1985). Habituation of attention as a measure of visual information processes in human infants: Summary, systematization, and synthesis. In Measurement of audition and vision in the first year of postnatal life. (eds. G. Gottlieb & N. Krasnegor) Norwood, NJ: Ablex.

Cheng, K. (1986). A purely geometric module in the rat's spatial representation. Cognition, 23, 148-178.

Gallistel, C. R. (in press) The organization of learning, Bradford Books/MIT Press, Cambridge, MA.

Goldman-Rakic, P. S. (1987). Development of cortical circuitry and cognitive function. Child Dev., 58, 601-622.

Hofsten, C. von. (1983). Catching skills in infancy. J. of Exp. Psych.: Hum. Percep. Perf., 9, 75-85.

Katz, G. (1989). Infants' conception of inertia: Rectilinear motion in the absence of forms. Unpublished honors thesis, Cornell university.

Kim, I. K., & Spelke, E. S. (1989). Infants' conceptions of gravity and acceleration. Unpublished ms.

Piaget, J. (1952). The origins of intelligence in children. New York: International University Press.

Piaget, J. (1954). The construction of reality in the child. New York: Basic Books.

Premack, D. (1976). Intelligence in ape and man. Hillsdale, NJ: Lawrence Erlbaum Associates.

Spelke, E. S. (1985). Preferential looking methods as tools for the study of cognition in infancy. In Measurement of audition and vision in the first year of postnatal life. (eds. G. Gottlieb & N. Krasnegor) Norwood, NJ: Ablex.

Spelke, E. S., Kestenbaum, R., & Wein, D. (1989). Spatio-Temporal continuity and object identity in infancy. Unpublished ms.

Spelke, E. S., Macomber,J., & Breinlinger, K. (1989). Intuitive physics in infancy: Early conceptions of object motion. Unpublished ms.

Turner, A. S., Spelke, E. S., & Brunson, L. (1989). Infant conceptions of object motion: Aspects of the principle of inertia. Unpublished ms.

Wellman, H. M., Cross, D., & Bartsch, K. (1987). Infant search and object permanence: A meta-analysis of the A-Not-B error. Mono. Soc. for Res. in Child Dev., 51(3).

21
Opioid and Nonopioid Influences on Behavioral Development in Rat and Human Infants

Elliott M. Blass

INTRODUCTION

A desideratum of developmental psychobiology is to identify particular early natural events that guide behavioral development and to understand the specific mechanisms through which these events effect change. This approach makes explicit the assumption that early experiences act to delimit the range of objects within a domain that will elicit the species typical action patterns and corresponding affective change associated with that object domain (Blass, 1987). In the case of ingestive behavior, for example, experience influences what and where to eat (Galef and Henderson, 1972) and not how to eat (Hall, 1975).

This approach also provides a broad interface between behavioral and neurological development in delineating how particular early experiences can influence the developing nervous system. It can align those aspects of motivation and action systems (Hall, 1979) that are closed to modification, at a particular time, with their underlying neurologies. Moreover, this approach can match those aspects of action systems that can be modified, with their corresponding neurologies that are likewise open to change. Precision in identifying the events that underlie behavioral and motivational change allows equal precision in identifying the managing neurology. Thus, it was Pedersen and Blass's (1982) identifying the precise behavioral events underlying acquisition of olfactory control over suckling in rats that allowed Pedersen et al. (1983) and Leon and his colleagues (Coopersmith and Leon, 1988) to identify the functional olfactory neurologies underlying these changes in motivation and the direction of action.

My own research has focused on the mechanisms through which mother-infant interactions in general, nursing-suckling encounters in particular select the classes of stimuli that elicit species-typical behaviors and their associated affective states.

Suckling lends itself well to this task. It is unique among mammals. Suckling is the expression of specialized neurologies that manage specialized and reciprocal behavioral exchanges between mother and infant. Suckling reflects a unique time-limited gastrointestinal adaptation. It is matched to changes in maternal morphology, physiology neuroendocrinology and behavior. Yet suckling functionally disappears at weaning. The environment, therefore, casts its influence during a very restricted period of the lifespan and these suckling experiences influence action patterns that emerge after suckling has receded (Fillion and Blass, 1985, 1986).

The present chapter focuses on a salient feature of this relationship; maternal properties that change infant behavioral and physiological states during suckling and the enduring effects of these changes. The mechanisms underlying these changes utilize both opioid and nonopioid pathways that are engaged by different aspects of the maternal stimulus array.

Development of Behavioral Responsivity to Opioids

It is now well established that newborn mammals are behaviorally responsive to opiates despite the relatively slow morphological and pharmacological development of opioid systems (Kehoe, 1988 for review). Fetal rats can associate morphine (an opiate) with a particular flavor injected into the amniotic fluid and express this appreciation by preferring this solution at two weeks postpartum (Stickrod, et al., 1982). This demonstrates that the developing fetal neurology can: (1) respond in an adult-fashion to an opiate, (2) associate it with preceding and concurrent events, (3) retain this association for over three weeks, and (4) mobilize and direct behaviors that maintain contact with the associated substance. These findings were of particular interest to me because they provided a potential mechanism through which the mother, through contact and nursing, could effectuate enduring change in her infant's behavioral development.

In order to determine some of the behavioral characteristics of opioid systems of developing rats and to provide a behavioral assay against which the opioid-like activity of milk, its constituents and other substances could be evaluated, Kehoe and Blass (1986a) demonstrated that morphine injections (0.5 mg/kg BW i.p.) caused a substantial decrease in pain responsivity (i.e. paw withdrawal latency from a 48°C surface was markedly elevated by the injection) and in social isolation distress (as judged by reduced ultrasonic vocalizations) in rats isolated from mother and siblings. Figure 1 illustrates these changes and also demonstrates that they were fully reversed by naltrexone, an opioid antagonist. This is classic evidence for opioid mediation.

Morphine, in addition to relieving distress was also a

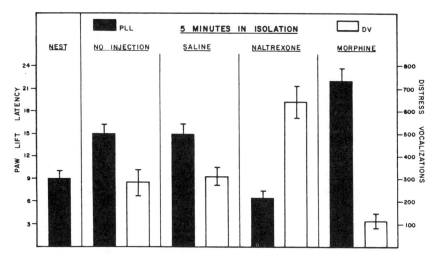

Figure 1. Effects of morphine or naltrexone administration on distress vocalizations and paw lift latencies of isolated 10-day-old rats.

rewarding agent that could become associated with predicting events. Kehoe and Blass (1986b, 1988) demonstrated that 5-day-old rats could associate an odor with morphine injection. Specifically pairing orange odor with morphine in 5-day-old rats led to a preference for that odor when these rats were 10 days of age. The association altered the motivational system mediating choice: animals overcame the aversive qualities of the orange scent. Preference formation was blocked by naltrexone pretreatment on Day 5 implicating an opioid basis for its establishment (Kehoe and Blass, 1986b). Preference expression was thwarted by naltrexone injection administered before testing (Kehoe and Blass, 1988). This implies that the preferred substance gained control over behavior because it caused a release of endogenous opioid. This was confirmed by demonstrating elevated paw lift latencies in morphine-odor conditioned rats that were exposed to the odor at the time of testing for pain withdrawal (Kehoe and Blass, 1988). Behavior may be sustained, therefore, by stimuli associated with a release of the endogenous peptide or transmitter by conditioned stimuli. Naltrexone caused a reversion to original choice because it prevented the endogenous opioid released by the conditioned stimulus to overcome the aversive sensory properties of the orange odor.

Evaluation of opioid-like properties of milk: In addition to demonstrating a functional opioid system in 5-day-old rats and a basis for overcoming aversive properties of stimuli, these studies have provided a metric against which to evaluate whether: (1) milk and its constituents altered behavior, (2) milk paired with different stimuli caused more lasting behavioral changes and (3) either or both of these alterations were realized through opioid pathways. Blass and Fitzgerald (1988) demonstrated an isomorphism between morphine injections and intraoral infusions of "half and half", a commercial product similar in its composition to rat's milk, on distress vocalizations and heat escape. Specifically, like morphine, milk elevated paw lift latency and markedly reduced distress vocalizations. Both of these changes were reversed by naltrexone injected prior to milk infusion. In comparison with intraoral sucrose infusions (Blass, et al., 1987), milk took longer to effectuate change in the vocalization pattern. This suggested a gastric or intestinal contribution to milk's mechanism of action as well as an oral component. Support for this idea has been provided by Weller and Blass's (1988) demonstration that the gut peptide cholecystokinin, effectively reduced distress vocalizations in isolated 10-day-old rats at a dose of 1 ug/kg BW.

Two classes of milk constituents, namely, fats (Shide and Blass, 1988) and sugars (Blass, et al., 1987) infused intraorally, have the same characteristics as morphine administered intraperitoneally or intracerebroventricularly (Kehoe and Blass, 1986c): (1) they immediately reduce distress vocalizations (2) they increase pain thresholds (3) both changes are sustained well past infusion termination, (4) both changes are normalized by the opioid antagonist naltrexone, (5) an odor can be classically conditioned to intraoral infusions of corn oil or sucrose, (6) conditioning can be blocked by pretreatment with naltrexone and (7) preference expression, for an odor associated with corn oil at least, can be blocked by naltrexone at the time of testing.

Thus, for rats, a direct opioid-mediated reciprocity between positive (taste and preference) and negative (pain and social distress) affective systems has been established. The reciprocity is of considerable interest concerning the development of motivational systems in general and feeding in particular because rats (Morley and Levine, 1980) and humans (Marks-Kaufman, 1982) selectively eat more sweets and fats when stressed and, as shown above, these substances appear to blunt distress through opioid mediation. The question arises, of course, are there classes of rewarding events that are nonopioid mediated—do these events have characteristics that differ fundamentally from those of opioid systems—and do the systems interact—if so, how?

Kehoe and Blass (1986d) demonstrated that contact with an anesthetized female immediately reduced distress vocalizations in totally isolated rats, and completely normalized paw lift latencies. In the first instance contact had the effect of opioid

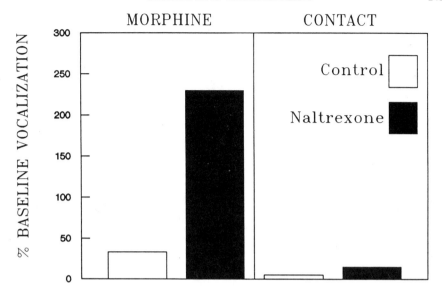

Figure 2. Comparison of morphine and maternal contact on distress
vocalization in rats following isotonic saline or naltrexone
treatment.

agonists; in the second, opioid antagonists. We have since found
that contact comfort in rats was nonopioid mediated. Figure 2
compares distress vocalizations of isolated rats receiving morphine
injections preceded by saline or naltrexone treatment with rats
that were returned to an anesthetized dam after these treatments
(right panel). Both morphine and contact markedly reduced
vocalizations (open columns), but through different mechanisms
(closed columns). Naltrexone reversed morphine's effect but did
not obviously influence contact quieting. This suggests that
contact utilizes nonopioid pathways, whose properties differ from
those of opioid systems. Data from human newborns support this
idea.

Opioid Mediation of State in Newborn Human Infants: The
range of moods exhibited by newborn humans and the standardization
of painful routines in U.S. hospitals have made it possible to
conduct studies in human newborns that closely parallel rat studies
concerning immediate effects of sugars on distress, mood and
affect.

Sucrose (12% w/v) given intraorally to spontaneously crying 1-
3 day old human infants arrests crying after only 0.2-0.4 ml are
delivered (Rochat et al., 1988). As with rats the soothing effects

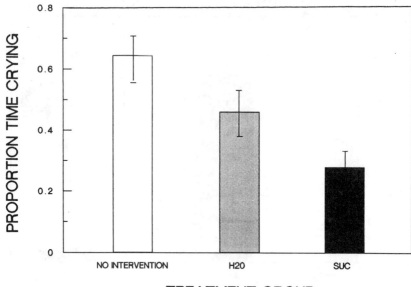

Figure 3. Modification of crying during circumcision in infants receiving no experimenter intervention, a pacifier dipped in water or a pacifier dipped in sucrose solution during the procedure.

persist well beyond sucrose termination. Both sucrose and glucose are powerful analgesics and interact additively with tactile stimulation as demonstrated on infants undergoing circumcision (Figure 3). Moreover, intraoral sucrose (2 ml 12%), administered 2 min. before blood collection for PKU tests, reduced crying in 1-2 day old infants by 50% during the collection procedure. In parallel with the rat findings, sucrose-induced analgesia endured: crying stopped within 1 min after blood collection and the quiet endured. Comparable states were not achieved by control (water infusion) infants until 5-6 min after the procedure (Hoffmeyer and Blass, unpublished observations).

State change caused by intraoral sugar, and that caused by pacifier are both immediate as judged by crying reduction. Yet they differ markedly in duration. Crying infants receiving 0.1 ml of sucrose/min for even 2 min. stop crying and remain calm upon sucrose withdrawal. In contrast, it requires 14-15 min of continuous sucking on a pacifier for calm to endure after pacifier removal. Temporal similarities and differences between oral sucrose stimulation and oral tactile stimulation suggest a unitary mode of action for sugars and a dual one for touch. Glucose and sucrose may act through endogenous opioid release that cause immediate and sustained effects. Calming is also an immediate response to proximate tactile stimulation. Unlike sucrose however, its effectiveness stops unless the infant has been sucking the pacifier for about 15 min. This suggests an immediate path distinguished by rapid onset with tactile administration and rapid offset upon its removal. A second pathway is characterized by a slow rise-time and, after threshold has been reached, a slow rate of decay upon removal of tactile stimulation.

GENERAL DISCUSSION

Mammalian mothers, during nursing, present their infants with a bewildering stimulus array. Included in this array are stimuli that uniquely define the mother, her odors for example, that do not elicit a particular initial response (Rosenblatt, 1983). In addition there are stimuli like touch or milk that elicit very stereotyped behavioral patterns such as rooting or sucking. One of my aims was to identify mechanisms that allow the infant to associate the mother's unique qualities with the tactile and nutritional consequences of sucking. This is an important step in identifying how early experiences influence later behavioral patterns. At least the effects of mother's milk are mediated through opioid pathways. Thermotactile qualities of the mother-- her skin and nipple--are effective through non-opioid mechanisms.

Figure 4 draws attention to both opioid and nonopioid consequences of suckling on stress and state systems and provides avenues of linkage to particular maternal features. This is a simplified version of present knowledge because it does not include postingestive mechanisms that affect state and does not show that state and stress affect suckling (see Shide and Blass, 1988 for emphasis on these aspects). Both opioid and nonopioid factors influence state and stress but with very different time courses of duration. Both can be conditioned to maternal stimuli but with potentially different consequences. The nonopioid factor has so far been identified as thermotactile. It has two components: one with a rapid rise time in pacifying infant rats and humans and in changing their state during proximate stimulation, the other has a slow rise time in causing more enduring state changes.

Fat and possibly sweet components of milk are detected by taste (and possibly olfactory) mechanisms which, in turn cause the release of endogenous opioids. The taste system in Figure 4 reflects stimulus duration taking adaptation and salivary dilution into account. The opioid component, however, endures well beyond taste offset and may be protracted further by gastric mechanisms. Opioid release reduces stress, calms the infant, changes state and serves as a reinforcing agent (the last three statements are subsumed as attributes of a state system for presentation simplicity).

Both tactile and opioid components of the system can be

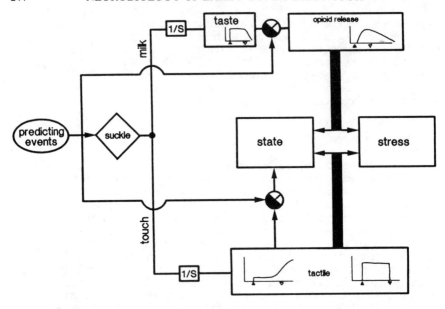

Figure 4. A model depicting relationships between opioid and nonopioid influences on stress and state systems, the engagement of these influences through milk and touch respectively arising from suckling and the opportunity of these events to become associated with predicting aspects of the mother.

associated with the events that predict suckling opportunity. We know more about the properties of stimuli associated with opioid changes. They become preferred environmental stimuli. They cause opioid release when presented in the absence of suckling. They calm and have analgesic properties. They direct available behavior patterns towards the associated stimulus.

The properties of stimuli associated with the tactile components are less well documented. They too become preferred (Sullivan and Leon, 1986) and may direct specific patterns of behavior (Alberts and May, 1984; Pedersen and Blass, 1982). I assume that this is due to their association with the rapid rise-time component of the tactile system. Beyond that, data are not available for the changes in state and pain reactivity that can be brought under control of the tactile system.

The figure guides specific experimental pathways for analyzing early experiences behaviorally, pharmacologically, and neurologically. It predicts differential outcomes of associating maternal cues with her specific rewarding properties. It predicts mediation at least in part by different pharmacologies and neurologies. The mother's simultaneously presenting both opioid and nonopioid classes of stimulation to their young makes our task of identifying the roots of ontogenetic influence on organizing and direct action patterns the more interesting and challenging.

ACKNOWLEDGEMENT

This research was supported by grants in aid of research DK18560 and HD19278 and Research Scientist Award MH00524 to the author.

REFERENCES

Alberts, J.R. and May, B. (1984). Nonnutritive Thermotactile Induction of Filial Huddling in Rat Pups. Dvptl. Psychobiol., 17, 161-181.

Blass, E.M. (1987). Critical Events During Sensitive Periods of Social Development in Rats. In Sensitive Periods in Development: Interdisciplinary Perspective. (ed. M. Bornstein). Erlbaum Assoc., New Jersey.

Blass, E.M. and Fitzgerald, E. (1988). Milk-Induced Analgesia and Comforting in 10-Day-Old Rats: Opioid Mediation. Pharma., Biochem. and Behav., 29, 9-13.

Blass, E.M., Fitzgerald, E. and Kehoe, P. (1987). Interactions Between Sucrose, Pain and Isolation Distress. Pharma., Biochem. and Behav., 26, 483-489.

Coopersmith, R. and Leon, M. (1988). The Neurobiology of Early Olfactory Learning. In Handbook of Behavioral Neurobiology: Developmental Psychobiology and Behavioral Ecology, Vol. 9. (ed. E.M. Blass). Plenum Press, New York.

Fillion, T.J. and Blass, E.M. (1985). Responsiveness to Estrous Chemostimuli in Male Rats (Rattus Norvegicus) of Different Ages. J. Comp. Psychol., 99, 328-335.

Fillion, T.J. and Blass, E.M. (1986). Infantile Experience Determines Adult Sexual Behavior in Male Rats. Science., 231, 729-731.

Galef, B.G. and Henderson, P.W. (1972). Mother's Milk: A Determinant of the Feeding Preferences of Weanling Rat Pups. J. Comp. Physiol. Psychol., 78, 213-219.

Hall, W.G. (1975). Weaning and Growth of Artificially Reared Rats. Science, 190, 1313-1315.

Hall, W.G. (1979). The Ontogeny of Feeding in Rats: I. Ingestion and Behavioral Processes to Oral Infusions. J. Comp. Physiol. Psychol., 93, 977-1000.

Kehoe, P. (1988). Opioids, Behavior and Learning in Mammalian Development. In Handbook of Behavioral Neurobiology: Developmental Psychobiology and Behavioral Ecology, Vol. 9. (ed. E.M. Blass). Plenum Press, New York.

Kehoe, P. and Blass, E.M. (1986)a. Behaviorally Functional Opioid Systems in Infant Rats: I. Evidence for Olfactory and Gustatory Classical Conditioning. Behav. Neurosci., 100, 359-367.

Kehoe, P. and Blass, E.M. (1986)b. Behaviorally Functional Opioid Systems in Infant Rats: II. Evidence for Pharmacological, Physiological and Psychological Mediation of Pain and Stress. Behav. Neurosci., 100, 624-630.

Kehoe, P. and Blass, E.M. (1986)c. Central Nervous System Mediation of Pleasure and Pain in Neonatal Albino Rats. Br. Res., 3, 61-82.

Kehoe, P. and Blass, E.M. (1986)d. Opioid-Mediation of Separation Distress in 10-Day-Old Rats: Reversal of Stress with Maternal Stimuli. Dvptl. Psychobio., 19, 385-398.

Kehoe P. and Blass, E.M. (1988). Conditioned Opioid Release in Ten-Day-Old Rats. Behav. Neurosci. (in press).

Marks-Kaufman, R. (1982). Increased Fat Consumption Induced by Morphine Administration in Rats. Pharmacol., Biochem. & Behav., 16, 949-955.

Morely, J.E. and Levine, A.S. (1980). Stress-Induced Eating is Mediated Through Endogenous Opiates. Science, 209, 1259-1261.

Pedersen, P.E. and Blass, E.M. (1982). Prenatal and Postnatal Determinants of the First Suckling Episode in Albino Rats. Dvptl. Psychobio., 15, 349-355.

Pedersen, P.E., Stewart, W.B., Green, C.A., and Shepherd, G.M. (1983). Evidence for Olfactory Function in Utero. Science, 221, 478-480.

Rochat, P., Blass, E.M. and Hoffmeyer, L.B. (1988). Oropharyngeal Control of Hand-Mouth Coordination in Newborn Infants. Dvptl. Psychol. 24, 459-463.

Rosenblatt, J.S. (1983). Olfaction Mediates Developmental Transition in the Altricial Newborn of Selected Species of Mammals. Dvptl. Psychobiol., 16, 347-375.

Shide, D. and Blass, E.M. (1988). Opioid-Like Effects of Intraoral Infusions of Corn Oil and Polycose on Stress Reactions in 10-Day-Old Rats. Behav. Neurosci. (in press).

Stickrod, G., Kimble, D.P. and Smotherman, W.P. (1982). Met-5-Enkephalin Effects on Associations Formed In-Utero. Peptides, 3, 881-883.

Sullivan, R.M. and Leon, M. (1986). Early Olfactory Learning Induces an Enhanced Olfactory Bulb Response in Young Rats. Dvptl. Br. Res., 27, 278-282.

Weller, A. and Blass, E.M. (1988). Behavioral Evidence for Cholecystokinin-Opiate Interactions in Neonatal Rats. Am. J. Physiol. (in press).

22
Telethermography in Measurement of Infant's Early Attachment

Keiko Mizukami, Noboru Kobayashi, Hiroo Iwata and Takemochi Ishii

INTRODUCTION

Recent infant behavioral research has proved infants to possess remarkable sensory abilities and to be able actively to forge ties of a social nature with people in their milieu from shortly after birth (Stone, et al., 1973; Field & Fox, 1985). It is reported that, from the neonatal period on, infants can distinguish their mother's voice (DeCasper & Fifer, 1980) and face (Field, 1985) from others' and that they react differently to their mother than they do to other people. It has not yet been quantitatively demonstrated, however, that from shortly after birth infants have any attachment to anyone in particular (specifically, to their mother).

Infant attachment research thus far has been based entirely on the theories and methods of Bowlby and Ainsworth. According to Bowlby (1969)'s theory of attachment, the infant forms attachments in the course of four developmental stages lasting several years after birth, and the first clearly identifiable attachment to the mother appears at 12 months. Ainsworth's Strange Situation System (1969), which draws on Bowlby's theory, defines attachment at 12 months as either secure or insecure.

To our knowledge, it has seldom been asked whether an infant's

This research was partially supported by a grant for maternal and child health research from the Ministry of Health and Welfare of Japan. The authors thank Hiroko Abo, Tamie Suemoto, Kumi Wada, Asako Hashimoto, Mami Ishibashi, student at Tokyo Woman's Christian University, and Takako Suzuki, doctorial course student at Ochanomizu University, for their help in our experiments and data arrangement. Correspondence and requests for reprints may be sent to Keiko Mizukami, Developmental Psychology Research Laboratory, NCMRC, Taishidoh, Setagaya-ku, Tokyo 154, Japan.

first personal attachments indeed begin to form about 7-8 months after birth (at about the time when, according to Piaget (1954), the child develops "object permanence") and whether they are indeed firmly established at 12 months.

We question neither the basic nature, nor the ethological function, nor the significance of attachment as described by Bowlby, Ainsworth, and others. We simply wish to propose with regard to its staging that attachment begins at an earlier age. Though infants' attachment toward specific persons has not yet been demonstrated earlier than 6 months of age, we believe that this failure is due to inadequacy of the indices used thus far: protest by the infant on separation from the mother and greeting following reunion. Separation protest is said to occur for the first time at about 5 months of age (Schaffer, 1963, Stayton et al., 1973), but almost all who study the development of attachment agree that neither this protest by the infant nor the infant's greeting the mother upon her return signify more than the infant's discrimination of the mother from other persons and the expression of the infant's pleasure at this recognition: "mere discrimination and preference do not constitute attachment[; ...] a baby must first have acquired at least a rudimentary concept of object permanence" (Stayton et al., 1973).

Assuming therefore that the traditional indices are inadequate, a new index might advance the study of infant's early attachment. By adequately demonstrating the presence of anxiety or stress in the infant upon separation namely "separation anxiety," we could confirm the existence of early attachment in the infant independently of object permanence.

With the purpose of studying infant attachment to the mother early in infancy, we used telethermographic measurements of facial skin surface temperature as overtly observable indices of reaction to stress (not of attachment behavior itself) to investigate how the presence or absence of the mother affected infants' behavior in a strange situation.

Infrared telethermography, the detection of skin surface temperature distribution at a distance, has been used for clinical diagnosis and research in dermatology and surgery (Fujimasa et al., 1986). This technique appears to be ideal for infant behavior studies as well, because it is noninvasive and does not restrict the subject's movement. Further, the thermographic device can be connected to a personal computer for image processing, enabling quantitative evaluation of thermal response.

It is a major premise of thermography in behavioral research that a change in skin surface temperature may indicate a change in the emotional state of the subject. In this study, we used a drop in the skin surface temperature as an index of stress, because it is known that stress has effects on changes in skin surface tem-

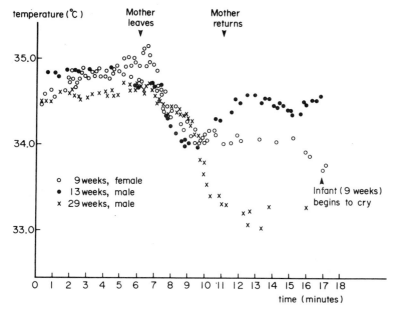

Fig. 1. Change in skin surface temperature of forehead area during mother-infant brief separation (Mizukami et al. 1987).

perature (Johnstone, 1974). Stress causes sympathetic nervous strain and contraction of shunt vessels (arteriovenous anastomoses) in the skin (Girling, 1952; Celander & Folkow, 1951, 1953). Because the skin has many shunt vessels which are sensitive to adrenaline secreted by the ends of vasoconstrictor nerves and by the adrenal medulla into blood vessels, skin temperature drops abruptly with shunt vessel contraction.

For several years, we have used infrared thermography in infant behavioral research to study changes in facial skin temperature as an index of stress. In a previous study (Mizukami et al., 1987), we showed using thermography that changes in the forehead skin temperature of infants aged 11 to 29 weeks separated from their mothers for a short time in a strange environment were similar to those observed in adults during stress, namely in that temperatures dropped (Fig. 1). In the previous study, however, which involved simple mother-infant separation without a control experiment, the observed temperature drop was a reaction to the stress of being left alone, and did not prove the infant's special attachment to the mother. The present experiment pursues the study a step further by providing two types of control to clarify the attachment to the mother by the infant at an early stage of development.

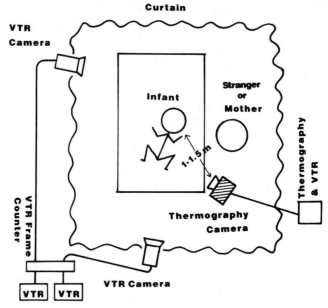

Fig. 2. Experimental setup

EXPERIMENT 1:   MOTHER IS REPLACED BY STRANGER

OBJECTIVE

    To test whether the infant feels stress when the mother leaves but a male stranger remains; in other words, whether a male stranger's presence is a substitute for the mother's.

METHOD

Subjects
    The subjects consisted of 11 pairs of mothers and healthy infants of both sexes aged 10–16 weeks, all infants born at term and appropriate for date.

Instruments
    Thermography Avionics Thermal Video System 1400, Sony SLO 420 video tape recorder, Sony CCD CS VTR camera, Houei VC–81 video counter.

Experimental setup (Fig. 2) and procedure
    The experiment was performed at the Developmental Psychology Research Laboratory, National Children's Medical Research Center.

The investigator and all equipment except the camera were hidden behind a curtain. Room temperature was between 24 and 26 degrees centigrade. Individual low thermographic temperatures were determined for each subject; sensitivity was set at 0.3 degrees.

Facial temperatures were thermographically video tape recorded in three consecutive situations: i) the mother placed the infant in bed then, seated in a chair beside the bed, played with the infant for about 6 minutes; ii) the mother left the room and a stranger entered and played with the infant for 5 minutes; iii) the stranger left the room, the mother returned and played with the infant for 3 to 5 minutes.

The experiment began at least 10 minutes after nursing at a time when the infant was cheerful and alert. A 3mm x 3mm piece of aluminum tape was placed on the right and left supraorbital regions to stabilize the point of analysis. A male pediatrician, the father of two children, played the stranger's part.

Analysis of the thermograms

The video-tape-recorded thermograms showing 16 degrees of brightness were analyzed using an NEC PC-9801 personal computer connected to the VTR. The thermogram was digitized in the image frame memory of the PC-9801. The degree of brightness corresponds to that of the temperature. Square windows were set manually using a pointer in the forehead area (1x1 on the midline of the forehead

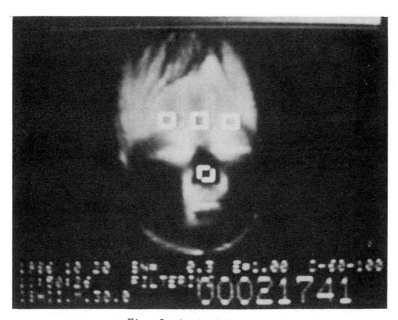

Fig. 3. Analyzed area

and 1x1 on the left or right supraorbital area) and the nasal area
(1x1 on the tip of the nose) (Fig. 3). We were not always able to
get all four items of data because of the face angle to the thermography camera. The frames which gave the most consistent angle
of the infant's face image between play period and separation
period were selected.

Mean temperatures were calculated from the mean brightness of
pixels in the analyzed windows.

RESULTS

Analysis could not be performed in 3 of 11 cases because a
thermogram could not be obtained from the desired facial angle or
because the infant began to cry while playing with the mother. The
data from the remaining 8 cases were analyzed. Because the midline
was analyzable in all 8 cases, the average temperature in the midline window was used. When the stranger replaced the mother in the
room, a significant drop in forehead temperature without crying was
observed in 5 cases (representative curves are shown in Fig. 4 and
Fig. 5); neither crying nor temperature change was seen in 2 cases
(Fig. 6); and crying was seen in 1 case (Fig. 7). In the crying
case, a significant temperature rise was seen; crying might cause
congestion of the blood vessels.

EXPERIMENT 2:   MOTHER AND STRANGER TOGETHER

OBJECTIVE

To test whether the infant's response to a stranger differs in
the presence and absence of the mother.

METHOD

Subjects
The subjects consisted of 9 pairs of mothers and healthy infants of both sexes aged 10-16 weeks, all infants born at term and
appropriate for date.

Experimental setup and procedure
The experimental setup was the same as in EXPERIMENT 1. The
experiment was performed at the Developmental Psychology Research
Laboratory, National Children's Medical Research Center.

Facial temperatures were thermographically video tape recorded
in three consecutive situations: i) the mother placed the infant in
bed then, seated in a chair beside the bed, played with the infant
for 5 minutes; ii) a stranger entered the room and played with the
infant for 5 minutes while the mother stood within view of the infant, watching without saying anything; iii) the stranger left the
room and the mother began again to play with the infant for 5
minutes.

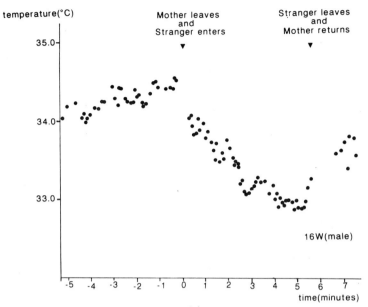

Fig. 4. Change in skin surface temperature of forehead area in a 16-week-old male who did not cry when his mother left and a stranger entered the room.

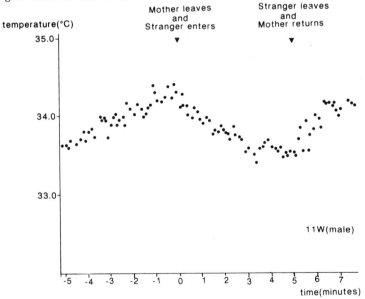

Fig. 5. Change in skin surface temperature of forehead area in a 11-week-old male who did not cry when his mother left and a stranger entered the room.

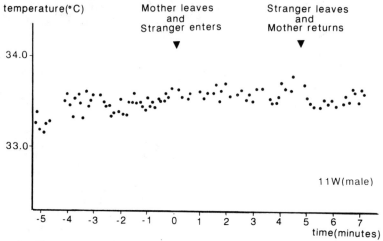

Fig. 6. Change in skin surface temperature of forehead area in an 11-week-old male who did not cry when his mother left and a stranger entered the room.

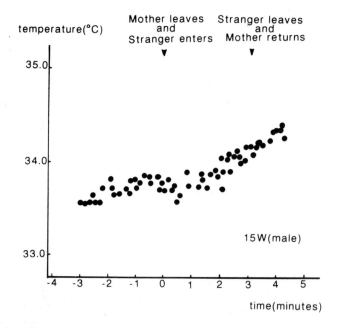

Fig. 7. Change in skin surface temperature of forehead area in a 15-week-old male who cried when his mother left and a stranger entered the room.

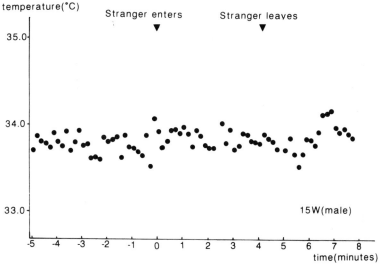

Fig. 8. Change in skin surface temperature of forehead area in a 15-week-old male who did not cry when a stranger played with him in his mother's presence.

Analysis
        Same as in EXPERIMENT 1.

RESULTS

        Seven of 9 cases were analyzable. Significant drops in temperature were not seen in any of the 7 analyzable cases. No infant cried. A representative curve is shown in Fig. 8.

DISCUSSION AND CONCLUSIONS

        The findings of Experiment 1 and Experiment 2 and of the previous study led us to the following conclusions: i) A mother's leaving her child alone in a strange place tends to be perceived by the infant as a stressful situation, even though the infant may not cry; ii) the perceived stress of being in a strange place without the mother is equal or greater in the presence of a male stranger; iii) however, the infant does not perceive stress from playing with a stranger if the mother is present.

        Viewed together, these findings indicate the infant's attachment to the mother from as early as the second to third postnatal month, although infants do not have an ability to express their anxiety and stressful feelings in the form of protest behavior. The findings also make us speculate further that at this very early age young infants may already be capable of self-regulation, since they apparently react to stress without crying.

Several remaining questions can be answered in a study involving a greater number of cases: i) how is response affected by order of birth (first-born, second-born, etc.) and the sex of infants? ii) do laughing, fretting, thumb-sucking, and other types of behavior correlate to simultaneously video-tape-recorded temperature changes? iii) do infants' responses to a female stranger differ from their responses to a male stranger and is the difference quantifiable? and iv) do infants show the same attachment to their father, grandmother, or grandfather as they do to their mother? We are investigating these questions in our laboratory.

REFERENCES

Ainsworth, M. D. S., & Witting, B. A. (1969). Attachment and exploratory behavior of one-year-olds in a strange situation. In B. M. Foss (Ed.), Determinants of Infant Behaviour (vol. IV) pp. 111-136. London: Methuen; and New York: John Willey.

Bowlby, J. (1969). Attachment and Loss: vol. 1, Attachment. London: The Hograth Press; and New York: Basic Books.

Celander, O., & Folkow, B. (1951). Are parasympathetic vasodilator fibres involved in depressor reflexes elicited from the barorecepter regions. Acta Physiologica Scandinavica, 23, 64-77.

Celander, O., & Folkow, B. (1953). The correlation between the stimulation frequency and the dilator response evoked by antidromic excitation of the thin afferent fibres in the dorsal roots. Acta Physiologica Scandinavica, 29, 371-376.

DeCasper, A. J., & Fifer, W. P. (1980). Of human bonding: Newborns prefer their mother's voice. Science, 208, 1174-1176.

Field, T. M.(1985). Naonatal perception of people: maturational and individual differences. In T. M. Field and N. A. Fox (Eds.), Social Perception in Infants, pp. 31-52. New Jersey: Ablex Publishing.

Field, T. M., & Fox, N. A.(Eds.). (1986). Social perception in infants. New Jersey: Ablex Publishing.

Fujimasa,I.(Ed.). (1986). Biomedical Thermography. The Japanese Society of Thermography.

Girling, F. (1952). Vasomotor effects of electrical stimulation. American Journal of Physiology, 170, 131-135.

Johnstone, M. (1974). Facial vasomotor behavior. British Journal of Anaethesia, 46, 765-769.

Mizukami, K., Kobayashi, N., Iwata, H., & Ishii, T. (1987). Tele thermography in infant's emotional behavioral research. The Lancet, 8549, 38-39.

Piaget, J. (1954). The construction of reality in the child. New York: Basic Books.

Schaffer, H. R. (1963). Some issues for research in the study of attachment behavior. In B. M. Foss(ed.), Determinants of Infant Behaviour (vol. II), pp. 179-199. London: Methuen.

Stayton, D. J., Ainsworth, M. D. and Main, M. B. (1973). Development of separation behavior in the first year of life. Developmental psychology, 9, 213-225.

Stone, L. J., Smith, H. T., and Murphy, L. B.(Eds.). (1973). The Competent Infant: Research and Commentary. New York: Basic Books.

23
Hemispheric Specialization for Face Recognition in Infancy

S. de Schonen, E. Mathivet and C. Deruelle

INTRODUCTION

We have been studying the development in infancy of hemispheric asymmetry in face processing with a view to answering the
following questions. Is the adult right hemisphere (RH) advantage
for face processing and recognition (for reviews, see Hecaen and
Albert, 1978; Moscovitch, 1979; Benton, 1980; Young, 1983; Ellis
and Young, 1988) already present when individual face recognition
emerges in infancy, or can this asymmetry be said to result from a
factor intervening later in development, such as the increasing
neural space allotted to language functions in the LH ? To what
extent may these hemispheric functional differences be related to
differences in the rates of maturation of homologous portions of
the two hemispheres ? Might the hemispheric differences in face
processing be totally prewired or might the particular features of
infants' visual sensory capacities contribute to shaping them ?

Small pieces of answer to this puzzle will be described here
together with some speculations. We shall first present some data
concerning the RH advantage for face recognition as well as data
concerning interhemispheric communication during the first year of
life. We shall thereafter outline a scenario which is an attempt
to tell how during the first few months of life the neural
networks involved in the process of individual face (physiognomy)
recognition in the RH are shaped by the particular kinds of visual
input they receive (de Schonen and Mathivet, in press).

THE RIGHT HEMISPHERE ADVANTAGE IN PHYSIOGNOMY RECOGNITION

The data available up to now converge to show that infants
process visual static physiognomic features in an individual face
at about the beginning of the 4th month of life. Before this age,
features such as hair style or hair colouring seem to be very

important cues for recognizing individuals. Familiar faces can be recognized from photographs at about the 4th month of age (for review, see Flin and Dziurawiec, 1988). In order to know whether this competence is controlled, from its onset, by the RH, we tested (de Schonen et al., 1986) the capacity of 4- to 9- month old infants to recognize their mother's face in the right visual field (RVF, LH) and in the left visual field (LVF, RH) with a divided visual field presentation technique similar to the technique used in adult studies. Infants were presented with color slides of their mother's face and a stranger's face. The pictures (for each infant the stranger was the mother of another infant) were taken in such a way as to suppress from the slides any differences between the two faces other than truly physiognomic features. A face was projected on the right or the left of a central fixation point with its inner boundary at a visual angle of 2° from the central fixation point. A face was projected when and only when the infant was fixating this central point. The exposure duration was 350 msec and 250 msec for infants aged 4 to 6 months and 7 to 9 months, respectively. The latencies of the first ocular saccade in response to the stimulus, measured from the onset of the stimulus, were subsequently analysed in terms of the identity of the faces and the visual fields tested.

The latencies of the responses to the mother's face became significantaly shorter during the experiment than those in res- ponse to the stranger's face. Since the stranger's face presented to an infant was the mother's face for another infant, it was con- cluded that the Ss recognized their mother's face and were thus processing the physiognomic features. The decrease in the saccade latencies in response to the mother's face occurred in the LVF but not in the RVF. As a result, the difference between the responses to the mother and to the stranger was greater in the LVF-RH, than in the RVF-LH. Neither a motoric bias, nor lateral differences in acuity, nor any attentional bias can account for the hemispheric difference observed in the responses to the mother. It was concluded that when the capacity to recognize the mother's face from a two-dimensional image develops, the RH reacts faster and/or more systematically and spontaneously to the identity of the face than the LH.

Data obtained in another study showed that this RH advantage in discriminating between familiar and unfamiliar faces is not restricted to the recognition of the mother's face but seems to occur also in responses to a photograph of a face with which the infant has been shortly familiarized (de Schonen et al., exp. 2, 1986). By contrast, when the infants are familiarized with one of several geometrical patterns and tested with the same procedure, a totally different response pattern occurs. These data support the conclusion that the RH advantage observed applies specifically to both more and less familiar individual faces, rather than to visual patterns in general.

The lack of a differential reaction to familiar vs. unfamiliar faces by the LH might have been due not to an incapacity
in the LH to discriminate between the two physiognomies, but to a
lack of spontaneous interest in the LH in producing different
behavior to different faces. In order to test this assumption, an
operant conditioning technique was used with 4- to 9-month old
infants in order to "instruct" or "constrain" each hemisphere to
discriminate between the mother's and a stranger's face (de
Schonen and Mathivet, 1987; de Schonen and Mathivet, submitted).
The stimuli were prepared and presented with brief exposure times
in a divided visual field technique as in the previous experiment.
The presentation of the mother's face in one visual field was the
signal to which the infant had to respond by looking up (operant
response) in the direction of a mechanical toy (placed above the
display panel), which was then activated as a reward. Presentation
of the stranger's face in the same visual field was the signal to
which the infant had to respond by looking down in the direction
of another toy (placed below the display panel), which was then
activated. After having completed the learning task in one VF (by
having either reached the learning criterion, or failed after 38
trials), all the Ss were immediately presented with the same
learning task in the contralateral VF. This procedure made it
possible to test whether interhemispheric communication occurred
by estimating the interhemispheric transfer from the number of
trials required in the second VF tested compared to the first VF.

This operant conditioning procedure was the same as that used
in two previous studies. In one of them, we tested the subjects'
ability to discriminate in each VF between two categories of
stimuli: schematic faces and scrambled faces (de Schonen and Bry,
1987). No differences were observed between the learning performances of the two VFs in infants aged 12- to 27- weeks. Transfer
was observed to occur however from the age of 19 weeks onward but
not before. Likewise, in the other study, where the Ss were required to discriminate between two visual patterns on the basis of
two of their constituent geometrical elements, infants learned
equally well whichever VF was used. Here, however, no transfer was
found to occur at the age of 27 weeks (de Schonen and Deruelle,
1988).

In contrast to the above results, a considerable RH advantage
was observed when the stimuli to be discriminated between were the
mother's face and a stranger's face, although the procedures were
identical. As can be seen in Table 1, significantly more Ss
reached the learning criterion when the first VF was the LVF than
when it was the RVF. Also, when the second VF tested was the LVF,
learning occurred in some Ss whereas no Ss reached the criterion
when the second VF tested was the RVF. Moreover, a significant
sex-related effect was observed: In the male group no Ss reached
the learning criterion in the RVF-LH, whereas in the female group
28% reached the criterion in the RVF-LH. This confirms the

sex-related factor observed in the two experiments mentioned above where a familiar individual face was reacted to faster than a stranger's face in the LVF-RH but not in the RVF-LH. This sex-related effect does not seem to vary with age. It was concluded that in males at least, the LH neither reacts spontaneously to the mother's face, nor discriminates between it and a stranger's face even when the task requirements specifically orient the infant's activity towards this discrimination. Moreover it seems to have been impossible for the LH to use the information processed by the RH. Indeed, only one subject (a female) reached the criterion in both VF and she did not exhibit any economy in the number of trials.

Table 1. The operant conditioning experiment: discrimination between the mother's and a stranger's face. Upper line: percentages of Ss reaching the criterion (Yes), failing after 40 trials (No), fussing after few trials (Rej.) when tested first in the LVF or the RVF. Lower line: scores in the second (contralateral) VF tested (not all the Ss could be tested in the contralateral VF)

First visual field: Left				First visual vield: Right			
Rej.	No	Yes	N=100%	Rej.	No	Yes	N=100%
25%	14%	61%	28	32%	54%	14%	28

Second visual field: Left				Second visual field: Right			
Rej.	No	Yes	N=100%	Rej.	No	Yes	N=100%
29%	29%	43%	14	50%	50%	0	12

Taken as a whole, these data show that: (i) the RH advantage observed concerns processes that are involved quite specifically in physiognomy recognition. The LH might have discriminated between the two physiognomies on the basis of non-physiognomic processing as if they were not faces. The results show however that the LH cannot even do this (at least within the number of trials allotted to learning). This suggests that in the great majority of the infants, the kind of processing required for fast discrimination between two such patterns to be possible emerges, from its functional onset in the first months of life, in the RH only, whereas the kind of processing required to recognize faceness as well as geometrical patterns develops in both hemispheres. This suggests that only the RH, and not the LH, can develop a specific system liable to process physiognomies and similar objects, or that this specific system develops earlier in the RH than in the LH. In both cases, the hypothesis that the RH advantage in physiognomic recognition is the direct result during development of the increasing neural space occupied by language during its acquisition can be excluded. It does not of course exclude the possibility that prewiring factors having allotted in the human species a great deal of LH space to the language acquisition device, the neural space allotted to physiognomy recognition and other related competences is consequently restricted to the RH before any language acquisition has taken place. (ii) At the age of 9 months, the activity of the RH in physiognomy recognition can still not be communicated to the LH. The fact that an interhemispheric transfer of learning occurs in the faceness recognition task only, supports once more the idea that phy- siognomy recognition is not controlled by the same neuronal structures as faceness recognition. This lack of interhemispheric communication might contribute to the stabilization of asymmetric synaptic organization. In this connection, one last result is worth mentioning. In the faceness situation as well as with the geometrical pattern discrimination situation, there exists a period of development during which, when one hemisphere has been learning a task successfully, the contralateral hemisphere cannot immediately thereafter learn this task, as if it were temporarily prevented for a few minutes from learning the same task. Indeed, before transfer can be observed there is an age period during which learning is impossible in the second VF tested (12 to 19 weeks in the case of the faceness discrimination, and 19 to 27 weeks in the case of geometrical patterns) despite the fact that each hemisphere can learn when tested first. This suggests that each hemisphere can have a temporary inhibitory effect on the other, preventing a double learning in the absence of on line interhemispheric communications. (iii) The lateralization of the advantage in face recognition appears to be related to sex. Males have a systematic RH advantage while females have a much less systematic advantage. It might be the case that the maturation rates differ between males and females (see Held, this volume). The perceptual competences investigated here might not develop at different rates in males and females. But in males the neural networks liable to control face recognition might become mature in the RH long before their left homologous counterpart. In females, the time lags between the right and left neural networks might be shorter, or even reversed.

Which aspects of the neural systems controlling physiognomy recognition are prewired, and which are shaped by experiential factors ?

A SCENARIO FOR THE DEVELOPMENT OF THE RH ADVANTAGE IN FACE RECOGNITION

Several authors have suggested that some portions of one hemisphere develop at a faster rate than their homologous counterparts (Corballis and Morgan, 1978; Netley and Rovet, 1983; Geschwind and Galaburda, 1985). Several arguments (for a review, Geschwind et al., 1985; Rosen et al., 1987) support the idea that some portions of the RH mature faster than their left homologues. It is not sure, however, whether after birth, when experience might be a shaping factor, there still exists a difference in the maturational rates. Rakic et al.'s data (1986; see also

Goldman-Rakic,* this volume) cannot be used as evidence against the idea that the RH and LH do not mature at different rates after birth. Small delays in synaptogenesis or at some later stage in synaptic functional development, may result in some synaptic organization being selected and stabilized rather than another. Stabilizing a network may take anything from a few minutes to a few hours or days (Fifkova and van Harreveld, 1977; Buisseret et al., 1978; Fifkova, 1985; Schechter and Murphy, 1976; Singer, 1987). The involvement of various cortical regions in their behavioral function does not occur at the same rate (Crowell et al., 1973; Best et al., 1982; Chugani and Phelps, 1986; Harwerth et al., 1986; Thatcher et al., 1987). In short, it is not at all impossible that even after birth, when visual experience is more liable to play a role, some portions of the RH and LH still mature at different rates. The RH advantage in physiognomy processing might result from the fact that the neuronal networks involved in this function might become functional in the RH before the LH.

Now, at the time when neuronal circuits in the RH reach the functional stage at which they are able to process physiognomies (at about 2-4 month), the infant's visual sensitivity is limited. The most closely documented approach to this limitation deals with the spatial frequency sensitivity. Numerous studies have shown that during the first few months of life, visual acuity and contrast sensitivity are limited (for review, Banks and Dannemiller, 1987). Around the age of 3 to 4 months which is of interest here, the contrast sensitivity functions have shown that visual acuity is 6 to 8 times lower then the adult level and the maximum contrast sensitivity, 10 to 20 times. Moreover the idea that different channels respond to different bands of spatial frequency seems to be valid from the age of 3 months onwards (Banks et al., 1985).

It is worth pointing out, however, that to describe the limitations of the visual sensitivity in terms of spatial frequency might not be the most relevant approach. Many other aspects of vision and of its possible limitation in infancy are not included in this description (see Held, this volume for instance). The main point of our argument is that the visual information which is conveyed to territories liable to process and recognize physiognomies around the age of 2 to 4 months is restricted. The RH physiognomy recognition device thus becomes functional on the basis of restricted visual information. If the neural networks which control physiognomic recognition stabilize their pattern of synaptic connections with afferents relating, for instance, to the lower rather than the higher spatial frequencies, then there is every likelihood that the RH physiognomic recognition device will become specialized in processing and memorizing the features that are present in the low spatial frequencies of individual faces or in poorly perceived faces.

---

* manuscript not submitted

From the above considerations, it might be predicted that in adults the specific RH way of processing individual faces keeps exactly the features it has acquired during its early functional history. To continue with our provisional description in terms of spatial frequencies, it might be predicted that in adults, the specific RH way of processing faces consists of processing the low spatial frequencies within a physiognomy. Indeed, Sergent (1982, 1983, 1986) has characterized the RH advantage over the LH as consisting of rapidly processing low spatial frequencies: the RH has an advantage over the LH when presented with defocused physiognomies comprising only low spatial frequencies (lower or equal to 2 cycles/d°). Michimata and Hellige (1987) have observed that visual features other than spatial frequencies might also play a role. Many data converge, however, to show that the differences between RH and LH do not lie in the first stages of spatial frequency processing, but are to be found at a pattern processing level (Beaton and Blakemore, 1981; Fiorentini and Berardi, 1980, 1984; Vassilev et al., 1985; Szelag et al., 1987). Some of the constituent features of the so-called "holistic" processing which was traditionally thought to be specific to the RH pattern processing might thus be related after all to its ability to process and organize shapes and patterns from the only features that are usable in poorly perceptible objects.

To assume that the neuronal networks involved in individual faces processing and memorizing are shaped in the RH by limited visual inputs experienced during the first months of life, does not imply that all RH neuronal networks involved in visual pattern processing will be characterized once and for all by the same shaping events. It depends on when the networks mature and become functional and whether their organization is rapidly stabilized. To go on with the example of the spatial frequencies, it is clear that after the first few months of life, high spatial frequencies will begin to be processed by the RH and will become in their turn constituents of visual information processing. Our hypothesis is that one, or the only, neuronal network in the RH which is liable to process physiognomies stabilizes fairly quickly because physiognomies, as well as some other body parts, are a category of visual patterns which fulfill the largest number of functions for infants, as well as being the most frequently encountered (see for a discussion, de Schonen et al., in press). Since they stabilize quickly, these neuronal networks will rapidly become specific and unable to be modified by the high spatial frequency pathways when these mature. Whereas other neuronal networks involved in visual patterns processing might change with age or might even develop later. These will process the whole range of spatial frequencies. Now, in the LH, no system for physiognomic processing similar to the RH one observed in the first months of life can develop because the delay in maturation results in a different synaptic organization. If some neuronal nets can still become specialized in physiognomic processing, they will include the inputs from the high spatial frequencies which will make them very different from the RH device. Moreover it is possible that the lack of interhemispheric communications and/or the temporary inhibition of the one hemisphere by the other (see above) contribute thereafter to preventing the LH from developing a similar face recognition device to that of the RH (Gazzaniga, 1970; Moscovitch, 1977; Doty and Negrao, 1973; Dennenberg, 1981). Finally, individual differences in hemispheric lateralization, such as sex-related differences (de Schonen and Mathivet, 1987; de Schonen et al., submitted), might be related to variations in the temporal relationships between the maturation rates of the two hemispheres.

REFERENCES

Banks, M.S. and Dannemiller, J.L. (1987). Infant visual psychophysics. In Handbook of Infant Perception (eds. P. Salapatek and L. Cohen). Academic Press, Orlando.

Banks, M.S., Stephens, B.R. and Hartmann, E.E. (1985). The development of basic mechanisms of pattern vision: spatial frequency channels. J. Exp. Child Psychol., 40, 501-527.

Beaton, A. and Blakemore, C. (1981). Orientation selectivity of the human system as a function of retinal eccentricity and visual hemifield. Perception, 10, 273-282.

Benton, A.L. (1980). The neuropsychology of facial recognition. Amer. Psychol., 35, 176-186.

Best, C.T., Hoffmann, H. and Glanville, B.B. (1982). Development of infant ear asymmetries for speech and music. Percept. and Psychophys., 31, 75-85.

Buisseret, P., Gary-Bobo, E. and Imbert, M. (1978). Ocular motility and recovery of orientational properties of visual cortical neurons in dark-reared kittens. Nature, 272, 816-817.

Chugani, H.T. and Phelps, M.E. (1986). Maturational changes in cerebral function in infants determined by FDG Positron Emission Tomography. Science, 231, 840-842.

Corballis, M.C. and Morgan, M.J. (1978). On the biological basis of human laterality. I. Evidence for a maturational left-right gradient. Behav. and Brain Sci., 2, 261-336.

Crowell, D.H., Jones, R.H., Kapuniai, L.E. and Nakagawa, J.K. (1973). Unilateral cortical activity in newborn humans: an early index of cerebral dominance ? Science, 180, 205-208.

Dennenberg, V.H. (1981). Hemispheric laterality in animals and the effects of early experience. Behav. and Brain Sci., 4, 1-48.

de Schonen, S. and Bry, I. (1987) Interhemispheric communication of visual learning: a developmental study in 3-6 month old infants. Neuropsychol., 25, 601-612.

de Schonen, S. and Deruelle, C. (1988). Communication inter-hémisphérique d'une discrimination de formes visuelles chez le nourrisson de 4 à 9 mois. Poster presented at the First Meeting of the Neuroscience Club, Marseille, April 1988 (paper in preparation).

de Schonen, S., Gil de Diaz, M. and Mathivet, E. (1986). Hemispheric asymmetry in face processing in infancy. In Aspects of Face Processing. (eds. H.D. Ellis, M.A. Jeeves, F. Newcombe and A. Young). Martinius Nijhoff, Dordrecht.

de Schonen, S. and Mathivet, E. (1987). Hemispheric asymmetry for face processing in 4- to 9-month old infants. Paper presented at the Second Conference of the European Society for Cognitive Psychology. Madrid, 7-11 September 1987.

de Schonen, S. and Mathivet, E. (in press). First come, first served: a scenario about the last stages in the development of hemispheric specialization in face processing. Europ. Bull. Cognit. Psychol., C.P.C. (to appear in 1989).

de Schonen, S. and Mathivet, E. (submitted). Hemispheric asymmetry and interhemispheric communication of face processing in infancy.

Doty, R.W. and Negrao, N. (1973). Forebrain commissures and vision. In Handbook of Sensory Physiology. (ed. R. Jung). Springer-Verlag, Berlin.

Ellis, H.D. and Young, A.W. (1988). Are faces special ? In Handbook of Research on Face Processing. (eds. A.W. Young and H.D. Ellis). North-Holland, Amsterdam.

Fifkova, E. (1985). A possible mechanism of morphometric changes in dendritic spines induced by stimulation. Cell. Mol. Neurobiology, 5, 47-63.

Fifkova, E. and Van Harreveld, A. (1977). Long lasting morphological changes in dendritic spines of granular cells following stimulation of the enthorinal area. J. Neurocytol., 6, 211-230.

Fiorentini, A. and Berardi, N. (1980). Perceptual learning specific for orientation and spatial frequency. Nature, 287, 43-44.

Fiorentini, A. and Berardi, N. (1984). Right hemisphere superiority in the discrimination of spatial phase. Perception,

13, 695-708.

Flin, R. and Dziurawiec, S. (1988). Developmental factors in face processing. In Handbook of Research on Face Processing. (eds. A. Young and H. Ellis). North Holland, Amsterdam.

Gazzaniga, M.S. (1970). The Bisected Brain. Appleton Century Crofts, New York.

Geschwind, N. and Galaburda, A.M. (1985). Cerebral lateralization. Biological mechanisms, associations, and pathology: I. A hypothesis and a program for research. Arch. Neurol., 42, 428-459.

Harwerth, R.S., Smith III, E.L., Duncan, G.C., Crawford, M.L.J. and von Noorden, G.K. (1986). Multiple sensitive periods in the development of the primate visual system. Science, 232, 235-238.

Hecaen, H. and Albert, M. (1978). Human Neuropsychology. Wiley, New York.

Michimata, C. and Hellige, J.B. (1987). Effects of blurring and stimulus size on the lateralized processing of nonverbal stimuli. Neuropsychol., 25, 397-407.

Moscovitch, M. (1977). The development of lateralization of language functions and its relation to cognitive and linguistic development: a review and some theoretical speculations. In Language Development and Neurobiological Theory (eds. S.J. Segalowitz and F.A. Gruber). Academic Press, New York.

Moscovitch, M. (1979). Information processing and the cerebral hemispheres. In Handbook of Neurobiology: Neuropsychology. (ed. M.S. Gazzaniga). Plenum Press, New York.

Netley, C. and Rovet, J. (1983). Relationships among brain organization, maturation rate and the development of verbal and nonverbal ability. In Language Functions and Brain Organization.(ed. S.J. Segalowitz). Academic Press, New York.

Rakic, P., Bourgeois, J.P., Eckenhoff, M.F., Zecevic, N., Goldman-Rakic, P.S. (1986). Concurrent overproduction of synapses in diverse regions of the primate cerebral cortex. Science, 232, 232-235.

Rosen, G.D., Galaburda, A.M. and Sherman, G.F. (1987). Mechanisms of brain asymmetry: new evidence and hypotheses. In Duality and Unity of the Brain. (ed. D. Ottoson). Plenum Press, New York.

Schechter, P.B. and Murphy, E.H. (1976). Brief monocular visual experience and kitten cortical binocularity. Brain Res., 109, 165-168.

Sergent, J. (1982). Methodological and theoretical consequences of variations in exposure duration in visual laterality studies. Percept. and Psychophys., 31, 451-461.

Sergent, J. (1983). The effects of sensory limitations on hemispheric processing. Canad. J. Psychol., 37, 345-366.

Sergent, J. (1986). Microgenesis of faceperception. In Aspects of Face Processing. (eds. H.D. Ellis, M.A. Jeeves, F. Newcombe and A. Young). Martinus Nijhoff, Dordrecht.

Singer, W. (1987). Activity-dependent self-organization of synaptic connections as a substrate of learning. In The Neural and Molecular Bases of Learning. (eds. J.P. Changeux and M. Konishi). Wiley, New York.

Szelag, W., Budohoska, W. and Koltuska, B. (1987). Hemispheric differences in the perception of gratings. Bull. Psychon. Soc., 25, 95-98.

Thatcher, R.W., Walker, R.A. and Giudice, S. (1987). Human cerebral hemispheres develop at different rates and ages. Science, 236, 1110-1113.

Vassilev, A., Verskaia, A.A., Manahilov, V., Mitov, D. and Leushina, L.I. (1985). Spatial vision in the left and right visual fields. Perception, 14, A38.

Young, A.W. (1983). Functions of the Right Cerebral Hemisphere. Academic Press, New York.

24

Factors Influencing Left-side Preference for Holding Newborn Infants

Peter de Château

Several studies have demonstrated the existence of a clear tendency for mothers to hold their infants on the left rather than on the right arm (Salk, 1960; Weiland, 1964; de Château, Holmberg, Winberg, 1978). In a limited number of societies this left bias in mothers child-holding techniques has been observed (Richards and Finger, 1975). Finger (1975), in a study of art works from European and American artists, found no significant side preference in pictures in which children were held by men. In contrast Harris and Fitzgerald (1985), using photographs from textbooks in developmental psychology, showed the same left-side holding in women and men. The development of side-preference for holding and carrying a doll (representing a newborn infant) was investigated in 305 children of both sexes (de Château and Andersson, 1976). Their ages ranged from 2 - 16 years. Preference was found to develop gradually during childhood. Girls held and carried on the left-side more than boys, both in the total sample and each group studied.

Direct observation of adult behaviour with newborns revealed that 80 per cent of all newly delivered mothers and fathers held their infant against a point to the left of the body mid line (de Château, 1983). Both new fathers and fathers with older infants displayed a significantly greater preference for holding the infant to the left than males without own children and with or without experience of other children. Greenberg and Morris (1974) found that fathers who had been present at the birth of their infants found themselves to be more comfortable in holding infants. The same fathers could distinguish their baby from other babies more easily as compared to a group of fathers who had not been present at delivery., Right-holding increases in separated mothers and is also related to more pre- and postnatal anxiety in their relationships to their infants (de Château, Mäki, Nyberg; 1982). Many men and women begin parenthood with great insecurity and with low estimates of their creditability as prospective parents. The reasons for this are complicated. Frequently, feelings of inadequacy go back to the individuals own early experiences and the relationships with one's own parents. Psychological, medical, and social information, as well as support, may neutralize part of this anxiety. However, adjustment to the parental role, sensitivity to the infant's needs, and the ability to meet the infant's demands may be less a cognitive function than an emotional, empathic one. If men in this respect are less well prepared than women, as indirectly indicated in their behaviour, perhaps more effort should be made to activate and promote their feelings.

Asymmetry in behaviour is of course something that fascinates us all. Trevarthen has in his presentation shown that indeed newborn infants also differ in behaviour depending on which side of the face one looks at and that the two sides of the brain have complementary roles. He describes for instance the early asymmetry of gestures with a dominating right-hand and a difference between boys and girls. The concept of a caretaker support and interplay between the adult brain and the infant's brain in the process of normal learning and development is certainly one that fits beautifully with the obvious need of newborn's and young infant's to gain more social knowledge. It seems however still difficult to understand what exactly the contribution of the young infant is. From our clinical experience we know of infants that fail to thrive within the setting of a given partnership. In bringing about changes in this partnership we many times seem to alter the course of events. But what is specific in the behavioural repertoire of the new partner that brings about a change to the better, and what happens to the mother-infant dyad after the change has been made? Certainly sensitivity to signals from the infant various greatly from adult to adult. Can we learn to read the needs of the newborn and act according to that new knowledge? Not all babies with failure-to-thrive come back to the hospital, in many cases the mother seems to manage on her own after a period of support and training.

One way of gaining more knowledge about signals between mother and infant might be the study of maternal and infant behaviour when they are together. The way, for instance, a mother holds her newborn baby may develop under the influence of mother-infant interaction. Nearly 80 per cent of all mothers hold their newborn infants against a point to the left of the body midline, irrespective of handedness and parity (de Château, Holmberg and Winberg, 1978). Salk (1960) first reported this side preference

and Weiland (1964) corroborated this finding in mothers
with older children in a well-baby clinic. Separation
of mothers and infants during the period immediately
after birth affected the extent of this preference (Salk,
1960; de Château, Holmberg and Winberg, 1978). Change
in holding behaviour may thus be an early sign of disturbed
mother-infant interaction. In a prospective study non-separated mothers holding to the left during the neonatal
period were over a three year period compared with mothers
holding to the right. Non-separated right-holding mothers
were in greater need for contact with the medical autho-
rities on account of their children (de Château, 1987).
During normal pregnancy, one month prior to delivery, 82
gravidae were interviewed. The way these mothers held their
infants was studied during the first postnatal week. Mothers
holding on the right had experienced a more negative perception of body changes and had made fewer preparations for
delivery of the expected baby during pregnancy (de Château,
Mäki and Nyberg, 1982).

Two theoretical explanations for this sidepreference
in holding infants have been put forward. Salk (1960) discussed the influence of the maternal heartbeat as an imprinting stimulant that has a soothing effect on the infant,
whereas Weiland (1964) postulated that the preference for
holding on the left primarily serves to relieve anxiety
in the adult carrier. However, the infant may very well
be able to play a key role in moulding maternal behavioural
patterns. Infant reactions to stimulation by sound, light
and touch, have proven to be asymmetrical under certain
conditions. Correlation has been found to exist between
the initial head-turning responses of infants two days
postpartum and maternal holding preference two to three
weeks later (Ginsburg et al, 1979). This could mean that
right-holding is appropriate in normal newborns showing
left-side preference in their behavioural reactions. In
sick, premature and/or separated newborns, this could be
a sign of disturbed neonatal behaviour, as the percentage
of atypical responses to stimuli increases.

References

de Château, P. (1983). Left-side preference for holding
and carrying newborn infants. Parental holding and carrying during the first week of life. J Nerv Ment Disease,
171, 241-245.

de Château, P. (1987). Left-side preference in holding
and carrying newborn infants. A three year follow-up
study. Acta Psychiat Scand, 75, 283-286.

de Château, P. and Andersson, Y. (1976). Left-side preference for holding and carrying newborn infants. II. Doll-holding and carrying from 2 to 16 years. Develop Med Child Neurol., 18, 738-744.

de Château, P., Holmberg, H. and Winberg, J. (1978). Left-side preference in holding and carrying newborn infants. Acta Paediatr Scand., 67, 169-175.

de Château, P., Mäki, M. and Nyberg, B. (1982). Left-side preference in holding and carrying newborn infants. III. Mothers' perception of pregnancy one month prior to delivery and subsequent holding behaviour. J Psychosom Obst and Gyn., 1, 72-76.

Finger, S. (1975). Child holding patterns in western art. Child Dev., 46, 267-271.

Ginsburg, H.J., Fling, S., Hope, M.L., Musgrave, D. and Andrews, C. Maternal holding preference: a consequence of newborn head-turning response. Child Dev., 50, 280-281.

Greenberg, M. and Morris, N. (1974). Engrossment: The newborn's impact upon the father. Am J Orthopsychiat., 44, 520-531.

Harris, L.J. and Fitzgerald, H.E. (1985). Lateral cradling preferences in men and women: results from a photographic study. J Gen Psychol., 112, 185-189.

Richards, J.L. and Finger, S. (1975). Mother-child holding patterns. A cross-cultural photographic study. Child Dev., 46, 1001-1004.

Salk, L. (1960). The effect of the normal heartbeat sound on the behavior of the newborn infant. World Ment Health, 12, 168-175.

Weiland, J.H. (1964). Heartbeat rhythm and maternal behavior. J Am Acad Child Psychiat., 3, 161-164.

25
Early Voice Discrimination

William Fifer and Christine Moon

INTRODUCTION

Newborn infants face the immense task of organizing a largely
novel perceptual world. From the earliest hours and days after
birth, babies come to approach some forms of stimulation and tune
out or avoid others. Researchers are attempting to understand how
fetal postnatal experience shapes these early behaviors and how,
in turn, these capabilities subserve later developmental
processes. In our laboratory, we have primarily focused our
investigative energies for the last several years on one aspect of
newborns' developmental agenda - the response to the sound of
voices.

There is abundant evidence that the sounds of speech are
salient to the neonate. Complex sounds in the frequency range of
voices have been shown to be more effective than either simple
tones or sounds out of the voice range in eliciting responses on a
variety of measures (Aslin, Pisoni & Jusczyk, 1983). Head and eye
orienting to the sound of a voice has been recognized as a marker
of behavioral competence of neonates (Brazelton, 1984). Moreover,
there is a growing body of research showing that even very young
infants respond selectively to particular voices, the most well-
documented being that of the infant's own mother. Mills and
Meluish (1974) showed that the maternal voice may be an important
stimulus for infants 20 to 30 days old. Amount of time spent
sucking and number of sucks per minute were greater when a brief
presentation of mother's voice followed initiations of sucking
bursts. In a study of one-month-old infants (Mehler, et al,
1978), sucking rate increased to presentations of mother's versus
a stranger female voice, but only when the voices were highly
intonated. Clinical observations suggested that newborn
infants preferentially orient to mother's voice (Andre-Thomas,

277

1966; and Hammond, 1970). Within two hours of birth, infants have been reported to be differentially responsive to their own mother calling their name in comparison to four other females (Querleu, et al, 1984). Thus, voices in general and mother's voice in particular appear to be selected by young infants from the array of available auditory stimuli.

METHODOLOGY

Most methods that have been effective in assessing neonatal responsiveness to auditory stimulation have not been applicable to the study of voice perception. Measurement of evoked potentials and habituation techniques are limited to studies of discrete, brief sounds. General body activation or quiescence during stimulation is difficult to quantify and interpret. Modifications of traditional learning techniques, however, have proven useful in obtaining reliable measures of the response of very young infants to the sound of voices. Newborns can make a change in their behavior when the consequence is hearing the sound of a human voice. One- and two-day-olds change sucking patterns to activate a recording of a singing group (Butterfield & Siperstein, 1972) or a recording of a single female vocalist (DeCasper & Carstens, 1981).

Using a temporal discrimination procedure, DeCasper and Fifer (1980) showed that babies can learn to activate a recording of their own mother's voice more than another mother's by changing sucking patterns. Newborn infants, forty-eight to seventy-two hours old, were presented with a contingency in which changes from baseline in rate of sucking resulted in differential presentation of recordings of mother's or stranger's voices. Eight of nine infants showing a preference chose their mother's voice; they produced their own mother's voice more often and for a longer total period of time. Four of the infants who demonstrated this preference subsequently encountered a reversal of the initial contingencies. All four newborns reversed their earlier pattern of sucking and thus again heard more of their own mother's voice. Thus with a limited number of infants and using a procedure which may be quite demanding for the infant, discrimination and preference for the maternal voice was demonstrated.

This work offered a promising methodological paradigm for further investigation of very young infants' ability and propensity to respond to complex auditory events. Over the past few years we have worked to develop and standardize this technique while applying it to questions about the relative reinforcing value of familiar and unfamiliar voices. The method has also proved useful in the investigation of newborn discrimination of syllables. It has generated information-rich data sets which allow conclusions about early organization of newborn behavior, and in addition, has generated enough questions and conundrums for years of future research.

All of our experiments have been conducted in the following manner. The subjects were between one and three days of age, and the experimental sessions were in a quiet hospital examination room near the newborn nursery, most often on the day the baby was discharged. Infants were brought to a quiet, alert state with eyes open in dim light by talking to them, holding them, swaddling or unswaddling, and elevating the head end of the bassinet. Babies not judged to have reached a quiet, alert state were returned to the nursery. This happened with about 1/5 of the infants. For the remaining subjects, a non-nutritive nipple was placed in the baby's mouth and headphones over the ears. A short period of adjustment, about two minutes, followed during which the baby's sucks were monitored for typical burst/pause patterns. Infants were rarely disqualified at this point in the procedure for failing to suck in measurable, discrete bursts. Auditory stimuli commenced and were presented for 18 minutes during which time the infant was attended by an experimenter who could not hear the stimuli. Sessions were terminated prematurely if an infant failed to emit measurable sucking bursts for two 45-second periods, due almost exclusively to fussiness or drowsiness. The attrition rate has been between 40 to 50 percent across experiments.

The sounds that were presented over the headphones were contingent upon the baby's sucking patterns. In the absence of a sucking burst, strings of syllables (the signals) were presented such that four seconds of one syllable alternated with four seconds of a second syllable, e.g. four seconds of /a/ ("ah") alternating with four seconds of /i/ ("ee"). If the infant initiated a sucking burst, the syllable string immediately ceased and one of two alternative sounds (a reinforcer) was presented. A reinforcer was presented for as long as the infant continued the sucking burst, on average about 7 seconds. At the termination of the burst, the reinforcer ceased, and the 4-second signal strings resumed. For example, in our first experiment, the syllables /pat/ and /pst/, spoken by a male voice, signalled the availability of either a recording of mother's voice or silence. For half of the subjects, initiating a sucking burst during the four seconds of /pat/ resulted in a presentation of mother's voice for the duration of the sucking burst. Sucking during /pst/ resulted in silence for the burst duration. For the other half of the subjects, /pat/ was paired with silence and /pst/ with

mother's voice. If mother's voice was reinforcing, a higher
frequency of bursts would be expected during the syllable which
signalled availability of the voice as compared to the signal for
silence, and there should be longer bursts during the voice than
silence. In addition to demonstrating greater responding to one
reinforcer than another, infants could also show the ability to
discriminate one syllable from another. Initially, we chose
syllables which we believed to be easily discriminable since the
focus of the experiments was on the reinforcing value of familiar
and unfamiliar voices.

SUMMARY OF RESULTS

The first question we asked of 12 newborns was (metaphorically
speaking), "Will you change your sucking patterns over the
18-minute session in order to hear a recording of your mother
talking to another adult?" (The other adult and extraneous
sounds and pauses were omitted from the tape.) The answer was,
"Yes". While there were no differences in the first or second six
minute periods of the session, during the final six minutes, 10 of
the 12 infants sucked longer during mothers voice than silence,
and 9 of the babies sucked with higher frequency during the signal
for her voice (Moon & Fifer, 1988a). Two-day-olds responded to
the sound of mother's voice, even when she was not speaking in
the special speech patterns reserved for them. This result was
subsequently replicated with a group of infants for whom the
signals were /pat/ and /tap/ (Moon, 1985, and Moon, Bever & Fifer,
1988).

Of the next two groups of babies we asked questions about the
reinforcing value of the voice of a woman who was not the mother
(Fifer & Moon, 1988a). In the first condition, the question was,
"If the voice is another baby's mother, will you change your
sucking patterns in order to listen to it?" A different voice was
used for each infant. Again, the answer was "Yes". During the
final 6 minutes, 11 of 12 subjects activated the voice for longer
durations than silence, and 10 of the babies sucked more
frequently during the signal for the voice. The sound of a
woman's voice in adult conversation was reinforcing for the
two-day-olds.

The second condition in the non-mother study was run as a
replication of DeCasper & Fifer's (1980) experiment in the context
of our standardized procedure and analysis. A group of 16
newborns was asked, "Will you activate your own mother's voice
more than another woman's voice?" The answer was a strong "Yes"
for the burst duration contingency (14 of 16 babies) but, in the

signal contingency, a non-significant number of the babies, 10 of 16, sucked longer during the signal for mother's voice. These results are similar to the pattern in DeCasper & Fifer (1980) in which the burst duration responses were stronger than the signal contingency responses, although in that study both measures were significant. There are a number of differences between the two mother/other voice studies including session length, type of voice recordings, and type of signals. We conclude that our results replicate the earlier finding of a preference for mother's voice, but in combination with our mother/silence results, it is clear that two-day-olds are also responding to other adult female voices.

What about male voices? DeCasper & Prescott (1984) found that for a group of 6 newborns, there was no evidence that recordings of stranger males' voices could induce a change in sucking patterns. We have just completed a similar study with 16 infants and have found that there is only weak evidence of a tendency to respond to the voices (Moon & Fifer, 1986). The male voices were recorded under the same conditions as the female voices. One explanation for the lack of clear response to the male voice is the possible role of familiarity with female voices from experience in the womb. Mother's voice is a prominent sound in the amniotic environment, dominating all other sounds. Other voices are transmitted with more attenuation, and male voices in particular may be masked by lower frequency vascular and digestive sounds (DeCasper & Prescott, 1984; Fifer & Moon, 1988b).

In addition to the results from studies with male voices, we have generated evidence that prenatal auditory experience influences postnatal responding. Using the same method, we asked 16 newborns, "Which will you activate more: a recording of your mother's voice altered to approximate its sound in the womb, or an unaltered recording of her voice? The "womb" version was low-pass filtered according to specifications from previous measurements made in the amniotic cavities of women about to give birth, with a recording of in utero maternal vascular sounds mixed in the background (Moon & Fifer, 1986). There was significantly more responding to the signal for the "womb" version as compared to the unaltered voice. We are currently conducting a replication of the study with mother's voice filtered as before, but without the background of vascular sounds. Thus far with 7 subjects, there is significantly more sucking during the syllable which is paired with the filtered voice. It is anticipated that these two studies, along with one by Spence & DeCasper (1987) will provide solid evidence that prenatal experience influences neonates' tendency to respond to mother's voice. A further line of experiments is planned to try to identify what aspects of the maternal and non-maternal speech signal are salient to newborns.

The two-day-olds have provided, along with the helpful answers, some perplexing questions for us. These questions have arisen primarily from patterns of results from several experiments taken together. For example, during the early parts of the experimental session when the response to the preferred reinforcer is being acquired, there appears to be a tendency for the infants to respond more to the alternative reinforcer, both in burst duration and signal contingencies (see Figures 1 and 2). This tendency becomes significant only when the data from several experiments are combined. We are optimistic that with a new, more powerful data collection system we will be able to test some of our hypotheses regarding this tendency. A second question involves an apparent interaction between the type of syllable signals and response to the reinforcers. In the experiments using /pat/ and /pst/ as signals (mother/quiet, other/quiet, mother/other), the burst duration contingency showed the stronger differential responding, even though the syllables should have been easily discriminable. In experiments using syllables which would seem to be less discriminable - /a/ versus /i/ (the male/quiet, utero/non-utero, and filtered/unfiltered experiments) or /pat/ versus /tap/ (the mother/quiet experiments) - the signal contingency provided stronger evidence of a differential response than did burst duration. This syllable/reinforcer interaction was especially evident in an experiment in which non- canonical syllables were used as signals (/pst/ versus /tsp/) and the infants paradoxically responded throughout the session to the signal for quiet more than mother's voice, contrary to the results of two other groups that showed a clear response in favor of mother over quiet (Moon, 1985)

For many years changes in heart rate have been used as an index of psychophysiological responsivity in newborn infants. We have hypothesized that a parasympathetic component of heart rate variability (HRV), respiratory sinus arrythmia (RSA), might provide another measure of CNS reactivity to external stimulation. We investigated whether infants would show a differential response in RSA to highly salient source of auditory stimulation - the maternal voice.

Eighteen healthy fullterm neonates were presented with alterations of a period of silence followed by a period of recorded mother's voice. Heart rate and sucking responses were recorded. The heart rate data were analyzed using spectral analysis which partitioned the HRV into frequency components. Our results show that newborns had significantly greater RSA during mother's voice as compared to periods of silence. Mean heart rate and sucking, traditional measures of stimulus responsivity, and HRV associated with frequencies other than the respiratory band

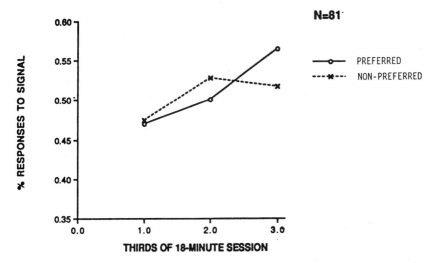

Figure 1. Average percent of responses to signals for the predicted preferred versus non-preferred voice. Data are from five experiments, with 18-minute sessions, reported in 6-minute periods.

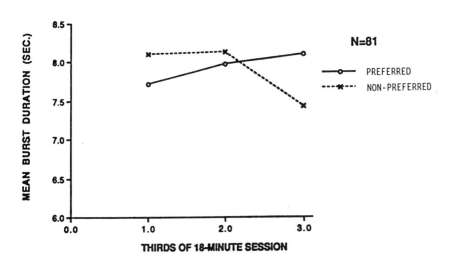

Figure 2. Average sucking burst durations during six-minute periods.

did not differ during the periods.

In addition to the behavioral data showing that newborns respond differentially to the maternal voice, the results of this study now provide us with psychophysiological data showing a differential response to voice. The use of RSA as a dependent measure of responsivity also provides us with another tool for further investigating newborn perceptual and learning capabilities.

DISCUSSION

Overall, the results from the choice procedure experiments demonstrate the infant's capacity to maintain an alert state for at least 18 minutes, to learn an active, differential response to two syllables shortly after birth, and to demonstrate preferences for auditory stimuli. An effort was made to more rigorously standardize several experimental variables across both of these experimental paradigms. Recordings of voices were of normal, adult-to-adult conversation which can serve as a standard for future comparisons to other patterns of speech. The length of the experimental sessions, i.e., 18 minutes in the choice procedure, 6 minutes in the autonomic procedure, was predetermined as were specifications for trial vs test periods. Criteria for exclusion were uniform and quantified. Data analyses were uniform. Standardization will facilitate individual and between-group comparisons in future, similar experiments with very young infants.

In our laboratory we plan to pursue the investigation of newborns' responses to familiar and unfamiliar voices and sounds of speech. Over the next months we will manipulate recordings of mother's voice to try to ascertain which aspects of the auditory signal are salient to newborns. The nature of the intrauterine maternal voice and older infants' responses to exaggerated intonation lead us to hypothesize that prosody is the key component in infant voice recognition. In addition, we plan to pursue the question of the interaction of syllable type and response to reinforcer by varying syllable signals. These results may have ramifications for meta-phonological development as well as contingency learning under different conditions.

Also currently underway are projects with three groups of infants who are considered at risk for mildly dysfunctional cognitive development: babies asphyxiated during birth and preterm and postmature infants. Using autonomic measures which are less demanding of the infant's awake, alert state than the sucking measures, we monitor responses to recordings of mother's voice which we know to be a potent auditory stimulus to neonates of uncomplicated deliveries. Autonomic indices in the presence or absence of the voice may provide an indication of subtle cognitive differences between the risk groups and normal newborns.

This early responsiveness to the speech signal creates a potential avenue into the investigation of several developmental domains. One obvious candidate is the area of speech perception. What aspects of the speech signal are salient to babies, and how do these preferences relate to later perception? Evolving responsiveness to voice provides a window into the exploration of very early memory. Infants need to retain information about mother's voice in order to respond selectively to it. A third line of investigation that suggests itself is in the study of social development. The voice is likely to be an important tool for the infant in organizing its behavior around the caretaker. Finally, voices carry much information about emotional state. The earliest interaction with these cues may be important in shaping the infants own "emotional" responses.

ACKNOWLEDGEMENTS

We gratefully acknowledge the assistance of Shahnaz Singh, Jodi Haiken and Danielle Moller in the preparation of this manuscript. Preparation of this paper was supported by PHS grants # HD22817 and # HD13063.

REFERENCES

Andre-Thomas, A.S. (1966). Locomotion from prenatal to postnatal life. London: Spastic Society, Heinemann.
Aslin, R.N., Pisoni, D.B. and Jusczyk, P.W.(1983). Auditory development and speech perception in infancy. In M.M. Haith & J.J. Campos (Eds.) Handbook of Child Psychology (vol.2). New York: Wiley.
Brazelton T.B. (1984). Neonatal Behavioral Assessment Scale (2nd ed.). Philadelphia: J.B. Lippincott Co.
Butterfield, E.C., & Siperstein, G.N. (1972). Influence of contingent auditory stimulation upon non-nutritional suckle. In J. Bosma(Ed.) Oral sensation and perception: The mouth of the infant. (pp. 313-343) Springfield, IL: Thomas.
DeCasper, A.J., and Carstens, A.A. (1981). Contingencies of stimulation:Effects on learning and emotion in neonates. Infant Behav. Dev., 4:19-35.
DeCasper, A.J. and Fifer, W.P. (1980). Of human bonding: Newborns prefer their mothers' voices. Science, 208, 1174-1176.

DeCasper, A.J. and Prescott, P.A. (1984) Human newborns'
    perception of male voices: Preference, discrimination, and
    reinforcing value. Developmental Psychobiology, 17, 481-491.
Fifer, W.P., & Moon, C. (1988a). Newborn discrimination
    learning: The value of voices. Manuscript submitted for
    publication.
Fifer, W.P. and Moon, C. (1988b) Auditory experience in the
    fetus. In W. Smotherman and S. Robertson (Eds.),
    Behavior of the Fetus. West Caldlwell, N.J.:Telford Press.
Hammond, J. (1970). Mother's voice. Developmental Medicine and
    Child Neurology, 12, 3-5.
Mehler, J., Bertoncini, J., Barriere, M., & Jassik-Gershenfeld,
    D. (1978) Infant recognition of mother's voice.
    Perception, 7, 491-497.
Mills, M., & Meluish, E. (1974). Recognition of mother's voice
    in early infancy. Nature, 252, 123-124.
Moon, C. (1985) Phonological universals and syllable
    discrimination in one-to-three-day old infants. Columbia
    University doctoral dissertation. Ann Arbor: University
    Microfilms International.
Moon, C., Bever, T. & Fifer, W.P. (1988). Syllable
    discrimination by newborn infants. Unpublished manuscript.
Moon, C. & Fifer, W.P. (1988a). Two-day-old infants change
    sucking patterns to hear mother's voice. Submitted for
    publication.
Moon, C. and Fifer W.P. (1988b) Newborn response to a male
    voice. Poster presented at biannual meeting of
    International Conference on Infant studies, Washington,
    D.C., May.
Moon, C., & Fifer, W.P. (1986) Newborns prefer the sound of
    mother's voice as experienced in the womb. Paper presented
    at International Society for Developmental Psychobiology,
    Annual Meeting, Annapolis, November.
Querleu, D., Lefebvre, C., Titran, M., Renard, X., Morillion,
    M., and Crepin, G. (1984). Reactivite du mouveau- ne de
    moins de deux heures de vie a la voix maternelle. In
    Gynecol. Obstet. Reprod., 13:125-34.
Spence, M.J. and DeCasper, A.J. (1987) Prenatal experience with
    low-frequency maternal-voice sounds influence neonatal
    perception of maternal voice samples. Infant Behavior and
    Development, 10,133-142.

26

The Early Development of Phonological Form

Michael Studdert-Kennedy

"The nervous system of man and animals is moulded structurally according to the modes of its functional exercise."
                                              – Henry Maudsley (1867, p. 41).
"Many if not most acquisitions of new structures in the course of evolution can be ascribed to selection forces exerted by newly acquired behaviors...Behavior, thus, plays an important role as the pacemaker of evolutionary change."
                                              – Ernst Mayr (1982, p. 612).

INTRODUCTION

The scope and flexibility of language, as a system of animal communication, depends on its dual structure. There are two levels of structure: phonology (or sound pattern) and syntax. Both depend on combinatorial rules by which a finite set of elements is repeatedly sampled, and the sampled elements combined, to produce novel utterances. At the level of phonology a small set of meaningless elements (consonants and vowels) is used to construct the very large set of meaningful (or syntactically functional) elements (words, morphemes) that constitute a speaker's lexicon. At the level of syntax a large, though finite, lexicon is used to construct an infinite set of utterances. Syntax is a hallmark of human language; so too is phonology. Indeed, syntax presupposes phonology, because the capacity to form words is logically, ontogenetically and, we must presume, evolutionarily prior to the capacity to form sentences. The present paper is entirely concerned with the development of phonological form.

In referring to consonants and vowels as primitive elements of phonological form, I am appealing to the reader's phonetic intuitions and knowledge of the conventions of alphabetic transcription. The fact that a spoken utterance can be transcribed as a sequence of discrete phonetic symbols by a writing listener, and regenerated as a more or less continuous articulatory-acoustic pattern by a reading speaker, is an important psychological datum, without which systematic study of either phonology or syntax would be impossible. Yet, as we have known for some forty years, discrete invariant segments, corresponding to consonants and vowels, cannot be isolated by purely physical measurement of either the articulatory or the acoustic record. The reason for this is that the concepts, consonant and vowel, are abstractions from what we actually observe in speech, namely, the acoustic consequences of repeated patterns of oral constriction and opening that form the basic metrical unit of speech, the syllable.

The syllable arises from complex, interleaved spatio-temporal patterns of gesture, executed by partially independent articulators (larynx, tongue, jaw, velum, lips). That the phoneme (consonant, vowel) has functional rather than merely descriptive status, as a gestural pattern within the syllable, is attested not only by the alphabet itself, and by the familiar poetic devices of alliteration, rhyme and assonance, but also by the systematicity of speech errors. Sub-syllabic metathetic errors ("spoonerisms") almost always entail exchange of elements with corresponding syllabic functions (onset, nucleus, coda). For example, bad dog might be erroneously executed as dad bog, bod dag or bag dod, but rarely as gad dob, never as bdd aog.

Thus, the sound pattern of every spoken language is hierarchically organized: syllable, segment, gesture. My goal in what follows is to sketch a possible course of development for this behavioral hierarchy (and, by implication, for its neural substrate) over the first two years of life.

THE FUNCTIONAL ORIGINS OF STRUCTURE

An entry into this issue is afforded, perhaps surprisingly, by recent studies of sign language "aphasia". Over the past twenty years or so we have learned that sign languages are not, as was once generally believed, adventitious mixes of pantomime and gesture, partly universal, partly parasitic on their surrounding spoken language. Rather, they are full-fledged, independent languages with dual structures of sign formation ("phonology") and syntax, analogous to the dual structures of spoken languages, though adapted to the oro-manual-visual rather than the vocal-auditory modality. I will not elaborate on the structure of sign languages (for which, see Klima and Bellugi,

1979). For the present discussion, it suffices to know that American Sign Language (ASL), the most intensively studied to date, is a heavily inflected language (analogous to, say, Russian or Greek), of which the inflections are elaborate modulations of the manual movements intrinsic to sign stems. In addition to its inflections, ASL syntax formally exploits the space in front of the signer to display complex spatio-temporal patterns that specify the arguments of verbs, and to maintain the anaphoric coherence of discourse. Very broadly, then, we may say that while the phonology and syntax of a spoken language are primarily instantiated in sequential acoustic patterns over time, those of a signed language are primarily instantiated in simultaneous optic patterns over space.

Given this contrast between the modalities of spoken and signed languages, the locus of brain specialization for a signed language, such as ASL, takes on a special interest. Does ASL, given its elaborate visuo-spatial structure, lateralize to the right hemisphere? Or do whatever perceptuomotor, or abstract linguistic, properties ASL shares with a spoken language ensure that it lateralize to the left hemisphere? The answer has come from the first systematic studies of ASL aphasia, conducted by Poizner, Klima and Bellugi (1986). They studied six brain damaged native signers of ASL, three with right hemisphere damage, three with left. Patients with right hemisphere lesions displayed normal perception and production of ASL, but were severely impaired on standard tests of visuo-spatial function. Patients with left hemisphere lesions displayed precisely the reverse pattern. Moreover, the patterns of ASL deficit in the three aphasic patients varied with the locus of left hemisphere lesion in a fashion strikingly similar to the variations described for such standard spoken language syndromes as Broca's and Wernicke's aphasia.

Further evidence for the effects on brain organization of learning ASL as a first language comes from the work of Neville (1985; in press). She studied evoked response potentials (ERP's) in normal hearing subjects and in literate, but profoundly deaf subjects whose first language was ASL. In one study she compared ERP's recorded over left and right occipital and anterior temporal sites, to words and signs briefly flashed in left and right visual fields. Words for normal hearing subjects, and both words and signs for native signers were more accurately recognized when flashed in the right visual field than when flashed in the left, indicating greater left than right hemisphere engagement by both words and signs. On the other hand, in normal hearing subjects, words yielded a characteristic pattern of ERP's that was absent in literate deaf subjects, suggesting different neural processes in word perception as a function of the language substrate on which reading was based. Yet signs yielded in deaf, but not in

hearing, subjects exactly the same ERP pattern as did words in
hearing subjects, suggesting an equivalence between processes of
word reading in hearing subjects and of sign perception in deaf
subjects. The results are evidently too complex, and the ERP
measures too gross, for easy interpretation.   But they do
indicate an intricate pattern of similarities and differences
between the neural processes that support the perception of
signs and words.   Interestingly, the   response   patterns
characteristic of the deaf subjects, all native signers of ASL,
were absent in bilingual English–ASL interpreters who had
learned ASL as a second language.

These studies of ASL argue that it is the activity of the
developing neural substrate for language, in response to the
environment, that determines its final organization.   Taken with
recent work on the early sensitivity of infants to speech, they
cast a new light on neonatal cerebral specializations.   Several
studies have shown that, in normal infants, the left hemisphere
is already at birth more sensitive to speech than the right, and
more sensitive to speech than to periodic or aperiodic nonspeech
sounds (for review, see Molfese and Betz, 1988).   However,
recent work suggests that this neonate bias may reflect prenatal
experience   no less   than   the   presumptive   structural
predispositions of the left hemisphere. Fifer (this volume) and
others (DeCasper and Fifer, 1980; DeCasper and Spence, 1986)
have shown that neonates prefer their mother's voice to that of
a stranger; Mehler and his colleagues (Mehler, Jusczyk,
Lambertz, Halsted, Bertoncini and Amiel–Tison, 1988) have shown
that neonates prefer the sounds of their maternal language to
those of another language, spoken by the same bilingual woman.
Since these preferences are present within days, or even hours,
of birth, it would seem that they reflect the infant's
intrauterine experience of its mother's voice.

The role of experience in shaping the neural substrate for
language is further evidenced by recent studies of babbling.
Oller, Eilers, Bull and Carney (1985) compared the vocalizations
of a deaf infant from 8 to 13 months of age with those of 11
hearing infants. The patterns of sound–making by the deaf
infant never advanced beyond those typical of 4–6 month old
hearing infants. The results demonstrated that the normal onset
and course of babbling development depend on exposure to the
sound patterns of a language. Yet, if a deaf infant is exposed
to ASL during the first months of life, "babbling" with the
fingers emerges around the age normal for speech babbling, that
is, roughly 6–7 months (Newport and Meier, 1985; Laura Petitto,
personal communication). Evidently, then, early exposure to the
acoustic or optic patterns of a natural language is necessary
and sufficient to precipitate the onset of "babbling" in the
appropriate modality.

Given the developmental continuity between babble and speech, now reported in several studies (e.g., Oller, Weiman, Doyle and Ross, 1975; Vihman, Macken, Miller, Simmons and Miller, 1985), and given that motor coordination of both the speech apparatus and the hands is normally vested in the left hemisphere, we may infer that the onset of babbling, whether spoken or signed, reflects the incipient growth of neuromotor support systems in that hemisphere. Evidently, the precise form of this early growth depends on the modality of the surrounding language.

In short, a diverse range of studies supports the principle that behavior (broadly understood as patterns of both perception and action) is the pacemaker of development, no less than of evolution (Mayr, 1982). We may therefore justly apply to the development of language in general, and of phonology in particular, the sound Darwinian principle that function determines form, rather than form function.

FROM MOUTH SOUNDS TO PHONEMES
Preliminary

Animal communicative displays often seem to arise by ritualization of motor routines that evolved for other purposes (Hinde, 1970). The change of function is presumably accompanied by a change in neuromotor control. For example, the topography of spreading wings in the African crane's courtship display may be identical with their topography immediately before flight, but we would not expect identity of underlying neural mechanisms. Indeed, in humans, dissociation of the capacity to use a tool from the capacity to imitate its use is sufficiently well known to have been given a diagnostic name, ideomotor apraxia. And recently, Poizner et al. (1986) have demonstrated, in ASL aphasics, dissociation of the capacities for linguistic and non-linguistic manual gesture. Thus, movements of identical topography, but different function, may come under different regimes, and even loci, of neural control.

I raise this issue here because in what follows I will sketch a speculative account of the process by which disparate and uncoordinated patterns of oral activity (and their correlated mouth sounds) are gradually harnessed to linguistic function, and so brought under specialized neural control. Most of what I have to say will concern production rather than perception because that is what we know most about. But this should not be taken to imply that perception is unimportant. On the contrary, it is obviously through perception that the infant gains access to the surrounding language.

At birth, as noted above, normal infants are already sensitive to at least the prosodic patterns of their maternal language (Mehler, et al., 1988). Within a few days or weeks they can discriminate virtually any speech contrast on which they are tested, and by six months (perhaps earlier, but we have no data) they can form sound categories based on the onset or coda of a consonant-vowel syllable -- a capacity they share with other animals (Kuhl, 1987), including Japanese quail (Kluender, Diehl and Killeen, 1987). Presumably, these capacities are somehow brought to bear on the language that infants hear around them. We have seen that some form of perceptual input is necessary for normal onset of babbling, around the seventh month. We also know that 6-month-old American infants are sensitive to acoustic correlates of clausal units in English utterances (Hirsh-Pasek, K., Kemler Nelson, D. G., Jusczyk, P. W., Cassidy, K. W., Druss, B., and Kennedy, L., 1987). We know too that, during the second six months, infants lose their sensitivity to certain subsyllabic contrasts that are not put to contrastive use in their native language (Best, McRoberts and Sithole, 1988; Werker and Tees, 1984). Finally, we know that around one year, before they have been heard to utter their first attempt at an adult word, infants may recognize the meanings of as many as 150 words (Benedict, 1979).

We can be quite confident then that the processes of differentiation and integration we observe in production are grounded in earlier, hidden processes of perception and memory. In short, without denying a possible role to articulatory exploration and its resulting feedback in refining infant perceptual skills, we may assume that perceptual growth generally precedes and guides production.

From mouth sounds to canonical babble: integration of movements

At birth the infant has two independent sound-making systems (Stark, 1986). The first, reflexive crying and fussing, has the obviously communicative, though not linguistic, function of signaling distress. The sounds are largely voiced "vocants" (Bauer, in press), sounds formed with an unconstricted vocal tract, displaying variations in duration, amplitude, pitch contour and rhythm. The second system, the vegetative movements and sounds associated with feeding and breathing, has no communicative function. The sounds may be voiced or voiceless vocants or "closants" (sounds formed with a constricted vocal tract) (Bauer, in press). Vegetative closants are typically voiceless clicks, stops, friction noises and trills (Stark, 1986).

Development over the first six months apparently entails the gradual harnessing and adaptation of these disparate phonatory and articulatory elements to what we might term protolinguistic use, in the closant-vocant, or "consonant-vowel" (CV) syllable of canonical babble. Particularly during the second trimester, the infant begins to superimpose movements of the velum, tongue, jaw and lips on the laryngeal actions associated with cry (Koopmans-Van Beinum and van der Stelt, 1986). Perhaps these combinations of cry and upper articulator action initially occur quite by chance. But the infant, already by 4-5 months (Kuhl and Meltzoff, 1982) and perhaps even earlier (Meltzoff, 1986), is inclined to imitate the actions of its conspecifics, and so to shape its sound-making to the rhythmic patterns of the surrounding language. Thus, the proportion of supraglottal to glottal articulations gradually increases (Holmgren, Lindblom, Aurelius, Jalling and Zetterström, 1986), and the fully voiced syllable emerges.

Oller (1986) has described the acoustic properties of a canonical CV syllable to which true babbling conforms. Salient among them are its temporal properties: the ratio of syllable opening (or release) to syllable nucleus drops, often quite suddenly around the seventh month, to the values typical of an adult stop-vowel syllable. The patterns of movement in early babble are not random. Partial closures, as in fricatives, affricates and glides, are less frequent than complete closures, as in stops. Points of closure are biased toward the front of the mouth, so that the "consonants" most often transcribed tend to be those formed with the lips or with tongue tip or blade (engaging muscle systems essential to sucking): /b,d,m,n,w,j/. During the open phase of the syllable the favored tongue positions are those associated with low-to-mid, front-to-central vowels, indicating that little or no upward movement of the tongue compensates for the lowering of the jaw. As would be expected, if these patterns were largely determined by the maturational state of the vocal anatomy and physiology, they have been observed (at least for the closants) in virtually every language studied (Locke, 1983).

The integration of simple movements into a more complex pattern may be facilitated by the emergence of rhythmic oscillations of the jaw (cf. Thelen, 1981; this volume). For much early canonical babble consists of strings of reduplicated syllables (/bababa, nenene, dadadada/, and so on), in which the infant seems to be running off a rhythmic sequence of stereotyped, undifferentiated syllables. In fact, MacNeilage and Davis (in press) propose that early babbling consists largely of rhythmic jaw opening and closing, with little or no active control over points of closure or over tongue position during the open phase.

If this is so, we may say that the principal achievement of the first half year is to integrate the mouth movements of feeding and breathing with the laryngeal actions of cry into the holistic spatio-temporal patterns of canonical syllables. Presumably this first step in the shift of function from nonlinguistic to linguistic use of movement is accompanied by an incipient shift in the underlying neural mechanisms and loci of perceptuomotor processing.

From canonical babble to early words: differentiation of gestures

Toward the end of the first year, full syllable reduplication begins to fade. "Variegated" sequences appear in which the consonant-like onset or vowel-like open phase, or both, may vary from one syllable to the next (Oller, 1980). The onset of variegated babbling seems to follow from two cognitive processes, already noted. First is the infant's growing capacity to recognize and store in memory syllables, or sequences of syllables, as units of meaning (words) (Benedict, 1979). Second is the infant's apparent capacity, around 10-12 months, to recognize the contrastive function of small sound variations within words, as evidenced by its loss of sensitivity to phonetic distinctions that are not put to contrastive use in the adult language (Best, et al., 1988; Werker and Tees, 1984).

These growing perceptual and memorial processes would not suffice to induce variegated babble were the child not able to recognize the equivalence or disparity between adult sound patterns and its own. Exploitation of this ability, essential to the development of imitation, seems to be fostered by babbling itself. Recently, Locke and Pearson (1988) have reported on a child deprived of babbling experience, from five to twenty months of age, by a tracheostomy, for bronchopulmonary dysplasia. The child's vocal output, upon removal of the cannula, was that of a child of less than six months of age. She vocalized, but showed little interest in vocalizing for communicative purposes. Only 2% of her utterances qualified as canonical syllables, according to the criteria of Oller (1986), and her consonant inventory was roughly one fifth of what would be expected in a normal 20-month old child. In fact, her level of vocal development was roughly that of a deaf child of the same age. Unlike the deaf, she had regularly heard adult speech around her since birth, perhaps permitting some degree of normal perceptual development; but the lack of vocal practice, with feedback from her own vocalizations, had blocked normal motor development. However, the effect was not permanent. On last report, at a chronological age of 4;4, her performance on a standard test of receptive and expressive language was at the level of 4;7. This, of course, as Locke and Pearson remark, testifies to the plasticity of the system rather than to the lack of any function for babbling in normal development.

Guided, then, by its growing apprehension of sound variation and function in the surrounding language, and by its growing perceptuomotor skills, the child launches into variegated babble at around the same time as it first attempts adult words. The two modes of output proceed concurrently, often for many months, with the words gradually coming to predominate. During this period the principal domain over which the child attempts to organize its articulations, whether of babble or speech, seems to be the syllable or disyllable. Within this "prosodic unit" (Macken, 1979 p. 11), the child strives to differentiate, and control the timing of, the component laryngeal and supralaryngeal gestures.

Evidence that an utterance (syllable, disyllable, word) is indeed a prosodic unit, and so planned as a whole (Menn, 1983), comes from gestural interactions: the child often fails to execute two different places or manners of articulation within the same utterance, thus maintaining some of the reduplicative tendencies of early babble. The most familiar examples are of consonant harmony (assimilation): gog for dog, guk or kuk for truck, and so on. Recently, Davis and MacNeilage (in press) have reported an extensive study of a child's concurrent babbling and speech over the period from 14 to 20 months of age. Their data are replete with instances not only of consonant, but of vowel and even consonant-vowel assimilation. The latter is revealed by the child's preference for high front vowels following alveolar closures, and for low, front-central vowels following labial closures. At the same time, these authors also report an inverse relation between consonant and vowel reduplication: where the child succeeds in combating assimilation in the open phases of a disyllable, she often fails to do so in the closing phases, and vice versa. This demonstrates an incipient segregation of consonants and vowels into phonetic classes.

The study by Davis and MacNeilage is particularly important because the child deployed an unusually large lexicon, growing from about 25 words at 14 months to over 750 words at 20 months. (A typical lexicon at 20 months would be from 1-300 words (Davis and MacNeilage, in press)). Evidently, a child may have a substantial lexicon long before it has fully mastered segmental structure. The principal phonological achievement of this period, then, is internal modification of the integrated syllable by differentiation of its gestural components.

From gestures to phonemes: integration

The final step in the path from mouth sounds to segments is the integration of gestural patterns of syllabic constriction and opening into the coherent perceptuomotor structures we know as consonants and vowels (Studdert-Kennedy, 1987). As we have seen, the status of the segment is problematic. For, on the one hand, we can neither specify the invariant articulatory-acoustic properties shared by all instances of a particular consonant or vowel, nor isolate any given segment as a discrete articulatory-acoustic entity within a syllable. On the other hand, across-word metathetic errors in speaking typically entail exchanges between consonants and vowels that occupy corresponding slots in their respective syllables. Since the exchanging elements may be physically quite disparate, it is evident that their exchange is premised on shared function (onset, nucleus, coda) in the formation of a syllable. There are therefore two aspects to the emergence of phonemes as elements of word formation in a child's lexicon. First is the grouping of all instances of a particular gesture-sound pattern into a single class (e.g., grouping the initial or final patterns of dad, dog, bed, etc. into the class /d/). Second is the grouping of these gesture-sound patterns into higher-order classes (consonants, vowels) on the basis of their syllabic functions.

Two possible selection pressures may precipitate formation of these classes. One pressure is toward economy of storage as the lexicon increases in size. We have seen that a child may accumulate an appreciable lexicon of some 750 words without showing signs of independent segmental control (Davis and MacNeilage, in press). But this lexicon is roughly one hundredth of the size that it will eventually become, and it seems reasonable to suppose that, as the lexicon increases, words should organize themselves on the basis of their shared gestural and sound properties. Recurrent patterns of laryngeal and supralaryngeal gesture would thus form themselves into unitary classes of potential utility for recognition and activation of lexical items (cf. Lindblom, 1988; Lindblom, MacNeilage and Studdert-Kennedy, 1983).

A second possible selection pressure is toward rapid lexical access in the formation of multi-word utterances. Several authors (e.g., Branigan, 1979; Donahue, 1986) have argued that the form of early multi-word combinations may be constrained by the child's limited ability to organize and execute the required articulatory sequences. One such constraint might be a child's inability to produce two successive words with different initial places of articulation. Donahue (1986), for example, describes two strategies adopted by her son in his first two-word utterances. One strategy was to attempt only those words that conformed to his preexisting rule of labial harmony: big book, big bird, big ball were all attempted, but big dog and big cooky were "adamantly refused" (p.215). The second strategy was to circumvent the consonant harmony rule by adopting vocalic words lacking consonants (e.g., where [ejʌ], want [wa]) as pivots that could be comfortably combined with many of the words already in his vocabulary. Such findings imply that the integration of gestures into independent phonemic control structures, or articulatory routines (Menn, 1983), may serve to insulate them from articulatory competition with incompatible gestures, and so facilitate their rapid, successive activation in multi-word utterances.

Finally, I should note that we have no reason to believe that this, or any earlier step in development, affects the child's entire speech repertoire at the same time. We have already seen that a child may be producing variegated, and even reduplicated, babble during the same period that it is producing a substantial number of words. We should also note that, although we may reasonably expect to see the same developmental progressions in different children, we should not expect to see all children develop at the same rate. Individual differences in style and rate of phonological development have become a commonplace of the field (e.g., Ferguson, 1979; Studdert-Kennedy, 1986; Vihman, Ferguson and Elbert, 1986). Children may vary widely not only in when their lexicon begins to take on segmental structure, but in when they first give evidence of that structure in speech errors.

Doubtless, many parents have anecdotal evidence of their young children's errors, but the only systematic data known to me come from Jeri Jaeger (personal communication). She reports her daughter's first across-word metathesis as occurring in her 27th month: ummy takes for tummy aches. This was followed in her 30th month by fritty pace for pretty face, sea tet for tea set, and Bernie and Ert for Ernie and Bert. Jaeger did not report data on the size of her daughter's lexicon at this time, nor on the complexity of her multi-word utterances. But the collection of errors suggests that both were well advanced. Further systematic diary data of this kind should throw light on the conditions under which phonemic structure emerges.

CONCLUSION

I have sketched the outline of a behavioral "embryology" of phonological development. The outline extends the principles of differentiation and integration observed in fetal growth to the postnatal development of behavior, and of its presumed neural substrate. Such an approach offers a way of accommodating both the enormous individual variability in developmental paths and the striking uniformity of outcome. This apparent paradox fits comfortably into a view of development as an epigenetic process, in which diverse environmental pressures combine with constraints from already established patterns of behavior, to guide the child toward a stable adult state.

Acknowledgement. Preparation of this paper was supported in part by NICHD Grant No. HD-01994 to Haskins Laboratories.

References

Bauer, H. (in press). The ethologic model of phonetic development: I. Phonetic contrast estimators. Clinical Linguistics and Phonetics.

Benedict, H. (1979). Early lexical development: comprehension and production. Journal of Child Language, 6, 183–200.

Best, C. T., McRoberts, G. W., and Sithole, N. W. (1988). Examination of perceptual reorganization for nonnative speech contrasts: Zulu click discrimination by English-speaking adults and infants. Journal of Experimental Psychology: Human Perception and Performance, 14, 345–360.

Branigan, G. (1979). Some reasons why successive single word utterances are not. Journal of Child Language, 6, 411–421.

Davis, B. L. and MacNeilage, P. F. (in press). Acquisition of correct vowel production: A quantitative case study. Journal of Speech and Hearing Research.

DeCasper, A. J. and Fifer, W. P. (1980). Of human bonding: Newborns prefer their mothers' voices. Science, 208, 1174–1176.

DeCasper, A. J. and Spence, M. J. (1986). Prenatal maternal speech influences newborns' perception of speech sounds. Infant Behavior and Development, 9, 133–150.

Donahue, M. (1986). Phonological constraints on the emergence of two-word utterances. Journal of Child Language, 13, 209–218.

Ferguson, C. A. (1979). Phonology as an individual access system: Some data from language acquisition. In C. J. Fillmore, D. Kempler and W.S-Y. Wang (eds.), Individual Differences in Language Ability and Language Behavior. New York: Academic Press, pp. 189–201.

Hinde, R. A. (1970). Animal Behavior. New York: McGraw Hill.

Hirsh-Pasek, K., Kemler Nelson, D. G., Jusczyk, P. W., Cassidy, K. W., Druss, B., and Kennedy, L. (1987). Clauses are perceptual units for young infants. Cognition, 26, 269–286.

Holmgren, K., Lindblom, B., Aurelius, G., Jalling, B. and Zetterstrom, R. (1986). On the phonetics of infant vocalization. In B. Lindblom, and R. Zetterström (eds.) op. cit., pp. 51–63.

Klima, E. S. and Bellugi,U. (1979). The Signs of Language. Cambridge, MA: Harvard University Press.

Kluender, K. R., Diehl, R. L., and Killeen, P. R. (1987). Japanese quail can learn phonetic categories. Science, 237, 1195-1197.

Koopmans-van Beinum, F. J., and Van der Stelt, J. M. (1986). Early Stages in the Development of Speech Movements. In B. Lindblom, and R. Zetterström (eds.) op. cit., pp. 37-50.

Kuhl, P. K. and Meltzoff, A. N. (1982). The bimodal perception of speech in infancy. Science, 218, 1138-1141.

Kuhl, P. K. (1987). Perception of speech and sound in early infancy. In P. Salapatek (ed.), Handbook of Infant Perception, Vol. 2. New York: Academic Press.

Lindblom, B. (1988). Some remarks on the origin of the "phonetic code". In C. von Euler (ed.) Brain and Reading. Basingstoke, England: MacMillan.

Lindblom, B. and Zetterstrom, R. (eds.). (1986). Precursors of Early Speech. Basingstoke, England: MacMillan.

Lindblom, B., MacNeilage, P., and M. Studdert-Kennedy. (1983). Self-organizing processes and the explanation of language universals. In B. Butterworth, B. Comrie, and O. Dahl (eds.), Explanations for Language Universals. The Hague: Mouton, pp. 181-203.

Locke, J. (1983). Phonological Acquisition and Change. New York: Academic Press.

Locke, J. and Pearson, D. M. (1988). Linguistic significance of babbling: Evidence from a tracheostomized infant. Report from the Neurolinguistics Laboratory at Massachusetts General Hospital (Whole Issue).

Macken, M. A. (1979). Developmental reorganization of phonology: A hierarchy of basic units of organization. Lingua, 49, 11-49.

MacNeilage, P. F. and Davis, B. L. (in press). Acquisition of speech production: Frames, then content. In M. Jeannerod (ed.), Attention and Performance, XIII: Motor Representation and Control.

Maudsley, H. (1867). The Physiology and Pathology of the Mind. New York: Appleton. (Reprinted in Significant Contributions to the History of Psychology, Series C: Medical Psychology, Vol. IV. Washington, DC: University Publications of America, 1977).

Mayr, E. (1982). The Growth of Biological Thought. Cambridge, MA: The Belknap Press.

Mehler, J., Jusczyk, P., Lambertz, G., Halstead, N., Bertoncini, J., and Amiel-Tison, C. (1988). A precursor of language in young children. Cognition, 29, 143-178.

Meltzoff, A. N. (1986). Imitation, intermodal representation, and the origins of mind. In B. Lindblom, and R. Zetterström (eds.) op. cit., pp. 245-265.

Menn, L. (1983). Development of articulatory, phonetic and phonological capabilities. In B. Butterworth (ed.). Language Production, Vol. II. London: Academic Press.

Molfese, D. L. and Betz, J. C. (1988). Electrophysiological indices of the early development of lateralization for language and cognition, and their implications for predicting later development. In D. H. Molfese, and S. J. Segalowitz (eds.), Brain Lateralization in Children. New York: The Guilford Press, pp. 171-190.

Neville, H. (1985). Effects of early sensory and language experience on the development of the human brain. In J. Mehler, and R. Fox (eds.), Neonate Cognition. Hillsdale, N.J., pp. 349-363.

Neville, H. J. (in press). Whence the specialization of the language hemisphere? In I. G. Mattingly and M. Studdert-Kennedy (eds.), Modularity and the Motor Theory of Speech Perception. Hillsdale, N. J.: Lawrence Erlbaum Associates.

Newport, E. L. and Meier, R. P. (1985). The acquisition of American Sign Language. In D. I. Slobin (ed.), The Cross-Linguistic Study of Language Acquisition, Volume I: The Data. Hillsdale, N.J.: Lawrence Erlbaum Associates, pp. 881-938.

Oller, D. K., Wieman, L. A., Doyle, W., and Ross, C. (1975). Infant babbling and speech. Journal of Child Language, 3, 1-11.

Oller, D. K. (1980). The emergence of the sounds of speech in infancy. In G. Yeni-Komshian, J. F. Kavanagh, and C. A. Ferguson (eds.). Child Phonology, Volume 1: Production. New York: Academic Press, 93-112.

Oller, D. K., Eilers, R. E., Bull, D. H. and A. E. Carney. (1985). Prespeech vocalizations of a deaf infant: A comparison with normal metaphonological development. Journal of Speech and Hearing Research, 28, 47-63.

Oller, D. K. (1986). Metaphonology and infant vocalizations. In B. Lindblom, and R. Zetterström (eds.) op. cit., pp. 21-35.

Poizner, H., Klima, E. S. and U. Bellugi. (1986). What the Hands Reveal About the Brain. Cambridge, MA: MIT Press.

Stark, R. E. (1986). Prespeech segmental feature development. In P. Fletcher, and M. Garman (eds.), Language Acquisition (second edition). New York: Cambridge University Press, pp. 149-173.

Studdert-Kennedy, M. (1986). Sources of variability in early speech development. In J. S. Perkell and D. H. Klatt (eds.), Invariance and Variability of Speech Processes. Hillsdale, N.J.: Lawrence Erlbaum Associates, pp. 58-76.

Studdert-Kennedy, M. (1987). The phoneme as a perceptuomotor structure. In A. Allport, D. MacKay, W. Prinz and E. Scheerer (eds.), Language Perception and Production. London: Academic Press, pp. 67-84.

Thelen, E. (1981). Rhythmical behavior in infancy: An ethological perspective. Developmental Psychology, 17, 237-257.

Vihman, M. M., Macken, M. A., Miller, R., Simmons, H., and Miller, J. (1985). From babbling to speech: A reassessment of the continuity issue. Language, 61, 397-445.

Vihman, M. M., Ferguson, C. A., and Elbert, M. (1986). Phonological development from babbling to speech: Common tendencies and individual differences. Applied Psycholinguistics, 7, 3-40.

Werker, J. F., and Tees, R. C. (1984). Cross-language speech perception: Evidence for perceptual reorganization during the first year of life. Infant Behavior and Development, 7, 49-63.

27
Role of Input in Children's Early Vocal Behavior

Björn Lindblom

Comparing the research reviewed in the present session with the ideas presented in the sixties by influential students of early communicative behavior such as Eric Lenneberg we observe a clear shift of emphasis. Whereas Lenneberg preferred to view the onset of language acquisition as an autonomous and largely endogenous process (Lenneberg 1967:125-142), the role of experience in modulating early development has now come much more to the fore. This trend was already apparent four years ago when, as mentioned by Rolf Zetterström, some of us met here to attend the Wenner-Gren symposium on **Precursors of Early Speech** (Lindblom and Zetterström 1986). It is further examplified to-day by Bill Fifer's work on in utero and post-natal auditory experience of the human voice and by Michael Studdert-Kennedy's account of the plasticity of the language learning mechanism.

If, as Fifer convincingly argues, children hear speech before birth, what is the nature of the signal that they hear? What are the transmission characteristics of the tissues surrounding them? How developed are their own auditory systems? Fifer suggests that sound reaching a fetus presumably contains predominantly low-frequency energy since speech waves generated by the mother or externally are likely to be transmitted in low-pass filtered form. Since the low frequency content of speech carries mainly prosodic features (intonation and rhythm) it makes sense to hypothesize, as he does, that prosody may be a key component in the infant's ability to recognize voices.

The study by Mehler, Jusczyk, Lambertz, Halstead, Bertoncini and Amiel-Tison (1988) indicates that four-day old infants are able to discriminate between

utterances from their native language and utterances
from a foreign language. Evidently they can do so also
when low-pass filtered stimuli are presented. These
findings would seem to be fully compatible with, and
lend strong support to, Fifer's interpretations.

Assuming that at an early stage prosody is indeed
more salient than segmental vowel and consonant
information what is the significance of that finding
for later speech development? Does a mastery of prosody
appear earlier in perception and production than that
of vowels and consonants? Although determining the
relative timing of segmental and prosodic competence
in production raises some difficult methodological
questions let us note the following.

Infants have been found to discriminate
contrasting stress and pitch contour patterns from 6
weeks on (Kuhl 1979). Crystal (1986:179) claims that
vocalizations "..come to resemble prosodic patterns of
the mother tongue - from as early as 6 months.." and (p
181) that "learned patterns of prosodic behavior are
characteristic of the output of the child during the
second half of the first year". What about the
production of segments? In his comprehensive (1983)
study Locke examined the babbled consonants from babies
with some 15 different mother tongues. He included data
also on hearing-impaired infants and children with
Down's syndrome. Across all three populations he found
a single phonetic repertoire which led him to conclude
that "the phonetic composition of babbling is shaped
primarily by internal factors" and can be seen, up to
about twelve months, as an expression of the child's
so-called "biological code" (p 38).

The cross-linguistic data and interpretations of
Locke (1983) seem more in line with Lenneberg's view of
babbling as a largely maturationally controlled
behavior than with the principle that is amply
supported by Studdert-Kennedy's presentation:
Perception guides and shapes production. Is the cross-
linguistic babbling data an exception to that
principle? No, taking another look at that data from a
slightly different perspective we shall make the
paradox disappear.

Stoel-Gammon (1988) compared babbling samples from
11 normally hearing subjects with vocalizations from 14
hearing-impaired children. The normal group was
followed from 4 to 18 months of age and the two groups
of hearing-impaired children from 4 to 39 months. There
was a much higher proportion of labial articulations in
the hearing-impaired population. Stoel-Gammon argues
that "since auditory cues are lacking, the hearing-
impaired subjects presumably attend to the visual cues
and reproduce the oral movements associated with
bilabial and labio-dental productions."

Mulford (1988) recorded the first 50 words of a group of 11 English-speaking blind children and made a comparison with the corresponding sets from a group of sighted children. The observations were classified according to place of articulation. The results indicate that normal children use significantly more labial consonants than blind children. Mulford suggests that the reason why labial words and segments are particularly salient to sighted children is because of their visual distinctiveness.

What do we conclude from these investigations? What have we learned that was not as evident at the time of the 'Precursors' meeting? First, the normal development of babbling presupposes a normal <u>auditory</u> system. You need to hear yourself and others adequately in order to exhibit normal babbling as well as normal vocabulary growth. This seems to be the message from the recent work on deaf children. It is also the conclusion we draw from the Locke&Pearson data on the tracheostomized girl mentioned by Studdert-Kennedy.

Second, there is a <u>visual</u> component in the normal development of early vocalizations. The importance of vision in this context is fully compatible with an observation of adult speech perception: Watching a speaker's face as well as hearing her/him facilitates the recognition of labial consonants in particular. The improvement for these consonants is equivalent to listening (without visual information) to an acoustic signal whose signal-to-noise ratio has been raised by about 10 dB.

All these results amplify Studdert-Kennedy's conclusion: Experience modulates early vocal behavior in subtle but important ways. But what about the finding that during the first year the repertoires of babbled consonants appear to be highly similar and independent of the linguistic environment? Why do we not find greater language-specific effects?

Some recent work on the phonetic inventories of 317 languages (Lindblom and Maddieson 1988) provides the clue to this paradox. The vowels and consonants of this database were classified into three categories: Basic, Elaborated and Complex segments. Complex articulations use combinations of Elaborated mechanisms. Elaborated segments superimpose some additional process on the elementary articulations of the Basic set. We found that the number of segments that a given language uses in each category is predictable from the total size of its inventory. Small vowel or consonant inventories recruit only Basic segments, medium-sized systems invoke Elaborated in addition to Basic articulations, and large inventories bring all three categories into play.

To understand why observed babbling repertoires do not show a stronger dependence on the linguistic environments we should note the following points: (i) All languages appear to share a core set of Basic segments whereas they may diverge in terms of Elaborated and Complex articulations; (ii) Children appear to acquire the Basic sounds early in their development and before the other types. And (iii) the above cross-linguistic comparisons - both of babbling and of phonetic inventories - are all based on counts of phonetic symbols derived from rather coarse-grained transcriptions. Bearing these circumstances in mind we should not be surprised to learn that a survey such as that of Locke (1983) fails to establish marked language-specific effects.

Consequently we are not entitled to agree with those who following Lenneberg see the absence of language-specific effects as suggesting that babbling is rather independent of experience and is therefore predominantly maturationally determined. There are now strong indications (Vihman 1988, Locke and Pearson in press) that from its onset the motor processes of canonical babbling, although traditionally considered as pre-linguistic, are already being shaped by the ambient language.

REFERENCES

Crystal, D (1986): "Prosodic Development", 174-197 in Fletcher, P and Garman, M (eds): Language Acquisition, Cambridge:Cambridge University Press.

Kuhl, P K (1979): "The Perception of Speech in Early Infancy", 1-47 in Lass, N J (ed): Speech and Language, Vol 1, New York:Academic Press.

Lenneberg E H (1967): Biological Foundations of Language, New York:Wiley.

Lindblom, B and Zetterström, R (1986): Precursors of Early Speech, New York:Stockton Press.

Lindblom, B and Maddieson, I (1988): "Phonetic Universals in Consonant Systems", 62-78 in Hyman, L M and Li, C N (eds): Language, Speech and Mind, London:Routledge.

Locke, J L (1983): Phonological Acquisition and Change, New York:Academic Press.

Locke, J L and Pearson, D M (in press): "Linguistic Significance of Babbling: Evidence from a

Tracheostomized Infant", Report from the
Neurolinguistics Laboratory at Massachusetts
General Hospital.

Mehler, J, Jusczyk, P,   Lambertz, G, Halstead, N,
    Bertoncini, J and Amiel-Tison, C (1988): "A
    Precursor of Language in Young Children",
    Cognition 29, 143-178.

Mulford R (1988): "First Words of the Blind Child", pp
    293-307 in Smith, M D & Locke, J L (eds): The
    Emergent Lexicon, New York:Academic Press.

Stoel-Gammon, C (1988): "Prelinguistic Vocalizations of
    Hearing-Impaired   and   Normally   Hearing
    Subjects: A   Comparison   of   Consonantal
    Inventories", J   of   Speech   and   Hearing
    Disorders 53(3), 302-315.

Vihman, M M (1988): "The Ontogeny of Phonetic Gestures:
    Speech Production", to appear in Mattingly, I
    and Studdert-Kennedy, M (eds): **Modularity and
    the Motor Theory of Speech Perception**,
    Hillsdale, NJ:LEA.

VI. Brain Activity Imaging

28

Positron Emission Tomography in the Study of the Brain of the Premature Infant

Joseph J. Volpe, A. Ernest and Jane G. Stein

Positron emission tomography (PET) has provided the capability of obtaining in vivo regional biochemical and physiological information about the human brain in health and disease (Volpe, 1987). This capability, not long ago considered an unattainable fantasy, is the product of four major developments in the necessary technology: (1) the apparatus for nuclear bombardment, i.e., the cyclotron, to produce positron-emitting isotopes, (2) techniques for rapid synthesis of radiopharmaceuticals necessary for biochemical and physiological studies, (3) the mathematical models and practical algorithms to obtain the critical information from the data, and (4) the PET instrumentation to detect safely the radiopharmaceuticals in vivo in a regional and quantitative manner.

In this presentation, I will review briefly the basic principles of PET, the principal measurements afforded by the technique, and some of our recent applications of PET to the study of the brain of the premature infant. In particular, I will illustrate the role PET has played (1) in elucidation of the basic nature of the major form of brain injury in the premature infant, and (2) in definition of the level of cerebral blood flow (CBF) required for brain viability in the premature newborn.

BASIC PRINCIPLES OF PET

The principle of PET is based on the events provoked by the emission of a positron within the tissue from the active isotope. The positron-emitting isotopes most suitable for in vivo measurements, oxygen-15 (^{15}0), nitrogen-13 (^{13}N), carbon-11 (^{11}C), and fluorine-18 (^{18}F), are incorporated into a chemical compound with desired biologic activity or distribution. The positron emitted from the isotope into the tissue is a low-energy particle which travels only a few millimeters before combining with an electron. The collision between them results in annihilation of the two particles with the emission of two high-energy x-rays in nearly exactly opposite directions. The x-rays are detected by the

external circumferential array of detectors which surround the head
in the PET scanner. The detectors are arranged in pairs, separated
by 180 degrees, and designed to register a signal only if both
sense high-energy x-rays simultaneously. This arrangement of
detectors in coincidence circuits provides the localizing
capability of PET. Computerized image reconstruction of the
regional data obtained from the detectors provides striking images.
Additionally, and of the greatest importance, because the images
represent the quantitative distribution of a radiotracer of
specific biologic importance, critical physiological and
biochemical measurements can be made.

The short half-lives of the isotopes utilized (^{15}O = 2 minutes,
^{13}N = 10 minutes, ^{11}C = 20 minutes, ^{18}F = 110 minutes) provide
three important advantages of PET. First, exposure time of tissue
to radiation is brief, and when this feature is coupled with the
highly sensitive modern PET scanner, the required radiation dose is
remarkably low. For example, in our recent studies of regional
cerebral blood flow (CBF) in the newborn with $H_2^{15}O$, calculated
radiation dose to brain was 75 mrads, to be contrasted with 1,300
to 1,500 mrads for the central slice of a computed tomographic (CT)
scan. Two additional advantages of the short isotope half-lives
are the ability to study the rapid metabolic and physiological
processes of brain, and the capacity to perform rapid serial
studies, since the radioactivity is cleared so quickly from the
previous study.

PRINCIPAL PET MEASUREMENTS

Despite the relatively restricted availability of PET scanning
facilities and the relative youth of the technique, a considerable
variety of important physiological and biochemical measurements
have been accomplished. The most commonly used and important of
these are determinations of regional CBF, metabolism and blood
volume.

Cerebral Blood Flow

Regional CBF has been measured by PET with a variety of labeled
tracers. It is beyond the scope of this discussion to review the
advantages and disadvantages of each approach. Suffice it to say,
recent developments in PET technology that allow an image to be
obtained in a relatively short period of time (e.g., 40 seconds
with the Washington University PET VI scanner) have led to highly
reliable and reproducible measurements of regional CBF. These are
accomplished with $H_2^{15}O$, an excellent tracer for CBF because water
is essentially freely diffusible.

Cerebral Metabolism

Regional measurements by PET of cerebral metabolism,

particularly the substrates utilized for energy production, i.e., glucose and oxygen, have been accomplished either with labeled substrate analogs, e.g., ^{18}F-2-deoxy-D-glucose, or with labeled substrates, e.g., ^{11}C-glucose, ^{15}O-oxygen. The relative advantages and disadvantages of the various approaches are beyond the scope of this discussion. Ideally, the labeled tracer should be identical with the substrate under study and should be quantifiable by PET within a very short measurement time, in view of the rapidity of substrate utilization in brain. Indeed, the use of a PET system capable of rapid, multislice imaging (e.g., the Washington University PET VI scanner) has allowed highly reliable and reproducible measurements of regional oxygen utilization with ^{15}O-oxygen. The radiopharmaceutical is delivered by inhalation of a single breath of ^{15}O-oxygen-labeled air.

Cerebral Blood Volume

Regional cerebral blood volume has been measured by PET most satisfactorily with ^{11}C-labeled or ^{15}O-labeled carboxyhemoglobin. The tracer (^{11}C- or ^{15}O-labeled carbon monoxide) is trapped in the vascular compartment after inhalation of air that contains trace amounts of the radiopharmaceutical. Measurements of regional cerebral blood volume are of particular importance, in part because they are necessary to determine the concentration of any radiopharmaceutical in the vascular compartment relative to the extravascular compartment. This distinction is necessary for the measurement of metabolism or tissue chemical composition by specific radiopharmaceuticals.

PERIVENTRICULAR HEMORRHAGIC INFARCTION IN THE PREMATURE INFANT

The single most important determinant of neurologic outcome in the premature infant is the presence of a characteristic periventricular parenchymal lesion, i.e., periventricular hemorrhagic infarction. Insight into the basic nature of this lesion was gained particularly by PET studies of CBF in premature infants with the periventricular lesion (Volpe et al., 1983), identified in vivo by cranial ultrasonography as a periventricular intraparenchymal echodensity (IPE) (McMenamin et al., 1984; Guzzetta et al., 1986).

PET and the Basic Nature of IPE

Because of the severity of the neurological deficits subsequently observed in patients with IPE (McMenamin et al., 1984), we suspected earlier that the true extent of the parenchymal lesion was greater than the extent suggested by the ultrasonographic appearance in vivo. We undertook a study of regional CBF in a series of such patients with the rationale that the extent of impairment of regional CBF would provide a more

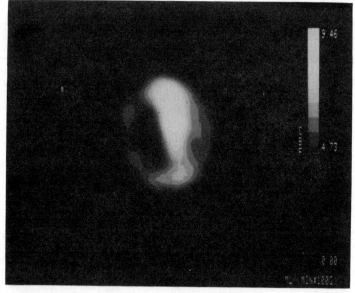

Fig. 1. PET scan from a preterm infant with IVH and periventricular hemorrhagic infarction, as manifested by IPE in the left
frontal region on cranial ultrasound. The scan represents a
horizontal section of cerebrum just above the lateral ventricles.
The gray scale is a linear representation of CBF values, with
highest flows at the top (i.e., white) and lowest at the bottom
(i.e., black). Actual values of CBF were obtained for this case
and, therefore, the gray scale numbers are in ml/100 g·min. Note
the markedly lower CBF in the entire cerebral white matter of the
left cerebral hemisphere, i.e., much more extensive distribution
than that of the IPE.

sensitive indication of the extent of parenchymal injury than
provided by the extent of abnormality by conventional imaging
techniques.

    Thus, in an initial series of six premature infants with IPE
localized by ultrasonography to the left frontal-anterior parietal
white matter, we determined regional CBF by PET with the $H_2^{15}O$
technique (Volpe et al., 1983). The results in these infants and
in 12 subsequently studied infants have been striking and
consistent (Fig. 1). First, anteriorly in the region corresponding
to the periventricular parenchymal echodensity, CBF was reduced
markedly (as expected). Second, and unexpectedly, markedly
diminished CBF was observed also in posterior cerebral (posterior
parietal and parieto-occipital) white matter in the same
hemisphere. Thus the impairment of CBF in the hemisphere

containing the IPE was much more extensive than could be accounted
for by the locus of the echodensity. This larger lesion presumably
accounts for the very serious neurologic deficits nearly uniformly
observed in the survivors of the lesion.

The PET data suggested that IPE marked only a portion of a
larger lesion. The basic nature of this larger lesion appeared
most consistent with an infarction, a portion of which is
characteristically hemorrhagic. Correlative neuropathological
study confirmed this postulate (McMenamin et al., 1984; Guzzetta et
al., 1986).

Neuropathology

Careful neuropathologic study of the periventricular lesion
reveals a relatively large region of hemorrhagic necrosis in
periventricular white matter, just dorsal and lateral to the
external angle of the lateral ventricle. The necrosis
characteristically is strikingly asymmetric – in the largest
ultrasonographic series reported (Guzzetta et al., 1986) 67% of
such lesions were exclusively unilateral and in virtually all of
the remaining cases, grossly asymmetric, even though bilateral.
Approximately one-half of the lesions are extensive and involve the
periventricular white matter from frontal to parieto-occipital
regions; the remainder are more localized. Approximately 80% of
cases are associated with large germinal matrix/intraventricular
hemorrhage (IVH), and commonly (and mistakenly) the parenchymal
hemorrhagic lesion is described by ultrasonography as "extension"
of IVH. That simple extension of blood into cerebral white matter
from germinal matrix or lateral ventricle does not account for the
periventricular hemorrhagic necrosis has been shown clearly by
several neuropathological studies (McMenamin et al., 1984;
Armstrong et al., 1987; Guzzetta et al., 1986; Flodmark et al.,
1980; Gould et al., 1987; Rushton et al., 1985).

Microscopic study of this periventricular hemorrhagic necrosis
indicates that the lesion is a hemorrhagic infarction. The careful
studies of Gould et al. (1987) and Takashima et al. (1986)
emphasize that (1) the hemorrhagic component consists usually of
perivascular hemorrhages which follow closely the fan-shaped
distribution of the medullary veins in periventricular cerebral
white matter, and that (2) the hemorrhagic component tends to be
most concentrated near the ventricular angle where these veins
become confluent and ultimately join the terminal vein in the
subependymal region. Thus, it appears likely that periventricular
hemorrhagic necrosis occurring in association with large IVH is, in
fact, a venous infarction. This lesion is distinguishable
neuropathologically from secondary hemorrhage into periventricular
leukomalacia, the ischemic, usually nonhemorrhagic, and symmetric
lesion of periventricular white matter of the premature infant.
However, distinction of these two lesions in vivo is very
difficult.

Table 1. Association Between Severity of Intraventricular Hemorrhage (IVH) and Occurrence of
Intraparenchymal Echodensity (IPE*)

Severity of IVH	Number (%)[+] with IPE
Grade III	58 (77%)
Grades I-II	13 (18%)
None	4 (5%)

*IPE was defined as periventricular intra-
parenchymal echodensity >1 cm in at least one
dimension on ultrasound scan.

[+]% of all infants with IPE.

Pathogenesis

The pathogenesis of the periventricular hemorrhagic necrosis
that appears to be a venous infarction is not entirely established.
However, a direct relation to IVH seems likely on the basis of
three recently defined facts (Guzzetta et al., 1986). First,
approximately 80% of the parenchymal lesions were observed in
association with large (and usually asymmetric) IVH (Table 1).
Second, the parenchymal lesions invariably occurred on the same
side as the larger amount of intraventricular blood (Table 2).
Third, the parenchymal lesions developed and progressed after the
occurrence of the IVH. The peak time of their occurrence was the
fourth postnatal day, i.e., when 90% of cases of IVH have already
occurred. These data raised the possibility that the IVH and/or
its associated germinal matrix hemorrhage led to obstruction of the

Table 2. Relation of Side of Intraparenchymal
Echodensity (IPE) with Side of Asymmetric
Intraventricular Hemorrhage (IVH)

Severity of IVH	IPE Homolateral*	IPE Contralateral*
Grade III	47	0
Grades I-II	5	4

*IPE "homolateral" when IPE on same side as
larger amount of intraventricular blood.

IPE "contralateral" when IPE on opposite side.

terminal veins and hemorrhagic venous infarction. A similar conclusion has been suggested from a recent neuropathological study (Gould et al., 1987). Nevertheless, experimental studies raise the possibility that the intraventricular blood could contribute to the periventricular necrosis by causing (1) impairment of periventricular blood flow secondary to increased intraventricular pressure (Batton and Nardis, 1987) and/or local release of K^+ from hemolyzed red blood cells (Edvinsson et al., 1986) or (2) local release by red blood cells of lactic acid (Pranzatelli and Stumpf, 1985) or perhaps other vasoactive or otherwise injurious compounds. On balance, however, we consider most probable the pathogenetic notion of obstruction of medullary and terminal veins by intraventricular and germinal matrix blood clot.

Thus, the pathogenetic scheme that we consider to account for most examples of periventricular hemorrhagic infarction is shown in

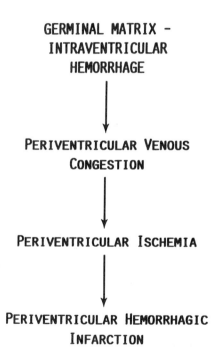

**GERMINAL MATRIX –
INTRAVENTRICULAR
HEMORRHAGE**

↓

**PERIVENTRICULAR VENOUS
CONGESTION**

↓

PERIVENTRICULAR ISCHEMIA

↓

**PERIVENTRICULAR HEMORRHAGIC
INFARCTION**

Fig. 2. Pathogenesis of periventricular hemorrhagic infarction. Formulation indicates a major role for germinal matrix and/or intraventricular hemorrhage in causation of the periventricular venous infarction.

Fig. 2. This scheme should be distinguished from that operative for hemorrhagic periventricular leukomalacia (Fig. 3), <u>although clearly the lesions could coexist</u>. The frequency of coexistence of the two lesions is not known. Additionally, the two pathogenetic schemes could operate in sequence, i.e., periventricular leukomalacia could become hemorrhagic (and perhaps a larger area of injury) when asymmetric germinal matrix or intraventricular hemorrhage subsequently causes venous obstruction.

CBF REQUIREMENT FOR BRAIN VIABILITY IN THE PREMATURE NEWBORN INFANT

CBF Thresholds in Adults

Because of the greater resistance of newborn vs. adult brain to hypoxic-ischemic insults, a basic difference in the CBF requirement for brain viability might be suspected. In adults, measurements of regional CBF in patients with cerebrovascular disease have demonstrated that CBF values below 17-18 ml/(100g·min) are associated with evidence of neuronal dysfunction (EEG slowing or hemiparesis) (Trojaberg and Boysen, 1973; Sundt et al., 1974) and that CBF below 10 ml/(100g·min) occurs only in areas of cerebral infarction (Powers et al., 1985; Baron et al., 1983). In contrast, recently Greisen and Trojaberg (1987) have reported normal visual evoked responses in preterm infants with mean CBF (measured by the 133-xenon technique) below 10 ml/(100g·min), an observation that

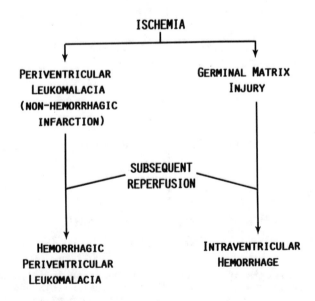

Fig. 3. Pathogenesis of hemorrhagic periventricular leukomalacia.

suggests neuronal viability is preserved at these low CBF levels. However, no neurological followup data on these infants was provided.

To obtain more insight into the level of CBF necessary to sustain neuronal viability in premature newborns, we have measured CBF with PET in 16 infants and determined the relationship between CBF and neurologic outcome. The results have been striking.

CBF and Outcome in Preterm Infants

Among 16 preterm infants studied by the $H_2^{15}O$ technique, the mean CBF ranged from 4.9 to 23 ml/(100g·min), with a mean of 11.5 ml/(100g·min) (Altman et al., 1988). There was no clear relation of mean CBF to neurologic diagnosis (principally intraventricular hemorrhage) or, more importantly in this context, to outcome. Thus, of the 10 infants with mean CBF > 10 ml/(100g·min), on followup four were normal, three had neurologic deficits and three died. Of the six infants with mean CBF < 10 ml/(100g·min), on followup three were normal, two had neurologic deficits, and one died. Interestingly, the two infants with the lowest mean CBF, i.e., 4.9 and 5.2 ml/(100g·min), were normal on followup.

CBF Requirement for Brain Viability

Our findings suggest strongly that: (1) values for mean CBF in the premature infant compatible with a normal neurological outcome are decidedly lower than normal values for mean CBF in the adult (i.e., approximately 50 ml/(100g·min) by the $H_2^{15}O$ technique in adults studied in this laboratory, and (2) the CBF requirement for brain viability in the premature infant is markedly lower than the CBF requirement in the adult.

Although the minimal CBF necessary to maintain neuronal viability in the premature newborn remains to be determined, our data indicate that the value must be below 5 ml/(100g·min). This observation is compatible with the recent demonstrations by Griesen et al. (1986, 1987) that values for mean CBF < 10 ml/(100g·min) are not uncommon in the premature newborn. Moreover, as noted above, Griesen and Trojaberg (1987) have shown that mean CBF as low as 4.3 ml/(100g·min) is sufficient to maintain neuronal function (assessed by visual evoked responses) in such infants. Our data now show that subsequent neurologic function can be normal with such low values of CBF in the neonatal period.

Mechanism(s) Underlying Low CBF in Premature Infants

The mechanism(s) underlying the low CBF in the newborn infant remain(s) unclear. The most likely hypothesis is that the metabolic requirements of premature brain are relatively low because of the anatomical and physiological immaturity of the tissue (Volpe, 1987). Considerable experimental data suggest that the latter mechanism is operative in developing animals (Volpe, 1987), and that this lower metabolic rate in large part underlies the apparent resistance of neonatal brain to energy depletion and tissue injury with hypoxic–ischemic insults. We have recently succeeded in determining regional cerebral metabolic rate for oxygen ($CMRO_2$) by PET with ^{15}O-oxygen (Altman et al., unpublished). Our preliminary data suggest that $CMRO_2$ is considerably lower in the human premature than in the adult. Thus, the same mechanism suggested to be most critical in animal studies to account for both the increased resistance of neonatal brain to oxygen deprivation and the relatively low neonatal values for CBF may also be operative in the human infant.

ACKNOWLEDGEMENT

This work was supported by a grant from the National Institutes of Health (PON506833D).

REFERENCES

Altman, D.I., Powers, W.J., Perlman, J.M., Herscovitch, P., Volpe, S.L. and Volpe, J.J. (1988). Cerebral blood flow requirement for brain viabilty in newborn infants is lower than in adults. Ann. Neurol., in press.

Armstrong, D.L., Sauls, C.D. and Goddard-Finegold, J. (1987). Neuropathologic findings in short-term survivors of intraventricular hemorrhage. Amer. J. Dis. Child., 141, 617–621.

Balton, D.G. and Nardis, E.E. (1987). The effect of intraventricular blood on cerebral blood flow in newborn dogs. Pediatr. Res., 21, 511–515.

Baron, J.C., Rougemont, D., Bousser, M.G. (1983). Local CBF, oxygen extraction and $CMRO_2$: Prognostic value in recent supratentorial infarction. J. Cereb. Blood Flow Metab., 3(S1), S1–S2.

Edvinsson, L., Lou, H.C., Tvede, K. (1986). On the pathogenesis of regional cerebral ischemia in intracranial hemorrhage: A causal influence of potassium? Pediatr. Res., 20, 478–480.

Flodmark, O., Becker, L.E., Harwood-Nash, D.C. (1980). Correlation between computed tomography and autopsy in premature and full-term neonates that have suffered perinatal asphyxia. Radiology, 137, 93–103.

Gould, S.J., Howard, S., Hope, P.L. and Reynolds, E.O.R. (1987). Periventricular intraparenchymal cerebral haemorrhage in preterm infants: The role of venous infarction. J. Pathol., 151, 197–202.

Greisen, G. (1986). Cerebral blood flow in preterm infants during the first week of life. Acta Paediatr. Scand., 75, 43–51.

Guzzetta, F., Shackelford, G.D., Volpe, S., Perlman, J.M. and Volpe, J.J. (1986). Periventricular intraparenchymal echodensities in the premature newborn: critical determinant of neurologic outcome. Pediatrics, 78, 995–1006.

McMenamin, J.B., Shackelford, G.D. and Volpe, J.J. (1984). Outcome of neonatal intraventricular hemorrhage with periventricular echodense lesions. Ann. Neurol., 15, 285-290.

Powers, W.J., Grubb, R.L., Jr., Darriet, D. and Raichle, M.E. (1985). Cerebral blood flow and cerebral metabolic rate of oxygen requirements for cerebral function and viability in humans. J. Cereb. Blood Flow Metab., 5, 600-608.

Pranzatelli, M.R. and Stumpf, D.A. (1985). The metabolic consequences of experimental intraventricular hemorrhage. Neurology, 35, 1299-1303.

Rushton, D.I., Preston, P.R. and Durbin, G.M. (1985). Structure and evolution of echodense lesions in the neonatal brain. Arch. Dis. Child, 60, 798-808.

Sundt, T.M., Jr., Sharbrough, F.S., Anderson, R.E. and Michenfelder, J.D. (1974). Cerebral blood flow measurements and electroencephalograms during carotid endarterectomy. J. Neurosurg., 41, 310-320.

Takashima, S., Mito, T. and Ando, Y. (1986). Pathogenesis of periventricular white matter hemorrhages in preterm infants. Brain & Develop., 8, 25-30.

Trojaberg, W. and Boysen, G. (1973). Relation between EEG, regional cerebral blood flow and internal carotid artery pressure during carotid endarterectomy. EEG Clin. Neurophysiol., 35, 59-62.

Volpe, J.J., Herscovitch, P., Perlman, J.M. and Raichle, M.E. (1983). Positron emission tomography in the newborn: extensive impairment of regional cerebral blood flow with intraventricular hemorrhage and hemorrhagic intracerebral involvement. Pediatrics, 72, 589-601.

Volpe, J.J. (1987). Neurology of the Newborn. W.B. Saunders, Philadelphia.

29

Metabolic Assessment of Functional Maturation and Neuronal Plasticity in the Human Brain

Harry T. Chugani, Michael E. Phelps and John C. Mazziotta

INTRODUCTION

In humans, a wide variety of chemical and physiologic processes in the brain can now be directly imaged and measured in vivo as a result of the development of positron emission tomography (PET) (Phelps et al., 1975). The noninvasive determination of local cerebral metabolic rates for glucose utilization (lCMRGlc), blood flow, oxygen utilization and protein synthesis, as well as neurotransmitter uptake and binding, and a number of other cerebral processes under both normal and pathological conditions have been successfully accomplished using PET (Phelps et al., 1979; Phelps and Mazziotta, 1985). Studies of lCMRGlc with PET in infants and children have been particularly enlightening in that they have provided us with a better understanding of the functional maturation of the normal brain (Chugani and Phelps, 1986; Chugani et al., 1987a). In addition, patterns of lCMRGlc disturbances can be used for improving diagnostic and prognostic accuracy, and optimizing management by the clinician involved in the care of children with neurologic dysfunction (Chugani and Phelps, 1988).

FUNCTIONAL MATURATION OF THE BRAIN

For ethical reasons, PET studies in completely normal children cannot be performed. However, a retrospective analysis of over 175 infants and children who had been studied with 2-deoxy-2[18F]fluoro-D-glucose (FDG) and PET at our institution disclosed 35 children (ages 5 days to 15 years) in whom neurologic disease was either relatively transient or eventually ruled out altogether. Since all 35 subjects continued to develop normally, detailed analysis of lCMRGlc in this population have allowed us to delineate the metabolic aspects of functional brain maturation, and to correlate lCMRGlc with neurobehavioral development in the infant (Chugani and Phelps, 1986; Chugani et al., 1987a).

Address correspondence and reprint requests to:
Harry T. Chugani, M.D.
Division of Pediatric Neurology
Room MDCC 22-464, UCLA School of Medicine
Los Angeles, CA 90024, USA

Our findings indicated that the pattern of lCMRGlc in the human neonate is markedly different from that of the adult; typically, four brain regions visualized on PET are metabolically prominent in newborns (Fig. 1A,B): sensorimotor cortex, thalamus, brainstem and cerebellar vermis. Phylogenetically, these are relatively old structures which dominate the behavior and participate in the primitive intrinsic reflexes of the normal newborn (Andre-Thomas and Saint-Anne Dargassies, 1960).

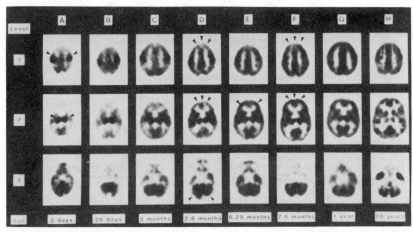

FIGURE 1.   FDG-PET images illustrating developmental changes in lCMRGlc with increasing age in the normal human infant, as compared with those of the adult.   Gray scale is proportional to lCMRGlc, with black being highest.   In each image, anterior portion of the brain is at the top of the image and left side of brain is at left   of image.   A: In 5-day-old, lCMRGlc is highest in sensorimotor cortex, thalamus, cerebellar vermis (arrows) and brainstem (not shown).   B,C,D: lCMRGlc gradually increases in parietal, temporal and calcarine cortices, basal ganglia, and cerebellar cortex (arrows), particularly during the second and third months.   E: In frontal cortex, lCMRGlc increases first in lateral prefrontal regions by approximately 6 months.   F: By approximately 8 months, lCMRGlc also increases in medial aspects of frontal cortex (arrows), as well as dorsolateral occipital cortex.   G,H: By 1 year, lCMRGlc pattern resembles that of adults.

As the infant matures in visuo-spatial and visuo-sensorimotor integrative functions in the second and third months of life (von Hofsten, 1984) and primitive reflexes become suppressed, increases in lCMRGlc are observed in parietal, temporal and primary visual cortical regions, basal ganglia, and cerebellar hemispheres (Fig. 1C,D). The last region in the human infant brain to undergo a maturational rise in lCMRGlc is the frontal cortex, where maturation of the lateral portion (Fig. 1E) precedes that of the phylogenetically newer dorsal prefrontal regions (Fig. 1F).   Increases of lCMRGlc in frontal cortex between 6 and 10 months are associated with rapid cognitive development during this period (Kagan, 1976).   By 1 year of age (Fig. 1G), lCMRGlc patterns resemble that of the normal young adult (Fig. 1H).   The general correlation between lCMRGlc and neurobehavioral development in infants supports the notion of Kennedy et al. (1982), that the metabolic maturation of a neuroanatomic structure indicates the time of onset of its contribution to behavior.

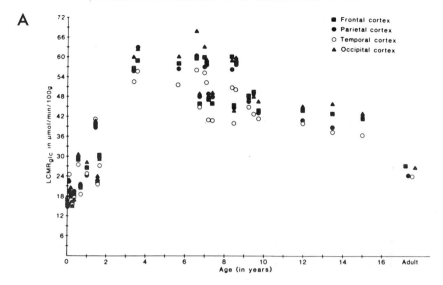

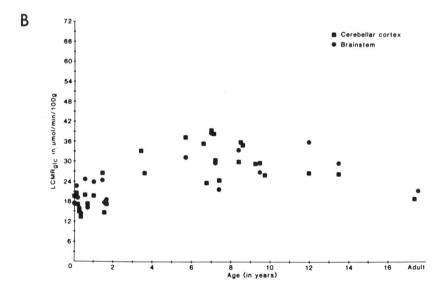

FIGURE 2. Absolute values of lCMRGlc for selected brain regions plotted as a function of age for 29 infants and children and seven young adults. In infants and children, points represent individual values of lCMRGlc; in adults, points are mean values from seven subjects, in which size of symbols equals standard error of mean. A: Cerebral cortex. B: Cerebellar cortex and brainstem.

Analysis of lCMRGlc in cerebral cortex during development indicates that lCMRGlc in newborns is about 30% lower than in adults; subsequently, lCMRGlc increases to adult values by about 2 years (Fig. 2A). By 3 to 4 years, lCMRGlc values are about twice those of adults, and continue to greatly exceed adult rates until about 9 to 10 years, when a slow decline is observed. Adult values are finally reached at the latter part of the second decade (Chugani et al., 1987a). Phylogenetically older areas of the brain, such as brainstem, are relatively mature metabolically even at birth (Fig. 2B), and lCMRGlc in these areas do not significantly exceed adult rates during development. The very early metabolic maturation of these neuroanatomic structures is not surprising in view of their mediation of basic life support functions.

The biological significance of the various segments of the lCMRGlc maturational curve is yet to be determined. It is probable that the high lCMRGlc observed in the developing human brain reflects the period of increased cerebral energy demand as a result of transient exuberant connectivity (Huttenlocher, 1979; Huttenlocher and de Courten, 1987). This period of excessive synapses and nerve terminals, which has also been observed in many other species, is a period of significant plasticity in the brain (Easter et al., 1985). It can be postulated that the ascending portion of the lCMRGlc development curve corresponds to the period of rapid production of synapses and nerve terminals, whereas that segment of the curve describing the lCMRClc decline corresponds to the period of selective elimination or "pruning" of excessive connectivity. Further studies will be required to test these hypotheses. Importantly, we believe that the in depth analyses of lCMRGlc maturational trends in humans can be accomplished noninvasively with PET, and ultimately yield an important index of brain plasticity. The association between lCMRGlc and brain plasticity is also being studied in the cat, where we have shown that, as in humans, the kitten also goes through a period during development when lCMRGlc exceeds adult values (Chugani et al., 1987b).

With a better understanding of normal maturational changes of various aspects of local cerebral metabolic activity (lCMRGlc, protein synthesis, receptor ontogeny, etc.), these data can be applied in the clinical management of children with neurologic disease, and in the study of brain response to injury and functional recovery following insult.

INTRACTABLE EPILEPSY IN INFANTS

In children with persistent seizures which begin in early infancy and are refractory to anticonvulsant medications, surgical excision of the epileptic focus often leads to complete seizure control and significant improvement in the function of the rest of the brain (Penfield, 1952; Verity et al., 1982). Localization of epileptogenic cortex is greatly enhanced with functional neuroimaging such as PET (Fig. 3).

Correlation of PET findings with cranial computed tomography (CT), magnetic resonance imaging (MRI) and neuropathology indicates that PET is a sensitive test capable of detecting epileptogenic cytoarchitectural disturbances, whereas CT and MRI often failed in this regard (Chugani et al., 1988a). In addition, PET has the unique capability of assessing the functional integrity of brain areas outside the epileptogenic region, thereby identifying those children with greatest potential for functional recovery following surgery.

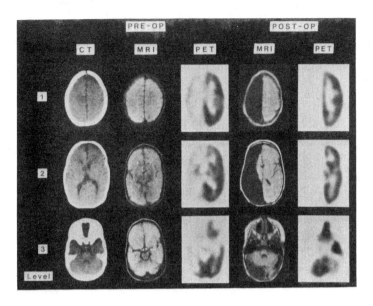

FIGURE 3. CT, MRI and FDG-PET brain images from an infant with idiopathic medically-refractory epilepsy beginning at 8 hours of age. At age 15 months, CT and MRI scans were normal, but PET revealed severe diffuse hypometabolism of all supratentorial structures in the left hemisphere. EEG showed diffuse left hemispheric spike-wave discharges. Left internal carotid infusion of sodium amytal during EEG monitoring resulted in suppression of left-sided spiking; no independent epileptiform activity was seen from the right hemisphere. Following left cerebral hemispherectomy (sparing basal ganglia and thalamus), all seizures ceased and the infant began to show rapid developmental progress. Pathological examination of left hemisphere revealed diffuse hamartomatous malformation. Postoperative MRI scan was normal for the remaining hemisphere, and 6 months later, PET revealed normal pattern of lCMRGlc in the right hemisphere.

lCMRGlc FOLLOWING CEREBRAL HEMISPHERECTOMY

Surgical procedures (focal cortical resection, cerebral hemispherectomy, and corpus callosotomy) performed for the control of intractable epilepsy in children are typically associated with remarkably little functional deficit (Wilson, 1970). The determination of lCMRGlc with PET in these children prior to and following surgery provides a unique assessment of the metabolic response to large cerebral resections as a function of age at surgery.

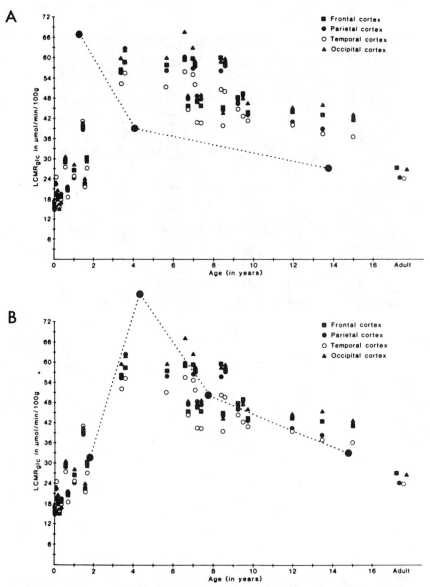

FIGURE 4. <u>Mean</u> cortical lCMRGlc of the intact hemisphere before and after cerebral hemispherectomy, shown against the background of normal developmental changes of lCMRGlc for cerebral cortical regions. (A) Prior to hemispherectomy, lCMRGlc values were outside the normal range for all 3 children. (B) Following hemispherectomy, lCMRGlc were in the normal range for 3 subjects, and in a fourth child (age 4 years), lCMRGlc exceeded normal values, possibly reflecting compensatory mechanisms in the remaining hemisphere.

In a limited number of such children (Fig. 4), we have demonstrated that the normal tendency of lCMRGlc to exceed adult rates between 3 and 16 years is maintained in the remaining hemisphere following unilateral cerebral hemispherectomy (Chugani et al., 1988b). Furthermore, in one child who had cerebral hemispherectomy at 4 years of age, we have observed very high lCMRGlc (exceeding the normally high values for age) following surgery (Fig. 4). Although preliminary, it is tempting to speculate that this "overshoot" of lCMRGlc may be related to compensatory mechanisms at work in the single remaining hemisphere.

CONCLUSION

Studies of local cerebral metabolic activity with PET offer a unique noninvasive approach in assessing functional maturation and developmental plasticity of the human brain. There are many other biochemical markers labeled with positron emitting isotopes that are potentially useful in elucidating the mechanisms of various neurologic disorders of childhood. When used in this clinical setting, such studies can be particularly rewarding in that not only is clinical management of these disorders improved, but our understanding of developmental processes is greatly enhanced.

REFERENCES

1.   Andre-Thomas, C.Y. and Saint-Anne Dargassies, S. (1960). The Neurological Examination of the Infant. Medical Advisory Committee of the National Spastics Society, London.

2.   Chugani, H.T. and Phelps, M.E. (1986). Maturational changes in cerebral function in infants determined by [18]FDG positron emission tomography. Science, 231, 840-843.

3.   Chugani, H.T. and Phelps, M.E. (1988). PET in children with seizures. Applied Radiol.,17,37-49.

4.   Chugani, H.T., Phelps, M.E., Mazziotta, J.C. (1987a). Positron emission tomography study of human brain functional development. Ann. Neurol., 22, 487-497.

5.   Chugani, H.T., Hovda, D.A., Phelps, M.E., Villablanca, J.R. (1987b). Metabolic maturation of the brain: A study of local cerebral glucose utilization in the cat. Soc. Neurosci. Abstr., 13,1139.

6.   Chugani, H.T., Shewmon, D.A., Peacock, W.J., Shields, W.D., Mazziotta, J.C., Phelps, M.E. (1988a). Surgical treatment of intractable neonatal-onset seizures: The role of positron emission tomography. Neurology, 38, 1178-1188.

7.   Chugani, H.T., Phelps, M.E., Mazziotta, J.C. (1988b). Local cerebral metabolic rates for glucose (lCMRGlc) following cerebral hemispherectomy. Neurology (Suppl. 1), 38,281.

8.   Easter, S.S. Jr., Purves, D., Rakic, P., Spitzer, N.C. (1985). The changing view of neural specificity. Science, 230, 507-511.

9. Huttenlocher, P.R. (1979). Synaptic density in human frontal cortex---developmental changes and effects of aging. Brain Res., 163, 195-205.

10. Huttenlocher, P.R. and de Courten, C. (1987). The development of synapses in striate cortex of man. Human Neurobiol., 6, 1-9.

11. Kagan, J. (1976). Emergent themes in human development. American Scientist, 64, 186-196.

12. Kennedy, C., Sakurada, O., Shinohara, M., Miyaoka, M. (1982). Local cerebral glucose utilization in the newborn macaque monkey. Ann. Neurol. 12, 333-340.

13. Penfield, W. (1952). Ablation of abnormal cortex in cerebral palsy. J. Neurol. Neurosurg. Psychiatry, 15, 73-78.

14. Phelps, M.E., Hoffman, E.J., Mullani, N.A., Ter-Pogossian, M.M. (1975). Application of annihilation coincidence detection to transaxial reconstruction tomography. J. Nucl. Med. 16, 210-224.

15. Phelps, M.E., Huang, S.C., Hoffman, E.J., Selin, C., Sokoloff, L., Kuhl, D.E. (1979). Tomographic measurement of local cerebral metabolic rate in humans with (18F)2-fluoro-2-deoxyglucose: validation of method. Ann. Neurol., 6, 371-388.

16. Phelps, M.E. and Mazziotta, J.C. (1985). Positron emission tomography: human brain function and biochemistry. Science, 228, 799-809.

17. Von Hofsten, C. (1984). Developmental changes in the organization of prereaching movements. Dev. Psychobiol., 20, 378-388.

18. Verity, C.M., Strauss, E.H., Moyes, P.D., Wada, J.A., Dunn, H.D., Lapointe, J.S. (1982). Long-term follow-up after cerebral hemispherectomy: neurophysiologic, radiologic, and psychological findings. Neurology, 32, 629-639.

19. Wilson, P.J.E. (1970). Cerebral hemispherectomy for infantile hemiplegia: A report of 50 cases. Brain, 93, 147-180.

30
Brain Circulation and Neurodevelopmental Disorders

Hans C. Lou

HYPOXIC-ISCHEMIC LESIONS AND PVH

Abnormal neurologic and intellectual development are common, with a prevalence of about 5-10 per cent in Western societies (Vanucci and Plum 1975). Hypoxic-ischemic brain damage and periventricular hemorrhage (PVH) are the main perinatal neurologic lesions (Pape and Wigglesworth 1979). The present chapter will deal with the following two items: 1) The pathogenesis of such lesions, and 2) their relation to subsequent neurologic and neuropsychologic development.

The character of these lesions is determined by postconceptional age, and the extension and duration of the insult. In general, ischemic lesions are located predominantly in border zones between vascular territories (Meldrum and Brierley 1971). Typical examples are periventricular leukomalacia and, in mature infants, parasagittal cortical infarcts. It is known from computerized tomographic (CT) studies and ultrasonography that approximately 40% of babies with birth weight below 1,500 g subsequently have PVH (Papile et al 1978) originating from the capillaries of the germinal matrix (Hambleton and Wigglesworth 1976). Larger hemorrhages are often fatal or may lead to the development of hydrocephalus. Hypoxic-ischemic lesions and PVH often occur in the same patient (De Reuck et al 1972, Fujimura et al 1979, Volpe et al 1983). Recent data permit the establishment of a comprehensive model of the pathogenesis of both these disorders.

Deficient Autoregulation in Perinatal Distress

Crucial to the understanding of the pathogenesis of perinatal hypoxic-ischemic lesions and of PVH is our finding of deficient autoregulation of cerebral blood flow (CBF) in the distressed fetus (Lou et al 1979b, Tweed et al 1983) and neonate (Lou et al 1979a, Tweed et al 1986). CBF was studied in utero in fetal sheep by the radioactive microsphere technique. In slightly hypertensive asphyxia, CBF increased five-fold, but it decreased proportionally in hypotension induced by bleeding, indicating arteriolar dilation and pressure-passive CBF. Autoregulation breaks down at an oxygen saturation of arterial blood (SaO_2) below 50%, not too far below the normal SaO_2 in utero of about 60%. Also after birth this limit seems critical (Tweed et al 1986). In other words, autoregulation is a fragile homeostatic mechanism which is particularly vulnerable in the hypoxic conditions of the intrauterine environment.

In 19 distressed newborns, we found a proportional relationship between arterial blood pressure and CBF measured by the ^{133}Xe clearance technique a few hours after birth. This relationship was also seen in subgroups defined by birthweight ($\leq$ 2,000 g or > 2,000 g) and by the degree of asphyxia at birth (Apgar score < 7 at 1 minute and Apgar score $\geq$ 7), indicating pressure-passive CBF in neonatal distress, as would be expected from our animal studies. In these infants, CBF was studied by the intra-arterial ^{133}Xe clearance technique (Lou et al 1979a). In a recent study using the intravenous ^{133}Xe clearance technique we determined CBF reactivity versus spontaneous changes in mean arterial blood pressure (MABP) in 62 preterm infants during the first 48 hours of life. 57 infants did not have ultrasound signs of intracranial hemorrhage or hypoxic ischemic encephalopathy at the time of measurement of autoregulation. Of these, CBF was about 25 per cent lower and pressure passive, as well as unresponsive to changes in PCO_2 in the ten who subsequently developed severe PVH and ischemic encephalopathy. In contrast, infants who never developed PVH had normal autoregulation of cerebral blood flow. The study has strengthened and refined the hypothesis that lost autoregulation of cerebral blood flow is crucial in the pathogenesis of cerebrovascular lesions in the newborn (Pryds et al, in preparation): When normal autoregulation is absent, even moderate hypotension may lead to a proportionate decrease in CBF and, hence, ischemia. Absent PCO_2 reactivity will block vasodilatation in response to metabolic activity and therefore contribute to ischemia. The effect of ischemia is further aggravated by hypoxemia. In <u>hypertension</u> the high pressure is transmitted unhampered to the capillary wall with the risk of rupture, as protective arteriolar constriction does not occur. Thus the frequent and often dramatic changes of MABP seen in newborns will become of prime pathogenetic relevance (Lou and Friis-Hansen 1979). Not only will ischemia facilitate the development of severe intraparenchymal hemorrhage. In its turn such hemorrhage may aggravate local ischemia by K^+ induced vasoconstriction (Edvinsson et al 1986) or venous compression (Volpe et al 1983).

NEONATAL CEREBRAL ISCHEMIA AND SUBSEQUENT DEVELOPMENT

Determinations of CBF by means of the intraarterial ^{133}Xe clearance technique in 19 asphyxic infants a few hours after birth have given low values ($\leq$ 20 ml 100 g/ min) in ten infants. Of these ten infants, three died in the neonatal period and showed signs of cerebral necrosis (periventricular leukomalacia). The surviving infants were studied at a follow-up examination at one year of age. Then cerebral atrophy was demonstrated in another three infants in the low-flow group, and in all except one abnormal neurologic signs had developed (Lou et al 1979c). In contrast, in none of the nine infants in the high-flow group did atrophic lesions or major neurologic impairment develop, with the exception of one infant who died with PVH.

At reexamination at the age of four years, poor articulation, dysphasia, attention deficit, and low IQ (Stanford-Binet) were found significantly more often in the group with low neonatal CBF (($p < 0.05$), Chi square test, Yates' correction). Dyspraxia, dyssynergia, spasticity, and short-term memory dysfunction were also seen more frequently in this group, although the differences were not statistically significant. By summarizing the abnormal findings in each of the two groups, the severe impact of neonatal ischemia on neurologic development became particularly striking: the difference between the groups was significant at the $p \ll 0.001$ level (Skov et al 1984).

Finally, at 9-10 years of age it was possible to study 12 of these children by means of detailed neuropsychologic tests and observations, and by ^{133}Xe emission computed tomography (SPECT). It was found that

performance on most neuropsychologic tests or observations correlated with neonatal CBF, but only excep-
tionally with other neonatal parameters (birth weight,
gestational age, Apgar score at 5 min.) Poor performance on each test or observation was in most instances
correlated to a distinct pattern of regional cerebral
dysfunction as assessed by SPECT. The dysfunctional
regions tended to be located periventricularly and in
the watershed regions between major cerebral arteries
(Lou et al, in preparation).

CONCLUSION

It is apparent from the present discussion that the
principal lesions of perinatal asphyxia - cerebral hypoxic-ischemic damage and IVH - are pathogenetically in-
terrelated, a concept that has long been suspected by
pathologists (Pape and Wigglesworth 1979). Prevention of
such lesions would ideally require measurements to re-
establish autoregulation of CBF. Circulatory support to
prevent hypotension, and on the other hand, means to
avoid excessive arterial pressure peaks in the early
neonatal period would be helpful. Neonatal ischemia is a
critical determinant for later neurologic and intellectual development, probably the most important single
factor at the present state of the art. Consistent with
this hypothesis is our finding of hypoperfusion and, by
interference, low metabolic activity and possible minor
structural changes in the white matter border zones between major arterial territories in children with severe learning disorders (Lou et al 1984).

References

De Reuck, J., Chatta, A.S., Richardson, E.P. (1972).
Pathogenesis and evolution of periventricular leukomalacia. Arch. Neurol., 27, 229-336.

Edvinsson, L., Lou, H.C., Tvede, K. (1986). On the pathogenesis of regional cerebral ischemia in intracranial
hemorrhage: A causal influence of potassium? Pediatr.
Res., 20, 478-480.

Fujimura, M., Salisbury, D.N., Robinson, R.O. (1979).
Clinical events relating to intraventricular haemorrhage
in the newborn. Arch. Dis. Childh., 54, 409-414.

Hambleton, G., Wigglesworth, J.S. (1976). Origin of intraventricular haemorrhage in the preterm infant. Arch
Dis. Child., 51, 651-659.

Lou, H.C., Lassen, N.A., Friis-Hansen, B. (1979a). Impaired autoregulation of cerebral blood flod in the distressed newborn infant. J. Pediatr., 94, 118-121.

Lou, H.C., Lassen, N.A., Tweed, W.A. (1979b). Pressure
passive cerebral blood flow and breakdown of the blood-
brain barrier in experimental fetal asphyxia. Acta
Paediatr. Scand., 68, 57-63.

Lou, H.C., Friis-Hansen, B. (1979). Elevations in arterial blood pressure during motor activity and epileptic
seizures in the newborn. Acta Paediatr. Scand., 68, 803-
806.

Lou, H.C., Skov, H., Pedersen, H. (1979c). Low cerebral
blood flow: A risk factor in the neonatal. J. Pediatr.,
95, 606-609.

Lou, H.C., Henriksen, L., Bruhn, P. (1984). Focal cerebral hypoperfusion in children with dysphasia and/or
attention deficit disorder. Arch. Neurol., 41, 825-829.

Meldrum, B.S., Brierley, J.B. (1971). Circulatory factors and cerebral boundary zone lesions. In Brain Hypoxia. (eds. J.B. Brierley and B.S. Meldrum). Spastics
International, London.

Pape, K.E., Wigglesworth, J.S. (1979). Haemorrhage, Ischemia, and the Perinatal Brain. Spastics International,
London.

Papile, L-A., Burstein, J., Burstein, R. (1978). Incidence and evolution of subependymal and intraventricular
hemorrhage. J. Pediatr., 92, 529-534.

Skov, H., Lou, H.C., Pedersen, H. (1984). Neonatal is-
chemia-impact on the four year-old child. J. Devel. Med.
Child. Neurol., 26, 353-358.

Tweed, W.A., Coté, J., Pash, M., Lou, H.C. (1983). Arterial oxygenation determines autoregulation of cerebral blood flow in the fetal lamb. Ped. Res., 17, 246-
249.

Tweed, W.A., Coté, J., Lou, H.C., Gregory, G., Wade, J.

(1986). Impairment of cerebral blood flow autoregulation in the newborn lamb by hypoxia. Ped. Res., 20, 516-519.

Vanucci, R.C.M., Plum, F. (1975). Pathophysiology of perinatal hypoxic-ischemic brain damage. In Biology of Brain Dysfunction. (ed. G. Garell). Plenum Press, New York.

Volpe, J.J., Herscovitch, P., Perlman, J.M., Raichle, M.E. (1983). Positron emission tomography in the newborn: Extensive impairment of regional cerebral blood flow with intraventricular hemorrhage and hemorrhage intracranial involvement. Pediatrics, 72, 589-601.

31
Electrophysiological Evidence for Gestational Age Effects in Infants Studied at Term: A BEAM Study

Frank H. Duffy

INTRODUCTION

The nature/nurture controversy has long stirred both scientific and philosophical debate. It is now firmly established that both an organisms genetic background and its environment during development have major impact upon adult neural structure and function. That these factors apply to human development is now also relatively non-controversial with the effects of extreme environmental or genetic deviation well catalogued. Clinical and developmental interest has recently turned to nature's natural "experiment", the prematurely born infant. Preterms, as we shall call them, have differing (poorer) behavioral profiles in the newborn period [Howard, Parmelee, Kopp, and Littman, 1976; Minde, Perrotta, and Marton, 1985] from their fullterm bretheren, and have, on the average, differing levels of overall academic performance in school aged years, being over-represented in the learning disabled population [Drillien, Thomson, and Bargoyne, 1980].

Interest now centers on why premies are "different". One explanation could be the high incidence of pathology that accompanies or follows premature birth. Intraventricular hemorrhage (IVH), hydrocephalus, seizures, necrotizing enterocotitis (NEC), **bronchopulmonary dysplasia (BPD)**, and retinopathy of prematurity (ROP) are frequently seen and have expected deleterious consequences. When free of such complications the fullterm/preterm difference in function diminishes. For example, Paludetto et al. [Paludetto, Mansi, Rinaldi, DeLuca, Corchia, De-Curtis, and Andolfi, 1982] report that preterms *without* any serious medical disorder when studied at their expected due date ("expected date of confinement" ["EDC"]) perform as well on the Brazelton Neonatal Behavioral Assessment Scale (NBAS) [Brazelton, 1973] as do fullterms. On the other hand, Piper et al. [Piper, Kunos, Willis, and Mazer, 1985] demonstrated significantly lower neurological scores for healthy preterms as a group than for fullterms. Moreover, Ferrari et al. [Ferrari, Grosoli, Fontana, and Cavazzuti, 1983], using the NBAS, confirm this finding for behavioral functioning, as do Sell et al., [Sell, Luick, Poisson, and Hill, 1980] using a pre-publication version of the Assessment of Preterm Infant Behavior (APIB) [Als, Lester, Tronick, and Brazelton, 1982-b]. Moreover, Als et al., [Als, Duffy, and McAnulty, in press] reported on three groups of infants (n=98) selected to be medically healthy and spanning the gestational age continuum from 28 to 41 weeks. Highly significant differences on the six summary APIB system scores were found among early born preterms (27-32 weeks), later born preterms (33-37 weeks), and fullterms (38-41 weeks) when studied two weeks after EDC (42 weeks post-conceptual age [CA]). Discriminant rules developed on this set of neonates correctly predicted the gestational age groupings of a previously studied population of healthy preterms and fullterms with over 90% accuracy. Thus, there is strong evidence to suggest that GA at birth plays a role in healthy infant behavioral competence even when CA is comparable and all infants are healthy, i.e., are free of major pathology.

There exist two viewpoints as to what might explain the important, residual fullterm pre-term difference that persists. The *first* approach emphasizes residual pathological influences resulting from the minor but inevitable medical complications of the premature extrauterine environment. Minor degrees of BPD may compromise brain oxygenation and NEC nutrition. Minor infections are not uncommon. Respiration may be intermittently compromised by excessive secretions. Tracheal suctioning may induce wide swings in blood pressure. Even minor medical manipulations, such as heel sticks for evaluation of blood chemistries, may induce behavior respones (e.g., prolonged weeping), which are regularly observed to transiently reduce blood oxygen content. The *second* point of view emphasizes the impact of differences of the overall premature environment from the dark, encompassing world of the third trimester uterus. This environmental perspective draws on the seminal work of Wiesel and Hubel [1963] which dramatically demonstrated the profound effects of environmental deviancy upon subsequent brain function. This perspective attributes much of the pre-term full-term difference to a developmentally inappropriate environment.

The current clinical debate vis a vis the premature human infant centers not about nature/nuture but about the cumulative effect of covert brain insult v.s. developmentally inappropriate extrauterine environment.

The current study was undertaken to extend the existing behavioral findings to a larger population and to examine this population for electrophysiological correlates of GA at birth.

SUBJECTS

To investigate this issue we studied a cohort of 135 infants at 42 weeks post-conceptual age (**PCA**) regardless of their gestational age (**GA**) at birth. All infants were selected to be appropriate for gestational age (**AGA**) in weight at birth, free of significant medical, genetic, or neurological problems (mother as well as infant), without documented social hardships, and without family history of substance abuse. None of the infants had suffered perinatal asphyxia at birth, IVH, BPD, seizures, hydrocephalus, ROP, or clinically significant NEC. All were singletons. Fifty-five were born with a GA of 27 to 32 weeks and were referred to as very early preterms "prepreterms" (**PPTs**) , 43 with a GA of 33 to 37 weeks referred to as preterms (**PTs**), and 37 with a GA of 38 to 41 weeks, referred to as fullterms (**FTs**). By 41 weeks all infants were home with their families. All were considered "normal" by both family and pediatrician. Details of the selection criteria and sample characteristics are available in Als et al. [Als, Duffy, and McAnulty, in press].

METHODS

All infants, accompanied by one or both parents, were studied at 42 weeks CA with the APIB [Als, Lester, Tronick, and Brazelton, 1982-a,b]. The APIB was developed to quantify not only the infant's skill repertoire, but primarily the modulation of response to controlled environment input [Als, 1983 1985; Als and Brazelton, 1981; Als and

Duffy, 1983]. It is described elsewhere in this volume [Als, this volume]. The assessment attempts to quantify the differences between, for instance, the infant who demonstrates alertness and shows visual following to animate and inanimate stimuli, but only with accompanying respiratory instability and motoric flaccidity, i.e., extreme stress to his autonomic and motor system, and the infant who has leeway and modulation to do so with animation and with stable autonomic and motoric functioning. The APIB uses the maneuvers of the NBAS [Brazelton, 1973] as a graded sequence of increasingly demanding environmental inputs or "packages", moving from distal stimulation presented during sleep to tactile stimulation which is gradually paired with vestibular stimulation, finally involving a face to face interaction with the examiner. During each "package" the examiner monitors the infant's reactions and behaviors along six systems of functioning, the autonomic system, the self-regulatory system, and the extent to which examiner facilitation is necessary to bring the infant to optimal performance and/or to help bring about return to an integrated, balanced state. This results in six operationally independent summary scores, one each for autonomic organization (**PHYSM1**), motoric organization (**MOTOM1**), state/organization (**STATM1**), attentional organization (**ATTNM1**), regulatory organization (**REGUM1**), and examiner facilitation necessary (**EXFAM1**). These scores are referred to as the "system scores" and identify the differential subsystem stability of the infant. They are considered to be the key parameters of the APIB and are the behavioral measures used in this study.

All examiners were blind as to the infant's GA at birth and were trained to APIB inter-rater reliability of over 90%. Every fifth examination was conducted with a senior investigator present and was scored independently by both examiners to assure continued maintenance of inter-rater reliability.

Electrophysiological Measures (BEAM)

The electroencephalogram (EEG) of the preterm has long been known to differ from that of the fullterm [Anderson, Torres, and Faoro, 1985; Dreyfus-Brisac, 1962] and most neonatal polygraphers agree that brain bioelectric development in healthy neonates is primarily a function of post-conceptual age with little or no influence from gestational age at birth. Nonetheless, Dreyfus-Brisac [1970] later recognized minor differences between preterms and fullterms when they reach CAs of 40 weeks. As a confounding factor, Lombroso [1975, 1985] cautioned that "transient dysmaturity" or "persistent dysmaturity" may be seen in response to pathology, with the latter having a worse prognosis. Accordingly, delay in EEG maturation seen in preterm infants - in comparison to fullterms of equivalent CA -is often suggested to be the product of past or present medical difficulty. Thus, EEG may be sensitive to the effects of both maturation and pathology [Lombroso, 1975; Parmelee and Stern, 1972]; however, the isolated effects of GA at birth taken separately are not yet satisfactorily established.

As our neurophysiologic technique we employed brain electrical activity mapping (BEAM), a method that combines quantified EEG analyses with topographic imaging. It was developed to overcome difficulties inherent in analysis of polygraphic data by visual inspection [Duffy, Bartels, and Burchfiel, 1981; Duffy, Burchfiel, and Lombroso, 1979]. In addition to spectral analyses of EEG, we performed evoked potential (EP) studies. The photic evoked response (PER) was chosen, since it is a measure known to be sensitive to neonatal maturation [Engel and Benson, 1968; Laget, Flores-Guevara, D'Allest, Ostre, Raimbault, and Mariani, 1977; Watanabe, Iwase, and Hara, 1972; Whyte, Pearce, and Taylor, 1987].

All infants were studied electrophysiologically during three behaviorally defined states, two waking and one sleep state. All examiners were blind as to subject GA at birth. EEG and EP data were gathered from 20 electrodes in the standard 10-20 format plus four additional electrodes placed so as to monitor vertical eye movement and blink, horizontal eye movement, muscle activity, and electrocardiogram (EKG). These additional channels were recorded, in order to be able to eliminate artifact, and to assist in sleep state estimation. Details of BEAM data management may be found in Duffy et al. [Duffy, Als, and McAnulty, in press].

Once formed the sets of 20 EEG spectra (one from each electrode) were topographically mapped by three point linear interpolation [Duffy, Burchfiel, and Lombroso, 1979] for each of six, four Hz wide EEG spectra ranging from 0.5 to 24 Hz: (delta = 0.5 - 3.75 Hz; theta = 4.0 - 7.75 Hz; alpha = 8.0 - 11.75 Hz; beta 1 = 12 - 15.75 Hz; beta

2 = 16 - 19.75 Hz; beta 3 = 20 - 23.75 Hz). Although BVR data (formed by signal averaging) could be viewed with maps every four msec, we customarily summated 10 data points, thereby averaging over forty msec, an interval derived from our clinical and research experience with infants and older children. Thus the BVR was broken into 37 forty-msec average intervals from 36 to 1536 msec. It needs to be kept in mind that BVR latency designations used in the results section reference the starting point of a latency range, yet extend over 40 msec epochs. The single exception is BVR 1368 which extends over 80 msec. In addition, traditional voltage and latency measures were taken from the BVR. Three recognizable components were measured for the BVR, recorded from the occipital midline electrode (OZ). A negative (N) wave was seen at 92 msec (N92), a positive (P) at 192 msec (P192), and another negative wave at 512 msec (N512). Peak voltages (V) were calculated for the intervals for P192 to N92 (**VP192-N92**) and from P192 to N512 (**VP192-N512**). Latencies (**LAT**) for each component (**LAT92, LAT192, LAT512**) were also recorded. In addition, the ratio of the peak voltage from the verex or central midline electrode (**CZ**) was formed with the P192 amplitude (**VCZ/VP192**) and taken as a measure of BVR spread from the occipital region, a factor believed to represent a maturational parameter [Umezaki and Morrell, 1970].

Photic stimuli were delivered during sleep via a Grass model PS 22 photostimulator set to intensity level 4 and placed at 30 cm from, and directly in front of, the infant's closed eyelids perpendicular to the facial plane. White noise was used to mask the characteristic phototube discharge sound. Great care was taken to maintain the phototube along an imaginary line drawn perpendicularly to the frontal plane half way between the eyes so as to avoid hemi-visual field stimulation. Details of the study protocol may be found in Duffy et al.[Duffy, Als, and McAnulty, in press]. A complete 26 channel polygraphic recording was performed during all states (waking, active sleep, quiet sleep).

The sleep state studied was the *trace alternant* state, referred to as **BTA** (Baby Trace Alternant) and defined according to usual criteria [Dreyfus-Brisac, Fischgold, Samson-Dollfus, Sainte-Anne Dargassies, Monod, and Blanc, 1957; Lombroso, 1981]. It is also referred to as "quiet sleep" or non-REM sleep. Waking states studied were "Alert

Processing", referred to as **BAP** (Baby Alert Processing), and "Awake Not Processing", referred to as **BNP** (Baby Not Processing). BAP was defined as full interactive alertness with bright shiny-eyed appearance, focussed attention on source of stimulation, appearing to process information actively. Motor activity was at a minimum, facial animation might include a slightly opened and rounded mouth, with eyebrows and cheeks mildy elevated. BNP was defined as noninteractive wakefulness, with eyes open or half open, with a glazed or dull look, giving the impression of little involvement; or, if focused, seeming to look through, rather than at, the examiner. Signs of active sleep were absent. Facial or finger twitches, eye movements and irregular respiration were not observed. BNP is somewhat similar to "drowsiness" but involves more than simple passive observation. The examiner continues to interact with the infant to actively maintain this state.

Group comparisons of BEAM data were performed using significance probability mapping (**SPM**) [Duffy, Bartels, and Burchfiel, 1981]. For each state and each electrode, among-group analysis of variance (ANOVA) was performed and the resultant F statistic imaged. This F-SPM process results in topographic maps of among-group differences, one map for each study condition or state. From F-SPMs, templates can be formed by eliminating regions not reaching a desired level of statistical significance. These templates are placed over each subject's data and the values beneath the templates summated so as to form numerical "features". Such features reflect the contribution of each subject to the corresponding among-group difference and are used for subsequent statistical evaluation [Duffy, Denckla, Bartels, Sandini, and Kiessling, 1980]. This established neurophysiological technique serves as a means to reduce the large number of variables that are produced by multi-electrode mapping studies.

Medical Measures

To assess the infant's degree of postnatal medical risk, all available medical records material were reviewed to obtain information as required for use of the Postnatal Complication Scale [Littman and Parmelee, 1974]. This scale assesses the occurrence of ten risk factors (respiratory distress, infection, ventilatory assistance, non-infectious illness or anomaly, metabolic disturbances, hyperbilirubinemia, temperature disturbances, failure to feed in first 48 hours, and surgery) and yields a standardized complication score (**PEDCO1**) with a mean of 100 and a standard deviation of 20, with higher scores reflecting fewer complications.

Statistical Analyses

Statistical analyses relied upon the BMDP software package [Dixon, 1985]. Analyses of Variance (**ANOVA**) was performed on the resultant electrophysiological parameters by gestational age group following assessment and correction for normality where indicated. Multivariate stepwise regression was performed as for the behavioral variables in a forward manner in order to assess the interrelationship among variables and GA. Path analysis [Duncan, 1966; Wright, 1921 1960] was used to investigate the influence of postnatal complications (PEDCO) upon the relationship of the behavioral and the electrophysiological outcome measures with gestational age. This technique allows one to calculate the partial effects of an independent variable on a dependent variable in the presence of one or more intervening variables. Using techniques of multiple regression one calculates coefficients representing both a direct effect for the independent variable and the indirect effects through one or more intervening variables. ANOVA was performed for the six APIB summary variables by GA group. Multivariate stepwise regression was performed next in a forward stepping manner in order to assess the interrelationship among the variables and GA. ANOVA was also performed for the postnatal complication score by GA groups.

RESULTS

The ANOVA among the three GA groupings revealed that all six summary variables were significant at the P<.00005 level with lower (better) mean scores for FTs than for PTs and better for PTs than PPTs. On the basis of group comparison t-tests with Bonferroni's correction, the FTs were significantly different on each variable from PTs and from PPTs. However, the PTs and PPTs differed significantly only for PHYSM1 and MOTOM1. Linear regresson against GA at birth was significant for all six APIB variables. In every instance direction of change indicated lower (better) scores for the later born infants. Stepwise regression against GA at birth, performed in a forward stepping manner, selected only one variable, PHYSM1. The linear regression of PHYSM1 against GA at birth explained 38.7% of the variance. Forcing other variables into the regression increased the percent variance explained by no more than one to two percentage points.

Path analysis was employed whereby the postnatal complications (PEDCO1) was assumed to be the single intervening variable between gestational age and all dependent (behavioral variables). STATM1, ATTENM1, and EXFAM1, did not demonstrate significant direct effects and were best explained on the basis of PEDCO1. REGUM1 showed a weak but significant direct effect (P<.05) but PHYSM1 and MOTOM1 each showed highly significant direct effects (P<.001).

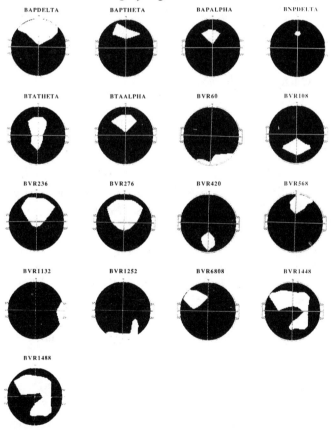

Figure 1 shows results of the F-SPM BEAM analysis among the three gestational age groupings. Seventeen operationally independent regions of among-group difference were delineated, six from EEG data (three from BAP, one from BNP, two from BTA) and 11 from evoked potential data (BVR). In no circumstance did artifact electrodes demonstrate significant between-group difference for the states and time periods illustrated in Figure 1. Note that the frontal region was implicated for 12 of the 17 F-SPMs. Involvement was largely symmetrical for 10, more right sided for six, and more left sided for two F-SPMs.

The statistically defined "regions of interest" (ROI) within the illustrated F-SPMs were used as templates to produce 17 corresponding neurophysiological variables or features. Results of the ANOVA between the three GA groupings revealed 16 significant at the P<.05 level or better, 14 of these at P<.01, five of these at P<.001, and one at P<.00005. Fourteen show significant FTxPPT differences, seven FTxPT differences, and three PTxPPT differences. There is somewhat more difference between FTs and PTs than between PTs and PPTs. All 17 BEAM features showed change in the direction of lower amplitude for earlier born infants.

Stepwise regression performed in a forward manner selected five variables in the following order: BVR1488, BVR108, BVR420, BNPDELTA, BVR1448. Four of the five were derived from EP and only one from EEG data. Two variables selected were frontal and right sided (BVR1488, BVR1448), two were symmetrically parietal (BVR108, BVR420), and one was symmetrical and frontal (BNPDELTA). The resulting regression equation explained 30.6% of the variance.

Despite similarities in the group mean mid occipital electrode waveforms, there was wide variation in appearance among individual subjects. Analysis of variance among the three groups for the six traditional EP measures was performed. Because the distributions were quite non-normal and difficult to bring into normality by simple correction, the non-parametric Kruskal-Wallis test was used. Only one significant finding was revealed, namely, increased 512 msec latency (LAT512) for the earlier born subjects. LAT192, V19V292, V192V512, and VCZ/VP192 failed to reach significance. Path analysis was performed for the 17 BEAM derived features, using PEDCO1 as the intervening variable as has been done for the behavioral variables. Of the 17 features, 13 failed to show significant direct effects and were best explained on the bases of PEDCO1. On the other hand, four continued to show significant direct effects, two weakly BVR276 (P<.05), BVR1448 (P<.05) and two strongly BAPALPHA (P<.01), BVR1488 (P<.01).

Stepwise regression was performed in a forward manner against GA at birth for all APIB and BEAM variables together. Five were selected in the order PHYSM1, BVR276, BVR108, BAPALPHA, and BVR1488. The resulting multivariate regression equation explained 48.4% of the variance.

A more detailed discussion of these results may be found in Duffy et al. [Duffy, Als, and McAnulty, in press].

DISCUSSION

Results of this study strongly support the notion that preterm infants differ from fullterm infants even when studied at the same post-conceptual age point, selected for current optimal health, and selected for historical absence of major medical risk factors. Behaviorally fullterm infants showed better autonomic, motoric, state, attentional, and self-regulatory organization and needed less facilitation than did either preterm group. Differences between the two preterm groups were present but less pronounced, with the middle-group preterms showing better autonomic and motoric organization than the early born preterms, but showing no difference on the remaining four summary scales. Automonic organization (PHYSM1) proved to be the most distinguishing variable and was chosen by multivariate stepwise regression as the only variable needed to explain 38% of the variance.

Exploratory analysis with BEAM revealed extensive regional electrophysiological differences among the three gestational age groups. All numerical features derived from these regions demonstrated a significantly linear relationship with gestational age at birth. Thus, these electrophysiological measures were more linearly related to gestational age than were the behavioral variables. Stepwise regression required five BEAM features and explained 31% of the variance, less than that explained by the best behavioral feature. Nonetheless, when multivariate regression was performed combining the behavioral variable and the electrophysiological features, 48% of the variance was explained. This suggests that the two measurements together provide more information than either one individually.

Not surprisingly all but one of the traditional PER voltage and latency measures failed to show significant gestational age effects. The large among-subject variability reported by others [Ellingson, 1970] was evident in this study and contributed to the negative findings. Thus the traditional measures were far less significant than the BEAM derived features.

The change for each BEAM feature was in the direction of lower amplitudes for earlier born infants. Spectral amplitudes of EEG were similarly reduced. Positive BVR components were less positive and negative BVR components less negative for infants of earlier gestational age at birth. The meaning of this across the board amplitude reduction is not readily explained. One explanation could be that the extrauterine experience of the preterms has "advanced" the normal maturational process. The EEG of the preterm studied before term has generally been found to be of higher amplitude than that of the term infant, suggesting EEG amplitude reduction as a normal maturational process. On the other hand, preterm EEG has also been found to have longer periods of amplitude suppression (*trace discontinue*), which is a sign of immaturity [Lombroso, 1985]. Similarly complex findings are reported for the traditional photic evoked response (PER). According to Umezaki and Morrell [Umezaki and Morrell, 1970], "The amplitudes of PERs of most of the premature infants were higher than those of older controls...". However, while earlier latency components show amplitude reduction as a sign of maturation, later components show an amplitude increase [Engel, 1970; Engel and Benson, 1968; Engel and Milstein, 1971; Hrbek and Mares, 1964; Laget, Flores-Guevara, D'Allest, Ostre, Raimbault, and Mariani, 1977; Lodge, Armington, Barnet, Shanks, and Newcomb, 1969; Umezaki and Morrell, 1970; Watanabe, Iwase, and Hara, 1972]. So "advanced maturation" is not a wholly satisfactory explanation. Indeed, our finding of a prolonged negative latency around 512 msec (N512) for earlier born infants when studied after term would suggest the opposite.

But four of six behavioral and four of 17 electrophysiological measures demonstrated a significant direct effect. Unfortunately results of path analysis are conditional upon model completeness. Alas we cannot argue that our model, which assumes the postnatal complication score as sole intervening variable, is complete. It may be that other toxic factors not yet considered could explain these apparently residual effects. Towbin [1970] was among the first to emphasize that our notions of mental retardation and cerebral palsy as arising primarily from birth injury constitute a major misconception. *Post mortem* studies have shown many instances of hypoxic damage "imprinted" upon the fetal brain weeks to months before delivery. Unfortunately, this appears to be a silent process not amenable to measurement. We cannot exclude, therefore, the presence of gestational age specific prenatal damage which could explain the residual behavior and neurophysiologic gestational age findings after the effects of postnatal complications are removed. Moreover, we cannot be sure whether a more fine grained and prospective measure of postnatal complications would have permitted the derivation of a more sensitive and all-encompassing measure.

On the other hand one must also wonder whether the simple fact of premature extrauterine experience may in and of itself have important consequences. Wiesel and Hubel [1963-a,b; 1965] have demonstrated the profound consequences of inappropriate environmental influence in the newborn kitten by their well known monocular deprivation paradigm. Equally profound effects can be seen with much less drastic environmental manipulation [Mower, Burchfiel, and Duffy, 1982]. Indeed, aberrant positive phenomena as well as deprivation can produce long term change in cat visual system physiology when implemented during early "critical periods" [Spinelli and Jensen, 1979]. Even the timing of critical period onset may be triggered by environmental stimuli [Mower, Berry, Burchfiel, and Duffy, 1981]. The basic mechanisms potentially underlying the unique mutability of the newborn brain were recently reviewed by Duffy et al. [Duffy, Mower, Jensen, and Als, 1984]. We question whether the extrauterine polysensory experience prior to term may trigger sensitive periods at a time when the preterm infant cannot appropriately incorporate such sensory influences thereby inducing less than optimal subsequent neural development.

The issue of whether preterm fullterm difference arises from noxious events or inappropriate environmental influence is of more than theoretical interest. For example, careful environmental and behavioral management of infants with broncho-pulmonary dysplasia has recently been shown to have a beneficial effect on the developmental outcomes of these high risk preterms [Als, Lawhon, Brown, Gibes, Duffy, McAnulty, and Blickman, 1986]. As one moves to further improve the care of such tiny, fragile infants it becomes important to know whether one should focus on reduction of subtle metabolic disturbance or upon more developmentally appropriate environments. It is likely that work in both areas would be appropriate.

REFERENCES

Als, H. (1983). Infant individuality: Assessing patterns of very early development. In F. Call, E. Galenson and R. L. Tyson (Eds.), *Frontiers in Infant Psychiatry* (pp. 363-378). New York: Basic Books.

Als, H. (1985). Patterns of infant behavior: Analogs of later organizational difficulties. In F. H. Duffy and N. Geschwind (Eds.), *Dyslexia: A Neuroscientific Approach to Clinical Evaluation* (pp. 67-92). Boston: Little Brown and Co.

Als, H., & Brazelton, T. B. (1981). A new model of assessing the behavioral organization in preterm and fullterm infants: Two case studies. *J. Amer. Acad. Child. Psychiat.*, *20*, 239-269.

Als, H., & Duffy, F. H. (1983). The behavior of the premature infant: A theoretical framework for a systematic assessment. In T. B. Brazelton and B. M. Lester (Eds.), *New Approaches to Developmental Screening of Infants* (pp. 153-174). New York: Elsevier, North Holland.

Als, H., Duffy, F. H., & McAnulty, G. B. (in press). Neurobehavioral competence in healthy preterm and fullterm infants: Newborn period to 9 months. *Dev. Psychol.*

Als, H., Duffy, F. H., & McAnulty, G. B. (1988). Behavioral differences between preterm and fullterm newborns as measured with the APIB system scores: I. *Infant Behav. Dev*, *11*, 305-318.

Als, H., Lawhon, G., Brown, E., Gibes, R., Duffy, F. H., McAnulty, G., & Blickman, J. G. (1986). Individualized behavioral and environmental care for the very low birth weight preterm infant at high risk for bronchopulmonary dysplasia: Neonatal intensive care unit and developmental outcome. *Pediatr.*, *78*, 1123-1132.

Als, H., Lester, B. M., Tronick, E., & Brazelton, T. B. (1982-a). Towards a research instrument for the assessment of preterm infants' behavior. In H. E. Fitzgerald, B. M. Lester and M. W. Yogman (Eds.), *Theory and Research in Behavioral Pediatrics* (pp. 35-63). New York: Plenum Press.

Als, H., Lester, B. M., Tronick, E. C., & Brazelton, T. B. (1982-b). Manual for the assessment of preterm infants' behavior (APIB). In H. E. Fitzgerald, B. M. Lester and M. W. Yogman (Eds.), *Theory and Research in Behavioral Pediatrics. Vol. I* (pp. 65-132). New York: Plenum Press.

Anderson, C. M., Torres, F., & Faoro, A. (1985). The EEG of the early premature. *Electroenceph. Clin. Neurophysiol.*, *60*, 95-105.

Brazelton, T. B. (1973). *Neonatal Behavioral Assessment Scale. Clinics in Developmental Medicine, No. 50.* Philadelphia: Lippincott.

Dixon, W. (1985). *BMDP Statistical Software (rev. ed.).* Berkeley: University of California Press.

Dreyfus-Brisac, C. (1962). The electroencephalogram of the premature infant. *World Neurology*, *3*, 5-12.

Dreyfus-Brisac, C. (1970). Ontogenesis of sleep in human prematures after 32 weeks of conceptional age. *Dev. Psychobiol.*, *3*, 91-121.

Dreyfus-Brisac, C., Fischgold, H., Samson-Dollfus, D., Sainte-Anne Dargassies, S., Monod, N., & Blanc, C. (1957). Veille, sommeil, réactivité sensorielle chez le prématuré, le nouveau-né et le nourrison. *Electroenceph. Clin. Neurophysiol.*, *6(Suppl.)*, 418-440.

Drillien, C. M., Thomson, A. J. M., & Bargoyne, K. (1980). Low birthweight children at early school-age: a longitudinal study. *Dev. Med. Child Neurol.*, *22*, 26-47.

Duffy, F. H., Als, H., & McAnulty, G. B. (in press) Behavioral and electrophysiological evidence for gestational age effects in healthy preterm and fullterm infants studied two weeks after expected due date. *Child Dev.*.

Duffy, F. H., Bartels, P. H., & Burchfiel, J. L. (1981). Significance probability mapping: An aid in the topographic analysis of brain electrical activity. *Electroenceph. Clin. Neurophysiol.*, *51*, 455-462.

Duffy, F. H., Burchfiel, J. L., & Lombroso, C. T. (1979). Brain electrical activity mapping (BEAM): A method for extending the clinical utility of EEG and evoked potential data. *Ann. Neurol.*, *5*, 309-321.

Duffy, F. H., Denckla, M. B., Bartels, P., Sandini, G., & Kiessling, L. S. (1980). Dyslexia: Automated diagnosis by computerized classification of brain electrical activity. *Ann. Neurol.*, *7*, 421-428.

Duffy, F. H., Mower, G. D., Jensen, F., & Als, H. (1984). Neural plasticity: A new frontier for infant development. In H. E. Fitzgerald, B. M. Lester and M. W. Yogman (Eds.), *Theory and Research in Behavioral Pediatrics II* (pp. 67-96). New York: Plenum.

Duncan, O. D. (1966). Path analysis: sociological examples. *Am. J. Sociol.*, *72*, 1-16.

Ellingson, R. J. (1970). Variability of visual evoked responses in the human newborn. *Electroenceph. Clin. Neurophysiol.*, *29*, 10-19.

Engel, R. (1970). EEG in prematures and subsequent development. In C. R. Angle and E. A. Bering (Eds.), *Physical Trauma as an Etiological Agent in Mental Retardation* (pp. 251-260). Washington, D.C.: U.S. Dept. of Health, Education and Welfare;U.S. Printing Office.

Engel, R., & Benson, R. C. (1968). Estimate of conceptional age by evoked response activity. *Biol. Neonat.*, *12*, 201-213.

Engel, R., & Milstein, V. (1971). Evoked response stability in tracé alternant. *Electroenceph. Clin. Neurophysiol.*, *31*, 377-382.

Ferrari, F., Grosoli, M. V., Fontana, G., & Cavazzuti, G. B. (1983). Neurobehavioral comparison of low-risk preterm and fullterm infants at term conceptual age. *Dev. Med. Child Neurol.*, *25*, 450-458.

Howard, J., Parmelee, A. H., Kopp, C. B., & Littman, B. (1976). A neurologic comparison of pre-term and full-term infants at term conceptual age. *J. Pediat.*, 995-1002.

Hrbek, A., & Mares, P. (1964). Cortical evoked responses to visual stimulation in fullterm and premature newborns. *Electroenceph. Clin. Neurophysiol.*, *16*, 575-581.

Laget, P., Flores-Guevara, R., D'Allest, A. M., Ostre, C., Raimbault, J., & Mariani, J. (1977). La maturation des potentiales évoqués chez l'enfant normal. *Electroenceph. Clin. Neurophysiol.*, *43*, 732-744.

Littman, B., & Parmelee, A. H. (1974). *Manual for Postnatal Complications Scale.* Unpublished manuscript.

Lodge, A., Armington, J. C., Barnet, A. B., Shanks, B. L., & Newcomb, C. N. (1969). Newborn infant's electroretinograms and evoked electroencephalographic responses to orange and white light. *Child Dev.*, *40*, 267-293.

Lombroso, C. T. (1975). Neurophysiological observations in diseased newborns. *Biol. Psychiat.*, *10*, 527-539.

Lombroso, C. T. (1981). Normal and abnormal EEGs in fullterm neonates. In Henry (Ed.), *Current Clinical Neurophysiology* (pp. 83-150). Holland: Elsevier North Holland.

Lombroso, C. T. (1985). Neonatal polygraphy in fullterm and premature infants: a review of normal and abnormal findings. *J. Clin. Neurophysiol.*, *2*, 105-155.

Minde, K., Perrotta, M., & Marton, P. (1985). Maternal caretaking and play with fullterm and premature infants. *J. Child Psychol. Psychiat.*, *26*, 231-244.

Mower, G. D., Berry, D., Burchfiel, J. L., & Duffy, F. H. (1981). Comparison of the effects of dark rearing and binocular suture on development and plasticity of cat visual cortex. *Brain Res.*, *220*, 255-267.

Mower, G. D., Burchfiel, J. L., & Duffy, F. H. (1982). Animal models of strabismic amblyopia: physiological studies of visual cortex and the lateral geniculate nucleus. *Dev. Brain Res.*, *5*, 311-327.

Paludetto, R., Mansi, G., Rinaldi, P., DeLuca, T., Corchia, G., De-Curtis, M., & Andolfi, M. (1982). Behavior of preterm newborns reaching term without any serious disorder. *Early Human Dev.*, *6*, 357-363.

Parmelee, J., A. H., & Stern, E. (1972). Development of states in infants. In C. D. Clemente (Ed.), *Sleep and the Maturing Nervous System* (pp. 199-219). New York: Academic Press.

Piper, M., Kunos, I., Willis, D. M., & Mazer, B. (1985). Effects of gestational age on neurological functioning of the very low-birthweight infant at 40 weeks. *Dev. Med. Child Neurol.*, *27*, 596-605.

Sell, E. J., Luick, A., Poisson, S. S., & Hill, S. (1980). Outcome of very low birthweight (VLBW) infants. I. Neonatal behavior of 188 infants. *Dev. Behav. Pediat.*, *1*, 78-85.

Spinelli, D. N., & Jensen, F. E. (1979). Plasticity: The mirror of experience. *Science*, *203*, 75-78.

Towbin, A. (1970). Central nervous system damage in the premature related to the occurrence of mental retardation. In C. R. Angle and E. A. Bering (Eds.), *Physical Trauma as an Etiological Agent in Mental Retardation*. Washington, D.C.: U.S. Department of Health, Education, and Welfare;U.S. Printing Office.

Umezaki, H., & Morrell, F. (1970). Developmental study of photic evoked responses in premature infants. *Electroenceph. Clin. Neurophysiol., 28*, 55-63.

Watanabe, K., Iwase, K., & Hara, K. (1972). Maturation of visual evoked responses in low-weight infants. *Dev. Med. Child Neurol., 14*, 425-435.

Whyte, H. E., Pearce, J. M., & Taylor, M. J. (1987). Changes in the VEP in preterm neonates with arousal states, as assessed by EEG monitoring. *Electroenceph. Clin. Neurophysiol., 68*, 223-225.

Wiesel, T. N., & Hubel, D. H. (1963-a). Receptive fields of cells in striate cortex of very young visually inexperienced kittens. *J. Neurophysiol., 26*, 994-1002.

Wiesel, T. N., & Hubel, D. H. (1963-b). Simple cell responses in striate cortex of kittens deprived of vision in one eye. *J. Neurophysiol., 26*, 1003-1017.

Wiesel, T. N., & Hubel, D. H. (1965). Comparison of the effects of unilateral and bilateral eye closure on cortical unit responses in kittens. *J. Neurophsyiol., 28*, 1029-1040.

Wright, S. (1921). Correlation and causation. *J. Agricultural Res., 20*, 557-585.

Wright, S. (1960). Path coefficients and path regressions: alternative or complementary concepts?. *Biometrics, 16*, 189-202.

32
Amplitude Integrated EEG Monitoring in Newborn Infants

N. W. Svenningsen

INTRODUCTION

Assessment of brain function in newborn babies is of major importance for evaluation of both shortterm and longterm outcome, especially in infants requiring neonatal intensive care. Topographical estimation of the brain by cranial ultrasound or advanced imaging techniques like computerized tomography or nuclear magnetic resonance techniques can be made even in newborn infants today. However, like cerebral blood flow measurements with Xenon-clearance or Doppler techniques, these measurements can only be made intermittently. Conventional EEG recordings have so far not become part of routine monitoring mainly because they require considerable expertise for their interpretation as well as voluminous paper recordings. An important advance has been EEG-recording onto cassette tape for prolonged periods as developed in recent years (Eyre et al. 1983a). However, the need to establish a technique simple enough to be convenient and applicable bedside also during incubator care and being compact for data collection is still required. In the clinical circumstances the necessity of data reduction must also be taken into consideration. Finally, the technique for continuous monitoring should be applicable during intensive care continuously with minimal interference.

In the Neonatal Intensive Care Unit in Lund we have applied a technique of amplitude integrated EEG (Prior 1979). In a collaboration between the Department of Clinical Neurophysiology and the Neonatal Intensive Care Unit in the University Hospital of Lund we have applied this technique for cerebral function monitoring (CFM) over an 8-year period studying the applicability of the technique in various clinical situations.

CONTINUOUS CEREBRAL FUNCTION MONITORING TECHNIQUE

The cerebral function monitor (CFM-TM monitor, Devices Ltd) gives a recording of an amplified integral encephalogram (EEG) obtained from two recording electrodes applied biparietally on the scalp. The electrodes are thin (0.1 mm) platinum needles placed intradermally. The needle position biparietally reduces muscle and movement artefacts and does not interfere with the nursing of the baby. The signals are filtered and amplitude integrated to attenuate the artefacts and passed through a special filter to reject frequencies outside the 2-15 Hz range. The signals are compressed logarithmically and rectified so both small and large amplitudes are shown without need for gained control. The signals are recorded on a slow running paper with two time-scales either 6 cm/h or 30 cm/h. As shown in figure 1 the tracings are shown as a band where the upper border represents maximum and the lower border minimum levels of electrical activity. In a later version of the CFM monitor (CFAM: Cerebral Function Analysing Monitor)(Maynard 1979, Prior et al. 1986) it is possible to obtain average peak, mean and average minimum voltages of processed EEG and the proportion of total activity in five frequency bands as well. In the CFM chart recording the quality of electrode to skin contact is recorded on a simultaneous impedance trace. This registers automatically artifacts from muscular activity, movement of the baby, loose electrodes, false calibration of the zero-lines. These factors must always be considered when interpreting the various CFM-patterns. As shown in figure 1 normal traces with sleep versus awake patterns and burst-suppression activity can easily be distinguished from periods with high voltage seizures shown as a saw-tooth pattern. Interpretation of the recordings can be made by the nurse or doctor in charge after some training, at least for specific changes as illustrated in figure 1. Thus, the presence of a neurophysiological technician is not required all the time, but only for intermittent check-ups. Raw EEG data can also be recorded on cassette tape from the CFM-device allowing reexamination of the CFM-traces by the neurophysiologists later on. All CFM recordings were performed in the Neonatal Intensive Care Unit or in the operation theatre during surgical procedures.

NEUROPHYSIOLOGICAL STUDIES AND CLINICAL APPLICATIONS

Continuous CFM registrations in newborn infants have been applied in the following situations: Normal infants in various gestational ages, newborns with con-

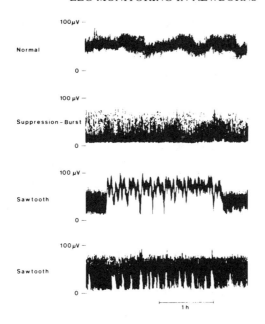

Figure 1. Typical CFM tracings showing normal pattern
with sleep-wakefulness fluctuations, suppression-burst
pattern, ictal seizure activity with saw-tooth patterns
(From Hellström-Westas et al. 1985).

vulsive disorders, effects of various medications and
treatments and in infants with hemorrhagic-ischemic
brain lesions. Previous studies have shown that the CFM-
tracings reflect conventional EEG activity accurately as
a diagnostic tool for convulsions, suppression of activity and for longterm monitoring for hours and days
(Bjerre et al. 1983). For localisation and quantifi-
cation of a morphological lesion conventional EEG and
imaging techniques like cranial ultrasound or computerized tomography are needed.

The studies performed so far in <u>normal babies</u>, both
preterm and fullterm, show <u>maturational CFM changes</u> in
sleep patterns over the conceptional age ranges from 30
to 43 weeks. In the first day of life there is an increase in voltage level and sleep/wakefulness fluctuations, more rapid in the fullterm infant than in the
preterm baby. Thus, transition of levels from around
5 mV to 10-15 mV is seen in fullterm infants after 37

weeks of gestation within one day of postnatal age. In moderately preterm infants of 33-37 gestational weeks this transition will occur after 3 to 6 days whereas in the very preterm infants at 30 weeks of less the transition will take more than 7 days (Viniker et al. 1984, Verma et al. 1984, Svenningsen et al. 1987). In collaboration with the Danish group in Rigshospitalet,Copenhagen, we have also made simultaneous registrations with CFM, EEG, cardiorespirography, clinical obsevations and cerebral blood flow measurements by Xenon-clearance after intravenous injections in healthy preterm infants of 29 to 34 weeks of gestation from 5 to 7 days of postnatal age (Greisen et al. 1985). In this study we found that cerebral blood flow was 22 % higher during wakefulness compared with quiet sleep. Yet, in these healthy preterm infants there was no increase in cerebral blood flow during active sleep suggesting that the neurophysiologic and neurometabolic mechanisms of rapid eye movement (active) sleep are not yet fully developed in preterm infants at these conceptional ages.

It is well known in neonatal medicine that convulsions are difficult to diagnose because they may occur with subtle, atypical signs with e.g. hypotonia or apnoea rather than obvious seizures which may also occur unrecognized even by experienced nurses and caretakers of the baby. On the other hand, some babies may show signs like jitteriness caused by extra cerebral factors such as hypothermia or electrolyte disturbances. The importance of continuous longtime monitoring for the diagnosis of neonatal seizures have been shown by several investigators (Eyre et al. 1983a, Hellström-Westas et al. 1985, Connell et al. 1987a). On the CFM recording cerebral ictal activity shows a typical sawtooth pattern (see figure 1), both in relation to clinical convulsions as well as to subclinical or so-called silent seizures as described by several authors in newborn infants (Rose et al. 1970, Hellström-Westas et al. 1985). Cerebral seizure activity can also be seen as a narrow high level activity around 25 mV or higher in the CFM registration. In our own studies we found a typical pattern of ictal epileptic activity on the CFM recording without clinical symptoms in about 16 % in sick newborn infants (Hellström-Westas et al. 1985, Svenningsen et al. 1987). As pointed out by other investigators (Perlman et al. 1983) such seizures may affect arterial blood pressure, cerebral blood flow velocity and intracranial pressure. Whether anticonvulsive treatment of silent seizures in newborn infants will reduce the rate of cerebral sequelae is still an open question.

Changes in <u>cerebral electrical activity during</u>
<u>various medications and treatments</u> in the newborn period
have also been studied, both by our group in Lund and
others as well (Eyre et al. 1983b, Hellström-Westas et
al. 1987). The effect of anticonvulsive treatment or the
lack of effect can be clearly illustrated with simultaneous continuous EEG monitoring. In intensive care
with e.g. paralysis of the newborn during ventilator
treatment continuous electroencephalographic recording
is necessary to detect seizure states. In recent unpublished studies <u>we have also shown significant effects</u>
<u>from treatment of extremely immature low birthweight</u>
<u>infants born between 24 and 29 weeks</u> from theophylline
treatment (Hellström-Westas et al. 1988, to be published). Further studies are needed within this field of
neonatal medicine.

Cerebrovascular disturbances with <u>ischemic-</u>
<u>hemorrhagic lesions</u> in fullterm and preterm infants have
also been shown to change the cerebral electrical activity when monitored continuously over longterm periods
of hours and days. The combination of very low or iso-
electric activity and/or permanent discontinuous activity when recorded over several hours by continuous EEG
monitoring has been proven by several authors to have a
predictive value for the longterm outcome (Bjerre et al.
1983, Archibald et al. 1984, Pezzani et al. 1986). For
fullterm infants with birth asphyxia flat CFM tracings
or suppression-burst and discontinuous activity remaining unchanged for more than 4 days always implied a
very poor outcome in these studies. On the contrary,
normalisation within the first two days and the presence
of sleep-wake pattern fluctuations and sleep state
organisation within the first two days of life had good
prognostic value.

In <u>preterm infants intraventricular and periventri-</u>
<u>cular hemorrhages and periventricular leukomalacia</u> are
the most important complications in perinatal life for
these infants. The introduction of non-invasive imaging
techniques with cranial ultrasound and computerized
tomography allow early diagnosis of intracranial pathology in newborn infants. It has been shown with continuous EEG monitoring that in cases where timing can be
established deterioration of the background EEG activity
always will precede ultrasound changes (Greisen et al.
1987, Connell et al. 1988). EEG abnormalities also
correlate well with the extent of hemorrhages according
to cranial ultrasound (Watanabe et al. 1983, Clancy et
al. 1984, Greisen et al. 1987). Furthermore, the EEG
changes have been found to be more prognostically
sensitive than imaging techniques (Lacey et al. 1986,

Connell et al. 1988). These results have been interpreted as EEG monitoring changes related to the original
insult causing the hemorrhage rather than to the effects
of the hemorrhage as such. In the same way, continuous
EEG monitoring in evaluation of lesions of ischemic
origin have also been shown to precede ultrasound evidence of parenchymal echodensities not only for hours
and days but for several weeks before cysts are seen in
cranial ultrasound (Connell et al. 1987b).

In summary, it can be stated that continuous EEG
monitoring in the newborn period has several advantages
whether registered by the CFM technique or other continuous ambulatory EEG monitors like the Medilog as described by Eyre et al. 1983a and Connell et al. 1987a.
In comparison to other methods CFM has the advantage of
being a bedside technique, with on-line display of
amplitude changes for immediate analysis and relatively
free of artifacts. It can be supplied also with raw EEG
monitoring on tape for later evaluation. The Medilog is
advantageous by being light, compact, giving raw EEG
from both hemispheres but slow to analyse (replaying of
24 hours data takes a minimum of 24 minutes by EEG-
specialist) and not on-line amplitude integrated like
the CFM. Later computerized versions of the Medilog may
allow earlier bedside evaluation as well. However, it
still requires a neurophysiological technician for the
interpretation (Wertheim et al. 1988). In newborn infants a normal EEG will most often imply a normal outcome. On the other hand, a severely abnormal EEG registered by continuous measurements over several hours
implies high risk of major cerebral sequelae. The best
correlation is obtained when the EEG is recorded as soon
as possible after birth or the cerebral insult as such.
Although the EEG changes are aetiologically non-specific
their extent, especially in background activity, duration and seizure activity, relates closely to the functional severity of the morphological lesion (Dreyfus-
Brisac 1979, Tharp et al. 1981).

CONCLUSIONS

In many clinical investigations precise information
about various aspects of the functional state of the
brain is needed. However, it is difficult to obtain
standardised objective measurements e.g. regarding
various sleep states, diagnosis of seizures or effects
of anticonvulsive and other medications. Conventional
EEG by visual assessment or computerized analysis will
remain a method of choice in many situations. However,
in neonatal care and monitoring this technique may add

unnecessarily complexed data difficult to quantify and
evaluate in short time recordings. The special skills
and expenses involved may not always be justifiable.
Simpler methods for routine monitoring during neonatal
intensive care as obtained with the CFM device is therefore preferable in such situations. According to our experience a modernised version of the CFM technique with
compressed chart recordings being interpreted at the
bedside immediately by the nursing personnel will be a
most useful monitoring device in future neonatal care.
It allows earlier and more accurate diagnosis and treatment beneficial for the individual baby. Further research
and development is important in this field.

ACKNOWLEDGEMENTS

     Supported by grants from Margaretahemmet, the Sven
Jerring Foundation, the Josef Carlsson Foundation and
the Swedish Medical Research Council, project no. 4732.

REFERENCES

Archibald, F., Verma, U.L., Tejani, N.A. and Handwerker,
S.M. (1984). Cerebral function monitoring in the
neonate. II. Birth-asphyxia. Dev. Med. Child. Neurol.,
26,162-168.

Bjerre,I., Hellström-Westas, L., Rosén, I. and
Svenningsen, N.W. (1983). Monitoring of cerebral
function after severe asphyxia in infancy. Arch. Dis.
Child., 58,997-1002.

Clancy, R.R., Tharp, B.R. and Enzman, D. (1984). EEG in
premature infants with intraventricular hemorrhage.
Neurology, 34, 583-590.

Connell, J.A., Oozeer, R. and Dubowitz, V. (1987a).
Continuous 4 channel EEG monitoring: a guide to
interpretation, with normal values, in preterm infants.
Neuropediatrics, 18, 138-145.

Connell, J.A., Oozeer, R., Regev, T., de Vries, L.S. and
Dubowitz, L.M.S. (1987b). Continuous EEG monitoring in
the evaluation of echodense ultrasound lesion and cystic
leukomalacia. Arch. Dis. Child., 62, 1019-1026.

Connell, J.A., de Vries, L.S., Oozeer, R., Regev, R.,
Dubowitz, L.M.S. and Dubowitz, V. (1988). Predictive
value of early continuous electroencephalogram moni-

toring in ventilated preterm infants with intraventricular hemorrhage. Pediatrics, 82, 337-343.

Dreyfus-Brisac, C. (1979). Neonatal electroencephalography. Rev. in Perinat. Med., 3, 397-471.

Eyre, J.A., Oozeer, R.C. and Wilkinson, A.R. (1983a).
Diagnosis of neonatal seizure by continuous recording
and rapid analysis of the electroencephalogram. Arch.
Dis. Child., 58, 785-790.

Eyre, J.A., Oozeer, R.C. and Wilkinson, A.R. (1983b).
Continuous electroencephalographic recording to detect
seizures in paralysed newborns. Br. Med. J., 286, 1017-
1018.

Greisen, G., Hellström-Westas, L., Lou, H., Rosén, I.
and Svenningsen, N. (1985). Sleep-waking shifts and
cerebral blood flow in stable preterm infants. Pediatr.
Res. 19, 1156-1159.

Greisen, G., Hellström-Westas, L., Lou, H., Rosén, I.
and Svenningsen, N.W. (1987). EEG depression and
germinal layer haemorrhage in the newborn. Acta
Paediatr. Scand., 76, 519-525.

Hellström-Westas, L., Rosén, I. and Svenningsen, N.W.
(1985). Silent seizures in sick infants in early life.
Acta Paediatr. Scand., 74, 741-748.

Hellström-Westas, L., Westgren, U., Rosén, I. and
Svenningsen, N.W. (1987). Lidocaine for treatment of
severe seizures in newborn infants. I. Clinical effects
and cerebral electrical activity monitoring. Acta
Paediatr. Scand., 77, 79-84.

Hellström-Westas, L., Svenningsen, N.W. and Rosén, I.
(1988). EEG-monitoring during the first week of life in
very low birthweight neonates born between 23 and 28
weeks of gestation. (In preparation)

Lacey, D.J., Topper, W.H., Buckwald, S., Zorn, W.A. and
Berger, P.E. (1986). Preterm and very low birthweight
neonates: relationship of EEG to intracranial
haemorrhage, perinatal complications and development
outcome. Neurology, 34, 1084-1087.

Maynard, D.E. (1979). Development of the CFM: The
cerebral function analyzing monitor (CFAM). Ann. Anesth.
Franc., 20, 253-258.

Perlman, J.M. and Volpe, J.J. (1983). Seizures in the preterm infant: effects on cerebral blood flow velocity, intracranial pressure and arterial blood pressure. J. Pediatr., 102, 288-293.

Pezzani, C., Radvayi-Bouvet, M.F., Relier, J.P. and Monod, N. (1986). Neonatal electroencephalography during the first twenty-four hours of life in fullterm newborn infants. Neuropediatrics, 17, 11-18.

Prior, P. (1979). Monitoring Cerebral Function. Longterm Recordings of Cerebral Electrical Activity. North Holland Biomedical Press, Amsterdam, pp 43-301.

Prior, P. and Maynard, D.E. (1986). Monitoring cerebral function. Elsevier, Amsterdam.

Rose, A.L. and Lambroso, C.T. (1970). Neonatal seizure states. Pediatrics, 45, 404-425.

Svenningsen, N.W., Hellström-Westas, L. and Rosén, I. (1987). Silent seizures in the newborn (Continuous cerebral function monitoring). In Physiological Foundations of Perinatal Care. (eds. Stern, Oh and Friis-Hansen), Elsevier, New York, pp 339-345.

Tharp, R.B., Cukier, F. and Monod, N. (1981). The prognostic value of the electroencephalogram in premataure infants. Electroencephalogr. Clin. Neurophysiol., 51, 219-236.

Watanabe, K., Hakamada, S., Kuroyanagi, M., Yamazaki, T. and Takeuchi, T. (1983). Electroencephalographic study of intraventricular haemorrhage in the preterm infant. Neuropediatrics, 14, 225-230.

Verma, U.L., Archbald, T., Tejani, N.A. and Handwerker, S.M. (1984). Cerebral function monitor in the neonate. I. Normal patterns. Dev. Med. Child. Neurol., 26, 154-161.

Wertheim, D.F.P., Connell, J., Brydon, J., Oozeer, R.C. and Dubowitz, V. (1988). A new computerised approach to the rapid analysis of the continuous EEG recording in the neonate (Abstract). Electroencephalogr. Clin. Neurol. (In press)

Viniker, D.A., Maynard, D.E. and Scott, D.F. (1984). Cerebral function monitor studies in neonates. Clin. Electroencephalogr. 15, 185-192.

Index

Trophic support activity-dependant p37 Jansen

<u>Neurotransmitters involved in aspects of developing brain</u>

Inhibition of breathing in foetus - somatostatin, endorphins, GABA, adenosine. 21-22
        perhaps via prostaglandins (?inhib by indomethacin, naloxone)

Adenosine & prostaglandins may cause pain thro placenta ··24

Nerve growth factor impt (trophic?) role in Cx devt ··32
     β NGF gene involved in hippocampal neurones — different effects in basal
   forebrain ·· 32

Activity dependent trophic influence seems essential for survival of motor neurones. 34
          from target (muscle fibres)

Acetylcholinesterase necessary to mediate/control opening time of channels and limit duration
  of action of NT at neuromuscle junctions 39